THE UNOFFICIAL GUIDE TO
SURGERY
CORE OPERATIONS

INDICATIONS, PRE-OP CARE, PROCEDURE DETAILS, POST-OP CARE, AND FOLLOW-UP

FIRST EDITION

Chief Editor

Katrina Mason BSc (Hons) MBChB MRCS (ENT)
Ear, Nose, and Throat Specialist Registrar
St George's Hospital, London, UK

Associate Editors

Gareth Rogers BSc (Hons) MBChB
Junior Doctor
Leeds Teaching Hospitals NHS Trust, UK

Madelaine Gimzewska BMedSci (Hons) MBChB MRCS MSc
ACF in Vascular Surgery
Imperial College London

Series Editor

Zeshan Qureshi BM MSc BSc (Hons) MRCPCH FAcadMEd MRCPS (Glas)
Paediatric Registrar
London, UK

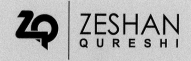

ZESHAN QURESHI

ISBN 978-0957149953

Text, design, and illustration © Zeshan Qureshi 2019

Edited by Katrina Mason, Gareth Rogers, Madelaine Gimzewska, and Zeshan Qureshi

Project Manager: Helena Qian

Published by Zeshan Qureshi. First published 2019

Original design by Zeshan Qureshi. Page make-up by Amnet. Cover design by Anne Bonson-Johnson. Cover image from Getty Images.

Illustrated by Francesca Corra (Cardiothoracics, Endocrine, ENT, Interventional Radiology, Lower GI, Opthalmology, Neurology, Orthopaedics, Paediatrics, Upper GI, Vascular, Surgical Position, Sutures, and Diathermy) and Caitlin Monney (Breast, Plastics, Neurology, Urology, Obstetrics, and Gynaecology).

Clinical photographs (scrubbing up) by Martin Burnett (UK Media Solutions). Modelling by Abiola Adeogun.

X-rays:
Angioplasty. Case courtesy of Dr Sajoscha Sorrentino. Radiopedia.org, rID: 14975.
Catheter-Directed Thrombolysis. Case courtesy of Dr Jeremy Jones. Radiopedia.org. rID: 6406.
Embolisation. Case courtesy of Dr Paresdh Desai. Radiopedia.org. rID: 12289.
IVC Filter. Cases courtesy of Dr Brino Di Muzio. Radiopedia.org. rID: 25103.
Percutaneous Biliary Drainage. Case courtesy of Dr Nitin Garg. Radiopedia.org. rID. 27563.
Percutaneous Nephrostomy. Case courtesy of Dr Omar Bashir. Radiopedia.org. rID. 18633.
TIPSS. Case courtesy of Dr A. Prof Frank Gaillard. Radiopedia.org. rID. 14292.
Gastrostomy. X-ray kindly provided by Brendan S Kelly.

Printed and bound by Jellyfish Print Solutions Ltd

Introduction

Whilst surgery is an incredibly challenging speciality, with a lot to learn, busier wards than ever, and long hours, I have no regrets about choosing this pathway. The combination of perfecting a practical skill and seeing sick patients get dramatically better makes it unique in its rewards.

I became involved in this project after my colleague Madelaine developed the initial idea of a book on core surgical operations. Editing this book alongside the invaluable efforts of Madelaine and Gareth, and working closely with my professional colleagues, has given me a great opportunity to refresh my wider surgical knowledge and to see surgery through the perspective of a student again. From speaking to students and trainees up and down the country, it is clear that everyone encounters universal challenges and common experiences that are worth reflecting upon.

A student enters theatre, and it is easy to forget that they may be seeing a surgical procedure for the first time. This entails seeing living, functioning organs working within a body before your very eyes, and it can be an overwhelming and humbling experience. You will not be the only one who has passed out in theatre. You will not be the only one who suddenly freezes when asked a difficult question. We as surgeons mustn't forget that what has become routine to us is regularly a novel experience to the people we teach.

Additionally, we must consider the details of the surgery. Whilst the anatomy is universally agreed upon, how to do the procedures themselves is not: there are many ways to skin a cat. What we have tried to do in this book is give safe and clear guidance on how to perform common surgical procedures. Remember, variations are based not only on the unit you might work in, but also your own personal preferences. The most important thing is to understand the principles behind the procedures and to be comfortable to perform them safely. There is also no substitute for clinical experience, so scrub in as often as you can, and let the words of this book come to life in the operating room.

Good luck with any upcoming exams. I look forward to calling you my colleague one day, should surgery be your passion.

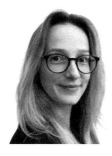

Katrina Mason
Chief Editor
The Unofficial Guide to Surgery: Core Operations

The Unofficial Guide to
Medicine Project

Additionally, we want you to get involved. This textbook has mainly been written by junior doctors and students just like you because we believe:

...that fresh graduates have a unique perspective on what works *for students*. We have tried to capture the insight of students and recent graduates to make the language we use to discuss this complex material more digestible *for students*.

...that texts are in *constant* need of being updated. *Every student* has the potential to contribute to the education of others through innovative ways of thinking and learning. This book is an open collaboration with you.

You have the power to *contribute* something valuable to medicine; we welcome your suggestions and would love for you to get in touch.

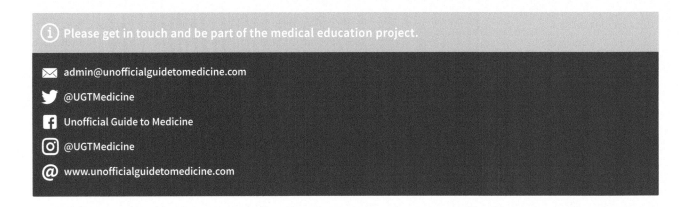

ⓘ **Please get in touch and be part of the medical education project.**

✉ admin@unofficialguidetomedicine.com

🐦 @UGTMedicine

fi Unofficial Guide to Medicine

⬡ @UGTMedicine

@ www.unofficialguidetomedicine.com

Foreword

The field of surgery has enchanted students for as long as it has existed, and today's medical students are no exception. Despite surgery being vital to our healthcare system, very few students are exposed to surgical teaching at a level of detail approaching that of their instruction in medicine or critical care. This textbook seeks to excise the mystery around the operating theatre and to equip students with a thorough understanding of the principles of common operations.

The Unofficial Guide to Surgery: Core Operations is a practical guide to common surgical operations, and it would be a useful resource for any medical or nursing student undertaking a rotation in surgery. Whether you're a surgeon-to-be at the cutting edge of your cohort and hoping to wow your senior colleagues, or a budding psychiatrist unexcited about standing in theatre for hours on end, this textbook has something for you. It is detailed enough to serve as a study resource for the Christina Yangs of tomorrow, but organised and concise so that even the least surgically inclined student can feel more prepared for their obligatory stint in theatre after reading through an operation report while changing into their scrubs.

The textbook features an introduction to the principles of surgery, followed by detailed operation reports for an extensive array of common procedures, organised in chapters based on speciality. Helpfully, each operation report includes the definition of the procedure being performed, its indications, high-quality illustrations of relevant anatomy, a step-by-step guide to the procedure at a level appropriate for students and junior doctors, and interesting trivia on the operation or associated condition. Students will be prepared for a niche question from even the most esoteric consultant!

This textbook is a testament to the hard work of the Unofficial Guide to Medicine team. As reviewers of this book, we cannot take credit for the immense amount of time and effort that the authoring and editing teams have spent developing this resource. We commend Zeshan and his team for their dedication to this book, and the international medical education project that is the Unofficial Guide to Medicine series more broadly. Finally, we are thrilled to have contributed to a project that reflects the more diverse and egalitarian future of surgery and its workforce.

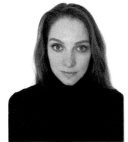 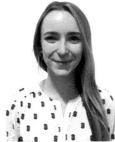

Imogen Thomson and Stella Harris
Final Year Medical Students
University of Sydney

Foreword

Let's get it straight. I enjoyed reading this book.

Any medical student or surgical trainee will benefit from reading the relevant chapter before an attachment to one of these surgical specialties. The opening chapter that covers the culture of the operating theatre, including 'gowning and gloving' is a great start. Each chapter follows a similar format with indications, applied anatomy and an operative outline supported by very high quality artwork. There is a consistency of style often lacking in multi-author texts. This makes for easy reading and both authors and editors are to be commended. The diagrams could easily be shown to patients to help them understand what is involved in a specific procedure. I particularly enjoyed the favourite question at the end of each procedure, though was regularly embarrassed by my lack of knowledge!

While this book is aimed at those directly involved with surgical patients. It would do no harm if those involved less directly, in primary care and hospital services that support surgery, could find the time to understand the basics of surgical interventions and appreciate the complexity of even the most straightforward of procedures.

As a final thought, you obviously don't need professors to write a really good book about surgery.

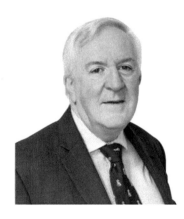

Derek Alderson MD FRCS
President
Royal College of Surgeons of England

Acknowledgements

We would like to thank all those who have made this possible, from the authors, to the reviewers, to the entire production and publication team that worked hard every step of the way. We are very grateful to our families and partners, who have supported us throughout the project. We would also like to dedicate the book to Sarah Prince, a well-loved and highly regarded surgeon at Belford Hospital in Fort William, who has been an inspiration to an entire generation of trainees and has brought both excellent clinical care and compassion to those she looked after.

Abbreviations

A&E: Accident and Emergency

AAA: abdominal aortic aneurysm

AC: alternating current

ACL: anterior cruciate ligament

ACTH: adrenocorticotrophic hormone

ADH: antidiuretic hormone

AIS: acute ischaemic stroke

AKA: above knee amputation

ALND: axillary lymph node dissection

AMI: acute myocardial infarction

ANC: axillary node clearance

AOM: acute otitis media

AP: anterior posterior

AR: aortic regurgitation

AS: aortic stenosis

ASD: atrial septal defect

ASIS: anterior superior iliac spine

AUB: abnormal uterine bleeding

AV: arteriovenous

AVM: arteriovenous malformation

BCT: breast conserving therapy

BKA: below knee amputation

BMI: body mass index

BPH: benign prostatic hypertrophy

B-PT-B: bone - patellar tendon - bone

BRCA: breast cancer gene

BSS: balanced salt solution

BXO: Balanitis Xerotica Obliterans

CABG: coronary artery bypass grafting

CBD: common bile duct

CCA: common carotid artery

CCAM: congenital cystic adenomatoid malformation

CDT: catheter-directed thrombolysis

CES: cauda equina syndrome

CFA: common femoral artery

CHA: common hepatic artery

CMLND: complete mediastinal lymph node dissection

CMV: Cytomegalovirus

CNS: clinical nurse specialist

COPD: chronic obstructive pulmonary disease

CPB: cardiopulmonary bypass

CPR: cardiopulmonary resuscitation

CRPS: complex regional pain syndrome

CRS: chronic rhinosinusitis

CSF: cerebrospinal fluid

CT: computed tomography

CTP: computed tomography perfusion

CTS: carpal tunnel syndrome

CUSA: cavitron ultrasonic surgical aspirator

CXR: chest X-ray

DCIS: ductal carcinoma in situ

DCR: dacryocystorhinostomy

DHS: dynamic hip screw

DIE: deep inferior epigastric

DIEA: deep inferior epigastric artery

DIEP: deep inferior epigastric perforator

DIEV: deep inferior epigastric vein

DIPJ: distal interphalangeal joints

DJ: duodenojejunal

DPNB: dorsal penile nerve block

DVT: deep vein thrombosis

EBV: Epstein-Barr virus

ECA: external carotid artery

ECG: electrocardiogram

EDC: extensor digitorum communis

EDM: extensor digiti minimi

EEG: electroencephalogram

EI: extensor indicis

ENT: ear, nose, throat

EOM: extraocular muscles

EPB: extensor pollicis brevis

EPL: extensor pollicis longus

ERCP: endoscopic retrograde cholangiopancreatography

ET: endotracheal tube

EUS: external urethral sphincter

EVAR: endovascular aneurysm repair

EVLT: endovenous laser treatment for varicose veins

F: French [sizing]

FCR: flexor carpi radialis

FDP: flexor digitorum profundus

FDS: flexor digitorum superficialis

FESS: Functional Endoscopic Sinus Surgery

FEV_1: forced expiratory volume (first second)

FPL: flexor pollicis longus

FSH: follicle stimulating hormone

FTSG: full thickness skin graft

GH: growth hormone

GHK: glenohumeral joint

GI: gastrointestinal

GORD: gastro-oesophageal reflux disease

GP: General Practitioner

GPA: Granulomatosis with Polyangiitis

GSV: great saphenous vein

GT: greater trochanter

GTN: glyceryl trinitrate

H Pylori: helicobacter pylori

HCC: hepatocellular carcinoma

HDU: high dependency unit

HIV: human immunodeficiency virus

HPT: hyperparathyroidism

HPV: human papillomavirus

HSV: herpes simplex virus

ICA: internal carotid artery

IDF: inferior duodenal flexure

IJV: internal jugular vein

II: image intensifier

IMA: inferior mesenteric artery

IMV: inferior mesenteric vein

INR: international normalized ratio

IOP: intraocular pressure

IP: infundibulo-pelvic

ITU: intensive treatment unit

IUD: intrauterine device

IUS: internal urethral sphincter

ABBREVIATIONS

IV: intravenous

IVC: inferior vena cava

LAD: left anterior descending

LCA: left coronary artery

LCIS: lobular carcinoma in situ

LD: latissimus dorsi

LDA: left posterior descending artery

LFT: liver function test

LGA: left gastric artery

LGE: left gastro-epiploic

LH: luteinising hormone

LLETZ: large loop excision of the trans-formation zone

LOAF: lateral lumbricals, opponens policies, abductor pollicis brevis and flexor pollicis brevis

LUTS: lower urinary tract symptoms

LV: left ventricular

MCL: medial collateral ligament

MCP: metacarpal-phalangeal

MDT: multidisciplinary team

MELD: model for end-stage liver disease

MEN: multiple endocrine neoplasia

MI: myocardial infarction

MPL: medial palpebral ligament

MR: mitral regurgitation

MRI: magnetic resonance imaging

MRM: modified radical mastectomy

MS: mitral stenosis

NAVY: nerve, artery, vein, Y fronts

NEC: necrotising enterocolitis

NG: nasogastric tube

NHS: National Health Service

NICU: Neonatal Intensive Care Unit

NOF: neck of femur

NSS: nephron sparing surgery

NSTEMI: non-ST elevation myocardial infarction

NVB: neurovascular bundle

OA: oesophageal atresia

OME: otitis media with effusion

OSA: obstructive sleep apnoea

OSNA: one-step nucleic amplification

PCA: patient controlled analgesia

PCI: percutaneous coronary intervention

PCL: posterior cruciate ligament

PDS: polydioxanone

PE: pulmonary embolism

PET: positron emission tomography

PFA: profunda femoral artery

PFO: patent foramen ovale

PH: potential hydrogen

PIP: proximal interphalangeal

PIPJ: proximal interphalangeal joints

POEM: per-oral endoscopic myotomy

PR: abdominoperineal resection

PTH: parathyroid hormone

RBMN: recurrent branch of the median nerve

RCA: right coronary artery

RCC: renal cell carcinoma

RGA: right gastric artery

RGE: right gastro-epiploic

RIG: radiologically inserted gastrostomy

RIGJ: radiologically inserted gastrojejunostomy

RL: recurrent laryngeal nerve

RM: radical mastectomy

SAM: systolic anterior motion

SCM: sternocleidomastoid

SDF: superior duodenal flexure

SFA: superior femoral artery

SFJ: saphenofemoral junction

SFV: superior femoral vein

SIEA: superior inferior epigastric artery

SIEV: superior inferior epigastric vein

SIGN: Scottish Intercollegiate Guidelines Network

SIT: supraspinatus, infraspinatus and teres minor

SLNB: sentinel lymph node biopsy

SM: simple mastectomy

SMA: superior mesenteric artery

SMV: superior mesenteric vein

SPA: sphenopalatine artery

SPA: superior pancreaticoduodenal artery

SSV: short saphenous vein

STEMI: ST elevation myocardial infarction

STSG: split thickness skin graft

SUI: stress urinary incontinence

T3: liothyronine

TAT: trans-anastomotic tube

TAVI: transcatheter aortic valve implantation

THR: total hip replacement

TKR: total knee replacement

TIPSS: trans-jugular intrahepatic portosystemic shunt

TM: tympanic membrane

TME: total mesorectal excision

TOE: transoesophageal echocardiography

TOF: tracheoesophageal fistula

tPA: tissue plasminogen activator

TRAM: transverse rectus abdominis muscle

TSH: thyroid stimulating hormone

TUR: transurethral resection

TURP: transurethral resection of the prostate

TURBT: transurethral resection of bladder tumour

TVT: tension-free vaginal tape

TWOC: trial without catheter

USP: US pharmacopoeia

VACTERL: vertebral, anal atresia, cardiovascular, tracheoesophageal, renal and limb defects

VAN: vein, artery, nerve

VATS: video-assisted thoracoscopic surgery

vCJD: variant Creutzfeldt Jacob Disease

VP: ventriculoperitoneal

VPI: velopharyngeal insufficiency

VTE: venous thromboembolic

WHO: World Health Organisation

WLE: wide local excision

Contributors

Chief Editor

Katrina Mason BSc (Hons) MBChB MRCS
(ENT)
ENT Surgery Registrar
St George's Hospital, London, UK

Series Editor

Zeshan Qureshi BM MSc BSc (Hons)
MRCPCH FAcadMEd MRCPS (Glas)
Paediatric Registrar
London, UK

Associate Editors

Madelaine Gimzewska BMedSci (Hons)
MBChB MRCS MSc
Academic Clinical Fellow in Vascular Surgery
Imperial College London, UK

Gareth Rogers MBChB BSc (Hons)
Junior Doctor
Leeds Teaching Hospital Trust, UK

Chapter Editors

Alison Bradley BSc (Hons) MBChB MRCSEd
Surgical Registrar
Glasgow, UK

Mathew Gallagher MBChB MRCS
Neurosurgery Registrar
The Walton Centre NHS Foundation Trust,
UK

Joanna Buchan MBChB BSc Hons
Surgical Trainee
NHS Tayside, UK

James Glasbey MBBCh BSc MRCS
Academic Clinical Fellow (Surgery)
University of Birmingham, UK

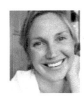

Laura Cormack MBChB BSc (Hons) MRCP
DTMH (Liv) FRCR
Consultant Radiologist
West Suffolk Hospital, UK

Brendan S Kelly MB BCh BAO MRCSI
ICAT HRB/Wellcome Trust Academic Fellow,
University College Dublin, Ireland.
Specialist Registrar in Radiology St Vincent's
University Hospital, Dublin, Ireland

Ganesh Devarajan MBBS MS (Ortho) FRCS
(Ortho)
Consultant Trauma and Orthopaedic
surgeon
Hull and East Yorkshire NHS Trust, UK

William B Lo MA (Cantab) MB BChir FRCS
(SN) FEBNS
Neurosurgery Registrar
Queen Elizabeth Hospital, Birmingham,
UK

Mary Patrice Eastwood MBChB PhD
MRCSed
Paediatric Surgical Registrar
Royal Belfast Hospital for Sick Children,
Belfast, UK

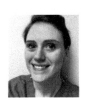

Greta McLachlan MbChB BSc (Hons)
MRCS (Eng)
General Surgical Trainee
Kent, Surrey and Sussex Deanery, UK

CONTRIBUTORS

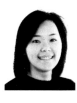 Lay Ping Ong MB BChir MA (Cantab) MRCS (Eng)
Wellcome Trust Clinical PhD Fellow.
Honorary RCS (Eng) Research Fellow
Cambridge, UK

 Farihah Tariq MBChB BSc (Hons)
Research Fellow, Oxford Eye Hospital
John Radcliffe Hospital, UK

 Esther Platt MA MBBS MRCS DTM&H
Speciality Registrar
Kent Surrey Sussex Deanery, UK

 Evgenia Theodorakopoulou BMedSci (Hons) BMBS MRCSEng
Plastic and Reconstructive Surgery Registrar.
St. Andrew's Centre for Plastic Surgery and
Burns, Broomfield Hospital, Chelmsford
Essex, UK

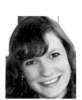 Jennifer Robertson BSc (Hons) MBChB (Hons)
Junior Doctor
Forth Valley Royal Hospital, Scotland, UK

 Mr Alexander Yao MBBS MA (Cantab)
ENT Registrar.
West Midlands Deanery, UK

Authors

 Stephen Ali BM MMedSc (Hons) PGCME MRCS (Eng)
Plastics, Burns and Reconstructive Surgery
Registrar
The Welsh Centre for Burns & Plastic Surgery

 Roberta Bullingham BMBS BSc (Hons)
BVSc MRCS
Core trainee
Guy's and St Thomas' Hospital. UK

 Stephanie Arrigo BSc (Hons) MD MRCS
Radiology Trainee
Mater Dei Hospital, Msida, Malta

 Ivana Capin
3rd Year Medical Student
University of Limerick, Ireland

 Richard D Bartlett
MB/PhD student
UCL, UK

 Darren KT Chan MBBS
Radiology Registrar
East Kent Hospitals University NHS Trust

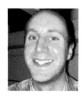 Jonathan Bialick BSc (Hons) MBBS
Junior Doctor
The Royal London Hospital, UK

 Tyson Chan Mb BCh BAO
Junior Doctor
Khoo Teck Puat Hospital, Singapore

 Carly Bisset MBChB
General Surgery Registrar
Royal Alexandra Hospital, Scotland, UK

 Christina Cheng MBBS (Hons)
Junior Doctor
Sydney, Australia

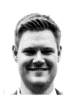 James Brooks
BMBS (Hons), BMedSci (Hons)
Anaesthetic trainee
University Hospital, Southampton NHS
Trust, UK

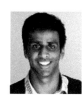 Abhishek Chitnis MBChB MClinEd
Junior Doctor
Tameside General Hospital, Greater
Manchester, UK

Luke Conway MBChB MRes MRCS
Surgical Trainee
Royal Liverpool and Broadgreen University
Hospital Trust, UK

 Angelina Jayakumar BSc (Hons) MBChB
MRCP DTM&H
Core Medical Trainee
The Royal London Hospital, Barts Heath
NHS Trust, UK

 James Cragg MBBCh MRCS PGDip
Vascular Registrar
West Midlands, UK

 John Kennedy BMSc (Hons) MBChB MRCS
Speciality Registrar Trauma and
Orthopaedics
West of Scotland Deanary, UK

 Alexander Dando BMBS, MMedSc (Hons)
Junior Doctor
University Hospital, Southampton NHS
Trust, UK

 Maria Knöbel MBBS BSc ARCS
Resident in ENT Surgery
Kantonsspital Aarau, Zurich, Switzerland

 Kirsty Dawson MBChB
Junior Doctor
North West Deanery, UK

 Nicholas Leaver MBChB
Junior Doctor
North West of England Foundation School,
UK

 Yasoda Dupaguntla
4th Year Medical Student
Southampton University, UK

 Jane Shujing Lim BMedSci (Hons)
Final Year Medical Student
University of Edinburgh, UK

 Stephanie Eltz Med Univ
Orthopaedic Registrar
North West London Deanery, UK

 Nigel Tapiwa Mabvuure BSc (Hons) MBBS
(Hons) MRCS
Plastics Registrar
Glasgow Royal Infirmary, Scotland, UK

 Lisa Grundy
4th Year Medical Student
Cardiff University, UK

 Huzaifa Malick MbCHb FRCOphth
Ophthalmology Registrar
Leicester Royal Infirmary, UK

 Louis Hainsworth BMBS MSc
Core Surgical Trainee
Musgrove Park Hospital, UK

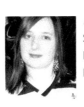 Andrea McCarthy MBBS BCh BAO
Surgical Tutor
Royal College of Surgeons in Ireland,
Republic of Ireland

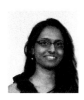 Nimeshi Jayakody BMBS MMedSc (Hons)
MRCS DOHNS MSc (Allergy) CST2
Junior Doctor
University Hospital, Southampton NHS
Trust, UK

 Sameena Mohamedally MBChB
Junior Doctor
William Harvey Hospital, Ashford,
Kent, UK

CONTRIBUTORS

 Dariush Nikkhah FRCS (Plast)
Trauma and Microsurgical Fellow
Royal Perth Hospital
Perth Hospital, Western Australia, Australia

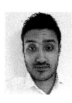 Georgios Pafitanis MD MSc (Hons)
Senior Microsurgery Fellow
Guys and St Thomas Hospital, London, UK
Group for Academic Plastic Surgery,
The Blizard Institute, Queen Mary
University of London, London, UK

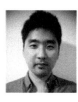 Joon Park MBBS
Medical Resident
The Prince Charles Hospital, Brisbane,
Queensland, Australia

 Conor Ramsden MA MRCP FRCOphth PhD
Ophthalmic Trainee
Moorfields Eye Hospital, UK

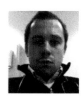 Paul Robinson MRCS MBBS BSc (Hons)
Surgical Registrar
Dorset County Hospital, UK

 Suhail Rokadiya MRCS
Oral and Maxillofacial Surgery Registrar
Scotland, UK

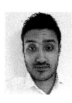 Shahab Shahid MBBS iBSc (Hons)
Junior Doctor
North Central, East Thames Deanery, UK

 Yashashwi Sinha MBChB MRes
Academic Foundation Doctor
Ealing Hospital, London, UK

 Rebecca Telfer BMedSci (Hons) MBCHB
Junior Doctor
Whiston Hospital, UK

 Sasha Shoba Devi Thrumurthy MBChB
MRCP(UK)
Specialist Registrar, Gastroenterology
and Hepatology
Tan Tock Seng Hospital, Singapore

 Chukwudi Uzoho
BM BSc BMedSci MRCS PgCert
Trauma and Orthopaedics Registrar
East Midlands Deanery, UK

 Nicholas Wroe MBChB (Hons) BSc (Hons)
Junior Doctor
Leeds Teaching Hospitals, UK

 Shiying Wu MBBS (Hons)
Junior Doctor
Albury-Wodonga Health, Australia

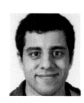 Muhamed Zuhair BSc
Medical Student
Hull York Medical School, UK

Senior Reviewers

CHAPTER 1 UPPER GASTROINTESTINAL

Richard Skipworth MD FRCS
Consultant Surgeon and Honorary Clinical Senior Lecturer
Royal Infirmary of Edinburgh, UK

Francis Hughes MB BS, MS, FRCS (England)
FRCS (General Surgery)
Consultant Upper GI Surgeon
Royal London Hospital, UK

Deepak Hariharan
Surgical Registrar (HPB)
Royal London Hospital, UK

CHAPTER 2 LOWER GASTROINTESTINAL

Jeff Garner MBChB MD MRCS (Glasg)
FRCS FRCSEd (Gen Surg)
Consultant General and Colorectal Surgeon
Rotherham NHS Foundation Trust, UK

Laura Arthur MBChB, MD, FRCS (Glasg)
Specialty Registrar
Glasgow, UK

CHAPTER 3 BREAST

S Chandrasekharan MS FRCS MSc
Consultant Breast Surgeon
Colchester General Hospital, UK

CHAPTER 4 EAR NOSE AND THROAT

Francis W Stafford MBBS FRCSEng FRCSEd
Consultant ENT and Head and Neck Surgeon
Sunderland Royal Hospital, UK

Christopher Pepper FRCS (ORL-HNS),
Consultant Paediatric ENT Surgeon
Evelina London Children's Hospital,
Guys and St Thomas' NHS Trust, UK

CHAPTER 5 ENDOCRINE

Wendy Craig FRCS
Consultant Endocrine Surgeon
University Hospitals of Morecambe Bay NHS
Foundation Trust, UK

Francis W Stafford MBBS FRCSEng FRCSEd
Consultant ENT and Head and Neck Surgeon
Sunderland Royal Hospital, UK

Christopher Pepper FRCS (ORL-HNS),
Consultant Paediatric ENT Surgeon
Evelina London Children's Hospital,
Guys and St Thomas' NHS Trust, UK

CHAPTER 6 VASCULAR

Tim Stansfield MSc FRCS
Consultant Vascular and Trauma Surgeon
Leeds General Infirmary, UK

Max Troxler MD FRCS FEBVS
Consultant Vascular Surgeon
Leeds Teaching Hospital Trust, UK

Sidhartha Sinha MA MSc MD (Res) MRCS FRCS
Vascular Surgery Registrar
King's College Hospital, London, UK

CHAPTER 7 UROLOGY

Sohier Elneil MRCOG
Consultant Urogynaecologist and Uro-neurologist
University College Hospital and the National Hospital
for Neurology and Neurosurgery, London, UK

CHAPTER 8 CARDIOTHORACICS

Simon Kendall MS, FRCS (C/Th), MB BS
Medical Director and Cardiac Surgeon, Honorary Secretary
Society for Cardiothoracic Surgery in Great Britain and
Ireland
James Cook University Hospital, UK

CHAPTER 9 NEUROSURGERY

William B Lo MA (Cantab) MB BChir FRCS (SN) FEBNS
Neurosurgery Registrar
Queen Elizabeth Hospital, Birmingham, UK

CHAPTER 10 ORTHOPAEDICS

Alexander Young MbChB MSc
MRCS PGCME
Trauma and Orthopaedic Registrar
Severn Deanary, UK

Ganesh Devarajan
MBBS MS (Ortho) FRCS (Ortho)
Consultant Trauma and Orthopaedic
surgeon
Hull and East Yorkshire NHS Trust, UK

CHAPTER 11 PLASTICS

Kallirroi Tzafetta MBBS FRCS (Plast) MPhil
Consultant Plastic Surgeon
Broomfield Hospital, Chelmsford, UK

CHAPTER 12 PAEDIATRICS

Professor Paolo De Coppi MBBS FRCS (Eng)
FRCS (Paed Surg)
Professor of Paediatric Surgery
Great Ormond Street Hospital, UK

CHAPTER 13 OBSTETRICS AND GYNAECOLOGY

Sohier Elneil MRCOG
Consultant Urogynaecologist and Uro-neurologist
University College Hospital and the National
Hospital for Neurology and Neurosurgery,
London, UK

CONTRIBUTORS

Asma Elissa MRCOG
Obstetric and Gynaecology Registrar
London, UK

CHAPTER 14 INTERVENTIONAL RADIOLOGY

Dr Andrew Hatrick MA BChir MRCP FRCR EBIR
Consultant Interventional Radiologist and
Chief of Service
Frimley Health Foundation Trust, UK

Dr Rory O' Donoghue MD FFR RCSI
Consultant Interventional and
Diagnostic Radiologist
Tallaght University Hospital, Dublin, Ireland

CHAPTER 15 OPHTHALMOLOGY

Marie Tsaloumas MBBS FRCOphth
Consultant Ophthalmologist
Queen Elizabeth Hospital, Birmingham, UK

Student Reviewers

Imogen Thomson
Medical Student
University of Sydney

Stella Harris
Medical Student
University of Sydney

Helena Qian
Medical Student
University of Newcastle

Contents

0 USEFUL THEATRE KNOWLEDGE

KATRINA MASON

SCRUBBING UP FOR THEATRE

Roberta Bullingham and Jonathan Bialick

AIM OF THE SURGICAL SCRUB

A systematic washing of the hands, forearms, and nails with an antiseptic wash with the aim of:

- Removing debris and transient microorganisms
- Reducing commensal microorganisms to a minimum
- Inhibiting "rebound" growth and release of bacteria under gloved hands

In case of puncture of the surgical glove, and the release of bacteria to the open wound, the scrub will reduce the risk of a surgical site infection (SSI) to an absolute minimum.

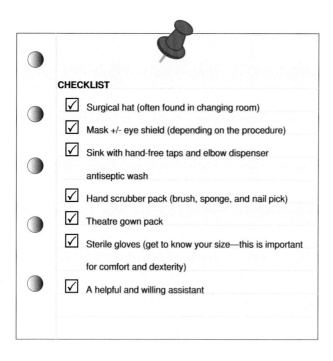

CHECKLIST

- ☑ Surgical hat (often found in changing room)
- ☑ Mask +/- eye shield (depending on the procedure)
- ☑ Sink with hand-free taps and elbow dispenser antiseptic wash
- ☑ Hand scrubber pack (brush, sponge, and nail pick)
- ☑ Theatre gown pack
- ☑ Sterile gloves (get to know your size—this is important for comfort and dexterity)
- ☑ A helpful and willing assistant

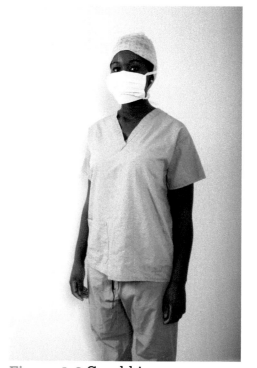

Figure 1.0 Scrubbing.

PREPARATION

- Keep nails short and clean, and do not wear artificial nails or nail polish.
- Remove all jewellery (rings, watches, bracelets) before entering the operating theatre.
- Wear scrubs, surgical hat, and theatre shoes to enter theatre.
- Wash hands and arms with a non-medicated soap, and dry before entering the operating theatre.
- Tie on face mask, covering nose and mouth (you will not be able to readjust when scrubbed).
- Open surgical gown packet, and gently tip it onto gowning trolley so that it faces upwards.
- Open the packet by pulling the edges outwards to unfold it (maintaining sterile field of the contents).
- Open the packet containing the gloves and tip them onto the open gown packet (just to the side of the paper towels).
- Open the hand scrubber and leave it on the edge of the sink (or within easy reach).

"SCRUBBING-IN"

The scrub procedure should last 5 minutes (this should be timed).

Phase 1

1 Turn on the water and regulate the flow and temperature of water (after this step, you must not touch the taps with your hands).
2 Wet hands and arms down to the elbow for a pre-scrub wash: use several drops of scrub solution, work up a heavy lather, then wash the hands and arms to the elbows (*Figure 1.1*).
3 Rinse hands and arms thoroughly, allowing the water to run from the hands to the elbows.
4 Use nail pick (from the hand scrubber pack) to remove dirt from under nails, and then discard into a sharps bin.
5 Use the elbow of one arm to dispense antiseptic wash onto the scrubber brush.
6 Lather fingertips with sponge side of brush; then, using bristle side of brush, scrub the spaces under the fingernails of the right or left hand. Repeat for other hand (*Figure 1.2*).
7 Lather fingers. Wash on all four sides of the fingers using the sponge side only. Discard the scrubber.
8 Rinse, always keeping hands above the elbows.

Phase 2

1 Dispense antiseptic wash into the palm of one hand (using the opposite elbow to press the lever).
2 Wash hands using the 6-step technique (WHO guidelines):
   a Palm to palm
   b Right palm over left dorsum and left palm over right dorsum
   c Palm to palm, fingers interlaced
   d Back of fingers to opposing palms with fingers interlocked
   e Rotational rubbing of right thumb clasped in left palm and vice versa
   f Rotational rubbing backwards and forwards with clasped fingers of right hand in left palm and vice versa
3 Rotationally rub the wrists, working down to the elbows with one hand and then vice versa.
4 Rinse hands and arms thoroughly from fingertip to elbow without retracing, allowing the water to drip from the elbow (*Figure 1.3*).

If the scrub practitioner's hands or arms accidentally touch the taps, sink, or other unsterile object during any phase of the scrub, they are considered contaminated and the process MUST begin again

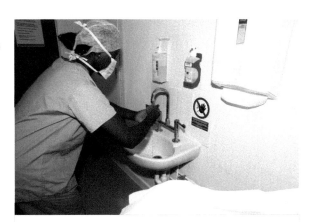

Figure 1.1 Wetting hands.

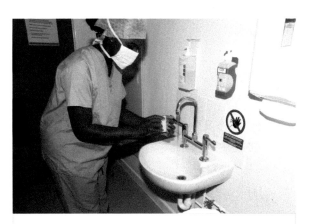

Figure 1.2 Cleaning fingertips.

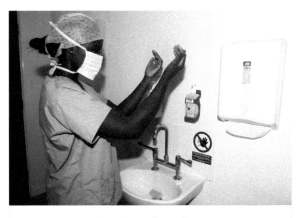

Figure 1.3 Rinsing hands.

USEFUL THEATRE KNOWLEDGE

Phase 3

1 Repeat phase 2, but stop halfway down the forearms.
2 Close the taps using elbows.
3 Return to gowning trolley, pick up one hand towel from the top of the gown pack, and step back from the table. Grasp the towel and open it fully (*Figure 1.4*).
4 Use an aseptic paper towel to dry using a patting motion. Start at fingers and work down arms; do not retrace any area. Each hand should only touch one side of the paper towel. Discard each paper towel after use (*Figure 1.5*).
5 Do not retrace any areas. Discard this towel in an appropriate receptacle.
6 Repeat with the other towel from the pack for the other hand/arm.

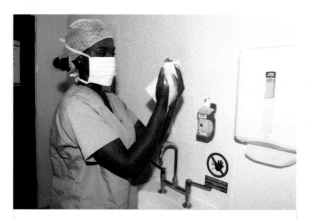

Figure 1.4 Drying hands.

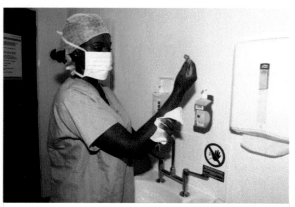

Figure 1.5 Drying arms.

GOWNING

1 Keep your hands close together with thumbs facing up and place hands into the arms of the gown (it will be facing this way in the pack).
2 Lift it off the trolley. Taking a wide step back (making sure you have enough space that you will not touch anything by mistake), extend your elbows, moving arms apart so that the gown unfolds (*Figure 1.6*).
3 Keep your hands within the sleeves (*Figure 1.7*).
4 Ask an assistant to fasten the Velcro and the ties at the back.

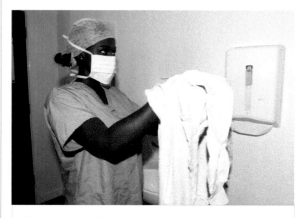

Figure 1.6 Putting on gown.

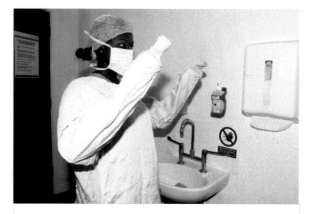

Figure 1.7 Keeping hands within sleeves.

DONNING GLOVES

1 Keeping hands tucked inside the sleeves of the gown, unfold the packet with the gloves inside.

2 Pick up one glove by the folded cuff edge with the sleeve-covered hand (opposite hand to glove labelled left or right). If you are right-handed, gloving your left hand first is easiest, but either way is fine (*Figure 1.8*).

3 Slip the fingers of the appropriate hand out of the sleeve of the gown into the glove (with the rest of the hand remaining covered) (*Figure 1.9*).

4 Use your still-covered opposite hand to fold back the rest of the glove so that it covers the wrist.

5 Pull and adjust the sleeves of the gown so that they cover a little more than the wrists under the gloves (*Figure 1.10*).

6 Follow the above steps for the opposite hand.

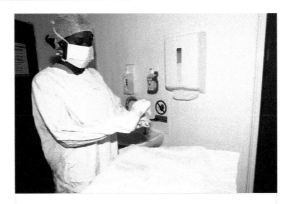

Figure 1.9 **Putting on gloves.**

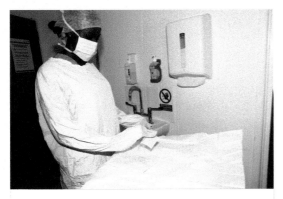

Figure 1.8 **Opening gloves.**

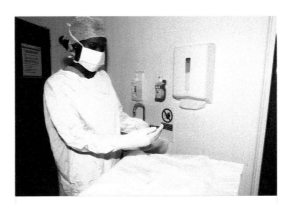

Figure 1.10 **Adjusting gloves.**

FINAL TIE OF THE GOWN

1 Take hold of the sterile card belt tab that secures the belt tie *(Figure 1.11)*.

2 Ask an assistant to take hold of the tab and walk all the way around you, ending in front of you (*Figure 1.12*).

3 Then take hold of the belt tie only (being careful not to touch the tab again) and pull on the tie, leaving the assistant with only the tab in their hand (*Figure 1.13*).

4 Tie the belt tie with a simple knot at the side of the gown.

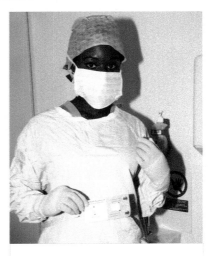

Figure 1.11 **Sterile card.**

USEFUL THEATRE KNOWLEDGE

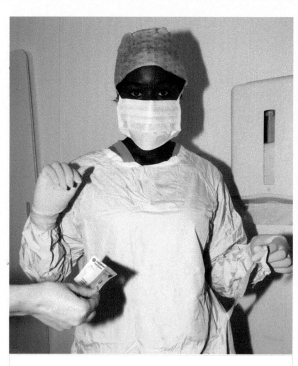

Figure 1.12 Assistant helping with final tie.

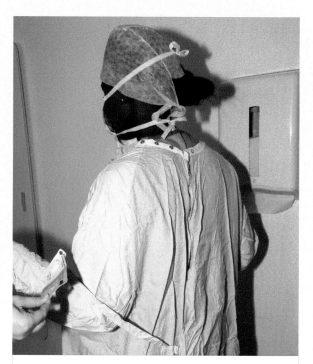

Figure 1.13 Rotating with tie held by assistant.

SURGEON'S TOP TIPS

1 When waiting for the procedure to start, keep your hands raised in front of your chest to maintain your sterile field.

2 If you have any questions during the scrubbing-in procedure, ask—there are always experienced people who can help.

3 If you do accidentally make contact with an unsterile object at any time, don't be afraid to say so. The surgical team and the patient will be glad you did!

WOUND CLOSURE AND DIATHERMY

Suhail Rokadiya

INTRODUCTION TO SUTURES

> The closure of a wound with sutures is known as healing by 'primary intention' and allows for the rapid and cosmetic closure of an open wound/other tissue.
> Sutures have been around for approximately 4,000 years. Linen, animal sinews, and a huge variety of other materials have been used. This chapter will help you further understand suture material types, suture examples, and their appropriate surgical uses.

CHOOSING THE APPROPRIATE SUTURE MATERIAL

> The ideal suture material should:
>> Be universally applicable
>> Be 'memory free' (i.e., limp and pliable)
>> Be inert and biocompatible
>> Have low drag when passing through tissues but good friction for knot-tying
>> Be free from stretch and not warp under tension
>> Be stable under sterilisation during manufacturing
> A suture material that is suitable for all closures does not exist. Therefore, the first question a surgeon will face when deciding on suture type is whether the suture needs to be absorbable or non-absorbable.
> Absorbable sutures undergo natural degradation through enzymatic action followed by hydrolytic action, or through hydrolytic action alone. Natural suture materials such as catgut (from animal intestines—monofilament) and collagen (from bovine tendons—multifilament) were traditionally used. In the main, however, synthetic materials are now utilised.
> Further considerations are whether the suture material is made from natural or synthetic material and whether the fabric of the suture is monofilament or multifilament (braided or twisted).
> Recently, barbed sutures have become available in a variety of absorbable synthetic materials, with the aim of avoiding knot-tying. They have not yet become widely utilised.
> The choice between multifilament and monofilament sutures is based on a variety of factors:
>> Multifilament sutures run a higher potential of bacterial contamination, as bacteria can adhere more easily to the crenulations in the material.
>> Multifilament sutures also have a wicking action, which has the potential to draw fluid into a wound and thus further increase the potential for wound infection. Monofilament sutures have a lower coefficient of friction, resulting in less drag than a multifilament suture. However, they are more sensitive to meticulous technique when knot-tying.
>> Thicker-grade sutures have 'suture memory', where the suture material retains the shape of its packing. Monofilament sutures often spring back to their original shape, making knot-tying more difficult.

ABSORBABLE SUTURES

Synthetic

1 Polydioxanone or PDS:
   a A monofilament suture hydrolysed (absorbed) in less than one year
   b Has memory and is thus sometimes difficult to manipulate without practice

2 Polyglycolic acid suture (e.g., Vicryl, Polysorb, Dexon)
   a Braided, although an ophthalmic monofilament suture is available
   b Generally absorbed within four weeks
   c Has generally good handling characteristics with little memory

3 Polyglecaprone (e.g., monocryl)

  a Available as either a clear or a dyed (purple) monofilament suture

  b Absorbed within 120 days

  c Has a degree of memory

4 Polyglyconate (Maxon)

  a A long-term monofilament suture absorbed within 210 days

  b Available as clear or green

  c Older versions were less pliable, but the material has good knot-holding capability

5 Polyglactin 910 (Vicryl rapide)

  a A white braided suture, absorbed within six weeks, but can be wiped off the skin within two weeks

  b Good handling characteristics

  c Made from 90% polyglycolic acid combined with 10% lactic acid

Natural

> Despite availability and good handling characteristics, natural absorbable sutures are rarely used due to concerns regarding the possible transmission of new variant Creutzfeldt-Jakob (VCJD) causing prions in patients.

> Catgut is a monofilament, rapidly absorbed, and available either plain (fast) or chromic coated to allow faster or slower enzymatic degradation depending on the site and the patient physiology.

NON-ABSORBABLE SUTURES

Synthetic

1 Nylon (e.g., Ethilon, Dafilon, Dermalon, Linex)

  a Monofilament, good tensile strength and minimal tissue reactivity

  b Inexpensive and widely used

2 Polypropylene (e.g., Prolene, Surgipro)

  a Very smooth monofilament suture but highly plastic and more difficult to tie securely than other materials

3 Polybutester (e.g., Novafil)

  a Elastic and thus can adapt to tissue oedema

  b Good handling and knot-tying properties

4 Polyester (e.g., Ticron, Dacron, Mersilene, Ethibond)

  a Braided suture, very strong with good handling and low tissue reaction

5 Stainless Steel

  a Used primarily in closure of the chest following cardiothoracic surgery and in orthopaedics for cerclage and tendon repair; can also be used for abdominal wall closure

  b High tensile strength, some elasticity and forms a secure knot

Natural

1 Silk

  a Braided treated suture

  b Has excellent handling and knot security

NEEDLES

Design and anatomy

> The needle should be made of high-quality stainless steel, be of the smallest possible cross-sectional area, and remain stable in the needle holder or hand.

> The anatomy of the needle can be separated into three parts:

  1 The point

  2 The body

  3 The swage/eye of the needle

> Needles are available in a variety of lengths, from 75 micrometres to 80 mm.

Point types *(Figure 1.14)*

> Cutting needles—designed to penetrate dense and thick tissues, including skin. They are triangular in cross section and have three cutting edges, either on the inside of the curve (conventional) or the outside of the curve (reverse cutting). Reverse cutting needles have a reduced risk of cutting through tissues and are therefore used in ophthalmic and cosmetic procedures where minimal tissue trauma is vital. Spatula needles were specifically designed for ophthalmic procedures, as the needle design splits/separates the layers of corneal tissue to create a plane through which the suture material can pass.

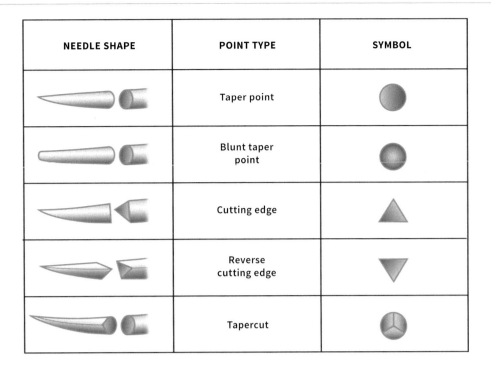

NEEDLE SHAPE	POINT TYPE	SYMBOL
	Taper point	
	Blunt taper point	
	Cutting edge	
	Reverse cutting edge	
	Tapercut	

Figure 1.14
Needle types.

- Tapered point needles—useful in subcutaneous layers and abdominal viscera where tissue can be stretched and penetrated without cutting. Sharpness is dictated by the taper ratio and tip angle.
- Blunt needles—pass through friable tissue (e.g., liver and kidney) without cutting.

Needle body types *(Figure 1.15)*
- Straight body—simple to use, but must be used with caution as the tissue is usually being manipulated by hand
- Curved body—can be used in tighter spaces and allow an even distribution of tension on rotation of the wrist

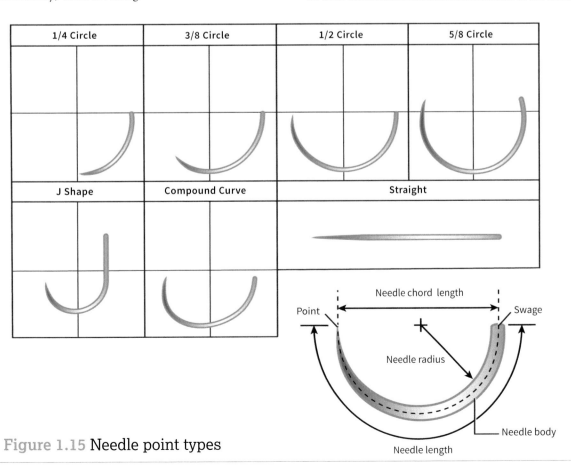

Figure 1.15 Needle point types

› Usually represented as fractions of a circle (e.g., 3/8, 5/8)
› Compound shape
› J-shaped

Swage types (the attachment of the needle to the suture)

› Channel—These needles have a larger diameter at the swage than at the needle point (a result of crimping the needle end around the suture).

› Non-swaged—Now unlikely to be used, as they result in more tissue trauma and suture handling, these needles require passing the suture through the needle's eye (such as in tailoring).

› Drill—The end of the needle is finely removed (often with a laser) during production, allowing the swage to be a smaller diameter than the needle. This results in less tissue trauma when being pulled through.

SUTURE SIZE

Sizes are listed here from smallest to largest (Figure 1.16). Although the European units are more closely related to the actual diameter of the suture, USP (US pharmacopoeia) units are more widely used in the UK.

USP designation	Synthetic absorbable diameter (mm)	Non-absorbable diameter (mm)	Uses
11-0		0.01	Ophthalmic surgery
10-0	0.02	0.02	Digital vessel anastomosis and nerve repair
9-0	0.03	0.03	
8-0	0.04	0.04	Vessel repair and anastomosis Facial skin closure
7-0	0.05	0.05	Vascular grafts following endarterectomy or larger vessel repair
6-0	0.07	0.07	
5-0	0.1	0.1	
4-0	0.15	0.15	Skin closure
3-0	0.2	0.2	Closure of muscle fascia/ tense skin
2-0	0.3	0.3	Bowel repair
0	0.35	0.35	Abdominal closure, joint capsule repair
1	0.4	0.4	Hip and back surgery
2	0.5	0.5	
3	0.6	0.6	Tendon repair and high-tension orthopaedic procedures
4	0.6	0.6	
5	0.7	0.7	
6		0.8	
7			

Figure 1.16 Suture sizes

ALTERNATIVE SKIN CLOSURE

Staples

Staples can be applied rapidly for large scalp closures and less aesthetically demanding sites (Figure 1.17).

Skin glue

Skin glue may be appropriate for small wounds with little or no wound tension, or following suturing to enable a hermetic seal (Figure 1.18).

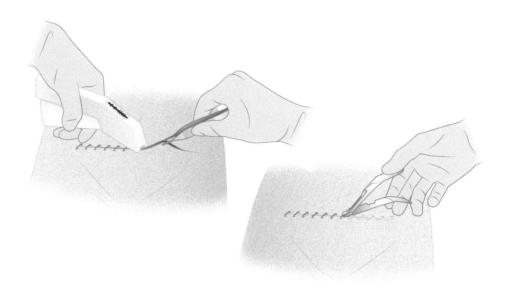

Figure 1.17 Staples

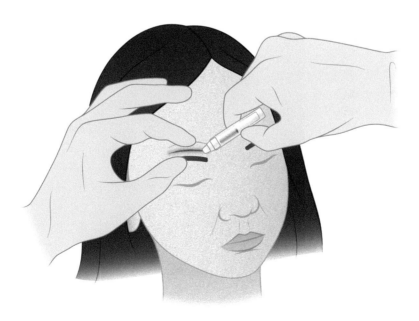

Figure 1.18 Skin glue

Steri-Strips

Wound sticky tape dressings, such as Steri-Strips, can be helpful in the apposition of skin edges following wound closure or as an adjunct to skin glue (Figure 1.19).

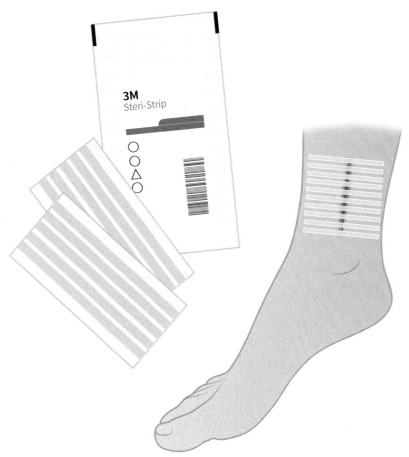

Figure 1.19 Steri-Strips

DIATHERMY

> Diathermy produces a localised heating effect through high-frequency AC electric current (400kHz–10MHz) by which tissue can be cut, cauterised, or destroyed.

> There are risks to the use of diathermy. To reduce these, it is important to ensure that flammable liquid (e.g., alcohol/chlorhexidine skin preparation) is allowed to dry prior to use of diathermy.

> Electrodes should be fully in contact with the patient's skin and not overlie bony prominences.

Monopolar

> From the generator, the current passes through the instrument, through the patient, and back out though a diathermy plate attached to the patient (usually the thigh) (Figure 1.20).

> Heat is concentrated at the tip and spread over the much larger surface area of the plate (>70cm2).

> Relatively high power and wattage are required.

Bipolar

> A conduction current is formed between the two limbs of the forceps so that a small amount of current passes through the tissue between the points of the forceps, locally producing heat (Figure 1.21).

> No plate is required, and thus a smaller wattage is required.

> It is safer for patients with pacemakers for this reason.

> Employed as one of three modes—**cutting** (a constant current), **coagulation** (intermittent pulses of current), or **blend** (a combination).

Figure 1.20 Monopolar diathermy

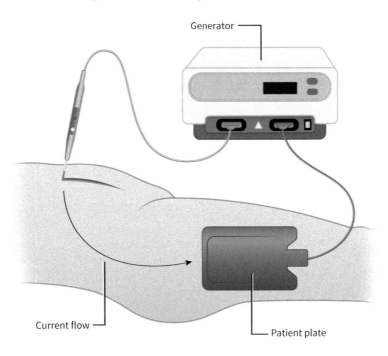

Figure 1.21 Bipolar diathermy

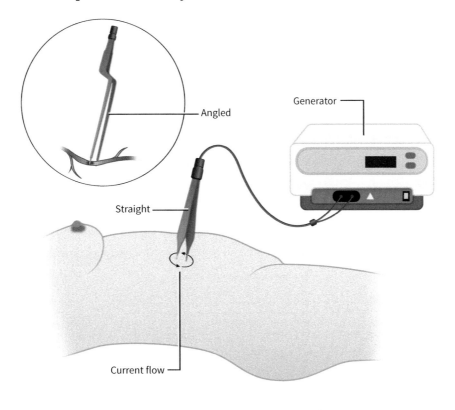

SURGICAL POSITIONS

Katrina Mason

In the images below we have summarised common surgical positions.

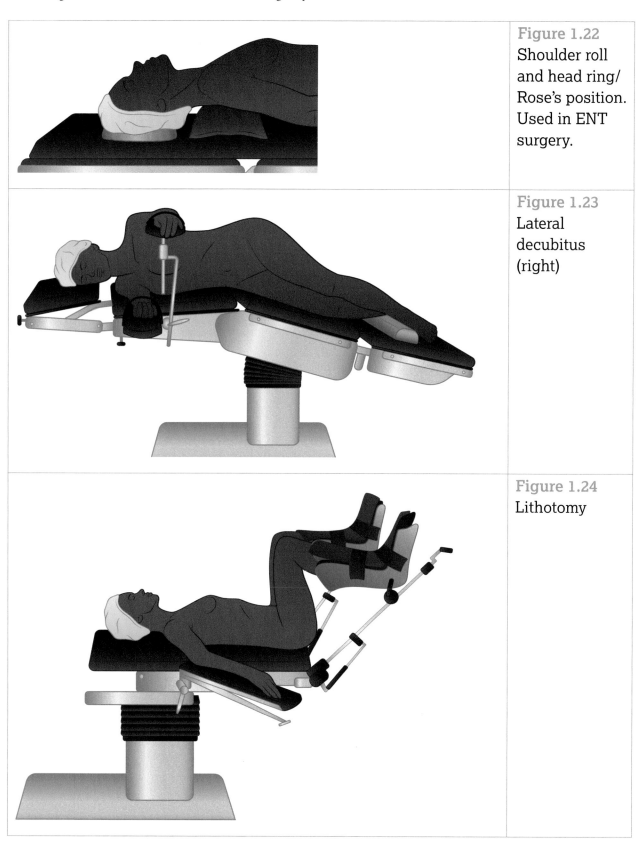

Figure 1.22
Shoulder roll and head ring/ Rose's position. Used in ENT surgery.

Figure 1.23
Lateral decubitus (right)

Figure 1.24
Lithotomy

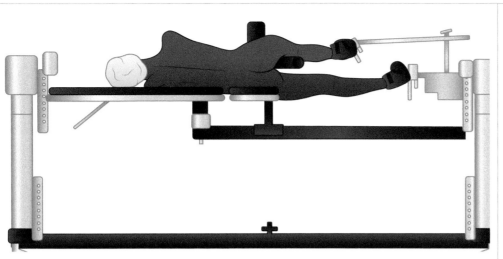

Figure 1.25
Orthopaedics trauma

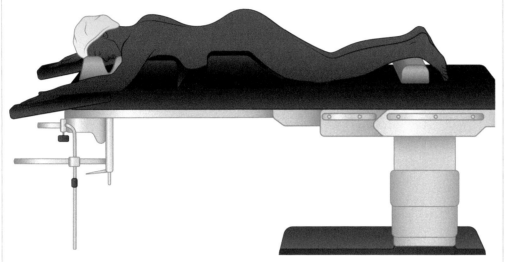

Figure 1.26
Prone

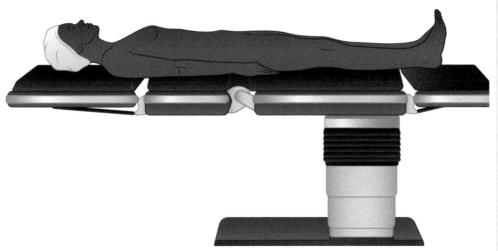

Figure 1.27
Supine

USEFUL THEATRE KNOWLEDGE

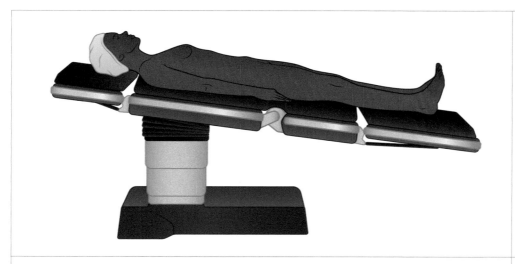

Figure 1.28
Reverse
Trendelenburg

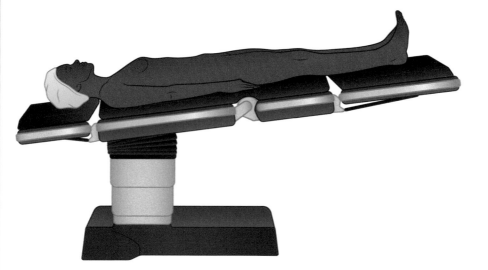

Figure 1.29
Trendelenburg

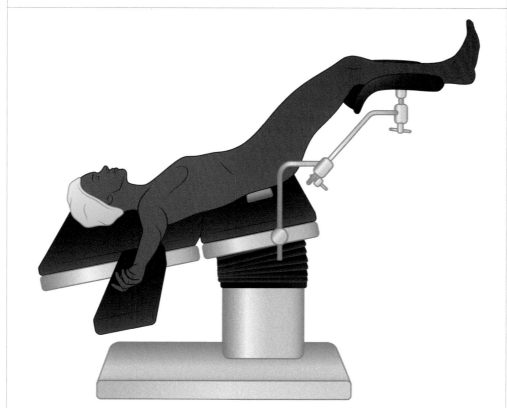

Figure 1.30
Lloyd Davies

1 UPPER GASTROINTESTINAL

JOANNA BUCHAN, GRETA MCLACHLAN

IVOR LEWIS OESOPHAGECTOMY

Andrea McCarthy

DEFINITION
The partial removal of the oesophagus and stomach with construction of a gastric conduit.

✓ INDICATIONS

- Oesophageal cancer—after multidisciplinary team (MDT) discussion and complete staging (CT chest, abdomen, and pelvis, staging laparoscopy, positron emission tomography (PET), endoscopic ultrasound).
- Severe strictures associated with reflux, lye ingestion, or end-stage achalasia.
- Para-oesophageal hernia.
- Gastric cancer involving the gastro-oesophageal junction.

✗ CONTRAINDICATIONS

- Oesophageal cancer T4b staged lesions—with invasion of the trachea, aorta, spine, or other crucial structures or with distant metastases and thus inoperable.
- Where the stomach is diseased or previously removed; other reconstructive options would need to be considered (e.g. colonic interposition).
- Those with significant comorbidities, poor performance status, or severe malnutrition.
- Poor lung function that precludes one lung ventilation.

ANATOMY

Gross anatomy

- The oesophagus extends from the lower border of the cricoid cartilage (C6) to the cardiac orifice of the stomach (T11).
- It is subdivided into three portions: cervical, thoracic, and abdominal.
  - The cervical portion extends from the cricopharyngeus to the suprasternal notch. Arterial supply is from the inferior thyroid artery, and venous drainage is to the inferior thyroid vein.
  - The thoracic oesophagus extends from the suprasternal notch to the diaphragm and lies in the posterior mediastinum. Arterial supply is from the bronchial and oesophageal branches of the thoracic aorta, and venous drainage is to the azygos and hemiazygos veins.
  - The abdominal portion originates at the diaphragm and runs into the cardiac portion of the stomach. Arterial supply is from the ascending branches of the left gastric artery with contribution from the inferior phrenic artery as well, and the venous drainage is to the left gastric (coronary) vein to the portal system (site of porto-systemic anastomosis).

Surgical relations

- Anterior to the oesophagus; the trachea and bronchi above and the pericardium and pulmonary veins below.
- The descending aorta lies posterior to the thoracic oesophagus.
- To the right of the oesophagus, the azygos vein, formed by the union of the ascending lumbar veins and the right subcostal vein at T12, drains the posterior walls of the thorax and abdomen. The azygos vein ascends in the posterior mediastinum along the right-hand side of the thoracic vertebral column to enter the superior vena cava.
- The angle of His (the cardiac notch) is the acute angle between the cardia of the stomach and the oesophagus. It is formed by the fibres of the collar sling and the circular muscles surrounding the gastro-oesophageal junction. It forms a sphincter that prevents reflux.
- The thoracic duct ascends from the cisterna chyli through the oesophageal hiatus in the diaphragm between the azygos vein and the aorta.

Figure 1.1 Anatomic relations of the oesophagus

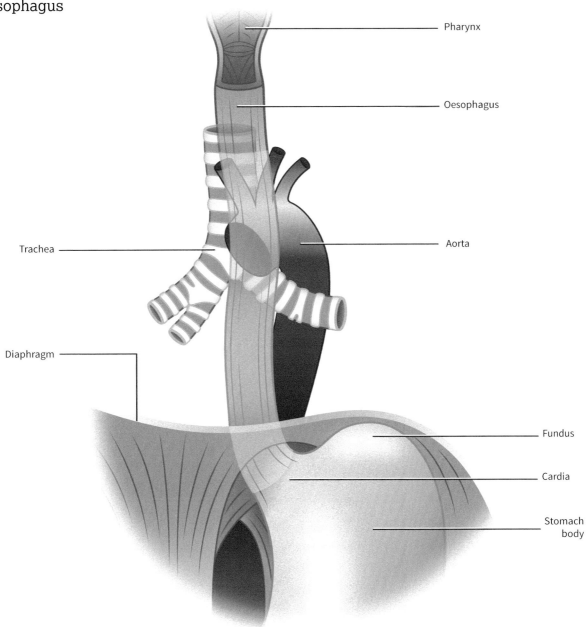

Pharynx

Oesophagus

Trachea

Aorta

Diaphragm

Fundus

Cardia

Stomach body

STEP-BY-STEP OPERATION

Anaesthesia: general with a double lumen endotracheal tube to allow deflation of the right lung. An epidural is also sited and a nasogastric (NG) tube inserted.

Position: reverse Trendelenburg with the surgeon positioned between the patient's legs.

Considerations: Ivor Lewis described a two-phase oesophagectomy involving an abdominal phase (laparotomy) and a thoracic phase (thoracotomy). This may be performed using laparoscopic and thoracoscopic approaches; many surgeons employ hybrid techniques. We describe the hybrid laparoscopic gastric mobilisation and right thoracotomy below.

Abdominal phase

1 Ports placed—in the midline 15 cm below the xiphisternum, right and left midclavicular lines, 5 cm below the costal margin, and a port for a liver retractor just below the xiphisternum.

2 The stomach is mobilised along the greater curvature, taking care to preserve the gastroepiploic arcade. Omental branches and the short gastric vessels are divided with a laparoscopic energy device. The fundus is mobilised. The lesser omentum is divided and the right gastric artery (RGA) divided. The left gastric artery (LGA) and vein are clipped and divided. Lymph nodes around the coeliac trunk are excised *en bloc*.

3 A cuff of crura is excised in continuity with the lower oesophagus and the plane developed into the mediastinum anterior to the aorta. The duodenum is mobilised as necessary to reach the diaphragm.

4 A feeding jejunostomy can be inserted at this point. Port sites are closed with absorbable sutures.

Thoracic phase

5 The patient is repositioned into the left lateral decubitus position. A right lateral thoracotomy is performed through the fifth intercostal space. Single-lung ventilation is used for oesophageal and mediastinal exposure.

6 The azygos vein is identified and divided, the mediastinal pleura incised medial to the azygos vein. The thoracic duct is ligated at the level of the diaphragm. A lymphadenectomy removes the para-tracheal nodes, posterior mediastinal, subcarinal, middle, and peri-oesophageal nodes *en bloc* with the specimen.

7 The gastro-oesophageal junction and the stomach are pulled through the oesophageal hiatus and into the chest.

8 The gastric tube is created with a linear stapler. The oesophagus is divided at least 5 cm proximal to the tumour. The specimen is removed.

9 An anastomosis is formed between the oesophagus and the remaining stomach. An NG tube is advanced into the distal stomach and two intercostal drains are placed. The ribs are approximated with non-absorbable sutures and the wound closed in layers.

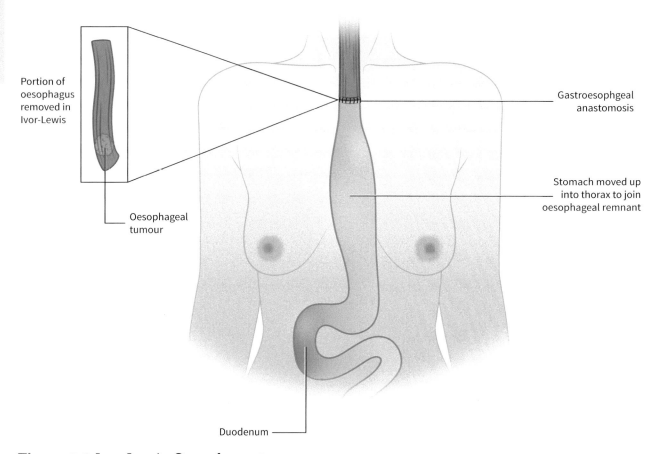

Portion of oesophagus removed in Ivor-Lewis

Oesophageal tumour

Gastroesophgeal anastomosis

Stomach moved up into thorax to join oesophageal remnant

Duodenum

Figure 1.2 Ivor Lewis Oesophagectomy

COMPLICATIONS

Early

- Haemorrhage.
- Injury to tracheobronchial tree.
- Recurrent laryngeal nerve injury—resulting in hoarseness of voice.
- Opening of the pleura during the laparoscopic phase—leading to capnothorax.
- Injury to surrounding organs—colon and splenic capsule.
- Pulmonary complications, including atelectasis, pneumonia, Acute Respiratory Distress Syndrome (ARDS).
- Thromboembolic complications.
- Cardiac complications, including arrhythmia, myocardial infarction, pericardial tamponade.
- Anastomosis leak (8–12%)—leading to mediastinitis or empyema.

Intermediate and late

- Gastric tube necrosis.
- Chylothorax.
- Herniation of the abdominal viscera through the diaphragmatic hiatus.
- Wound dehiscence.
- Complications related to feeding jejunostomy.
- Impaired emptying of stomach.
- Anastomotic stricturing.
- Post-vagotomy dumping syndrome.
- Reflux oesophagitis.
- Diaphragmatic hernia.
- Chronic pain in thoracotomy wound.

POSTOPERATIVE CARE

Inpatient

- Nutrition via a jejunostomy tube for the first few days.
- Water-soluble oral contrast swallow may be performed on day 5–7 post-op to assess anastomotic integrity. Oral intake can then be initiated if there is no anastomotic leak, commencing with liquids initially and progressing to a light diet as tolerated.
- Drains and NG tube removed when output is minimal.
- Patient discharged home once mobile and maintaining adequate nutritional intake.

Outpatient

- Outpatient dietetic follow-up.
- Surgical review at 6-week and 3-month intervals for the first year.
- Multidisciplinary discussion regarding adjuvant treatment for cancer patients.

 SURGEON'S FAVOURITE QUESTION

What provides the arterial supply to the stomach when it is relocated to the chest during an Ivor Lewis procedure?

Right gastro-epiploic artery.

NISSEN FUNDOPLICATION

Muhamed Zuhair

DEFINITION

A procedure where the fundus of the stomach is wrapped around the gastro-oesophageal junction to strengthen the sphincter and prevent herniation of the stomach through the diaphragm. It is undertaken in conjunction with repair of the diaphragmatic crura.

✓ INDICATIONS

- Surgery is considered in patients with a diagnosis of gastro-oesophageal reflux disease for whom:
  - Symptoms are controlled with acid suppression, but where the patient wishes to avoid long-term medication.
  - Medication side effects are not tolerable.
  - The predominant symptom is volume reflux.
  - Complications of Gastro-Oesophageal Reflux Disease (GORD) have developed, such as Barrett's oesophagus and peptic stricture.
  - Extra-oesophageal manifestations—asthma, hoarseness, cough, chest pain, and aspiration.

✗ CONTRAINDICATIONS

- Presence of poor gastric emptying and oesophageal hypomotility.
- Failure of impact of medical management.
- PH studies that do not confirm pathological acid reflux that correlates with patient's symptom.
- Patients with excessive belching or bloating.
- Patients who qualify for bariatric surgery should be considered for this first.

ANATOMY

Gross anatomy

- The oesophageal hiatus is at level T10 (vena cava T8, oesophagus T10, aortic hiatus T12).
- Components of the stomach:
  - Cardia—the area of stomach adjacent to the oesophagus.
  - Fundus—the most superior aspect of the stomach.
  - Body—the main region of the stomach.
  - Pylorus—the area proximal to the duodenum.
- The lesser curvature forms the smaller concave border of the stomach and serves as the attachment of the lesser omentum.
- The lesser omentum has two separate ligaments: the gastro-hepatic ligament, which connects the stomach and the liver, and the hepato-duodenal ligament, which connects the first part of the duodenum and the liver and contains the hepatic artery proper, the portal vein, and the common bile duct.
- The greater curvature forms the long, convex portion of the stomach and serves as the attachment to the greater omentum, which descends anterior to the abdominal viscera to then fold back over itself to insert into the transverse colon.
- The diaphragm consists of two components: the central tendon, which fuses with the pericardium, and the peripheral muscular part that arises from the xiphisternum, the lower six costal cartilages, the vertebral column, and the arcuate ligaments.
- The crura originate from the lumbar vertebrae and arch anteriorly over the lower oesophagus with a potential space posteriorly for herniation.
- The vagus nerves lie anterior and posterior to the oesophagus as it passes through the diaphragm at T10, with branches of the left gastric vessels.
- The aorta lies posterior to the oesophagus, passing through the diaphragm with the azygos vein and the thoracic duct at T12.
- The vena cava passes through the diaphragm at T8, with the right phrenic nerve. The left phrenic nerve pierces the left dome of the diaphragm.
- The above levels can be remembered using the mnemonic "I ate ten eggs at twelve": I (IVC) ate (T8) ten, (T10) eggs (oesophagus), at (aorta) twelve (T12).

Neurovasculature

- The coeliac trunk is the main blood supply to the stomach. It has three main branches: the left gastric artery, the hepatic artery proper, and the splenic artery.
- The fundus of the stomach is supplied by short gastric arteries (originating from the splenic artery).

> ‣ The pylorus of the stomach and the first part of the duodenum are supplied by the gastroduodenal artery (a branch of the hepatic artery proper).
> ‣ The lesser curvature of the stomach is supplied by the left gastric artery and the right gastric artery (a branch of the hepatic artery proper).

> ‣ The greater curvature of the stomach is supplied by an anastomosis between the right gastro-epiploic artery (a branch of the gastroduodenal artery) and the left gastro-epiploic artery (a branch of the splenic artery).

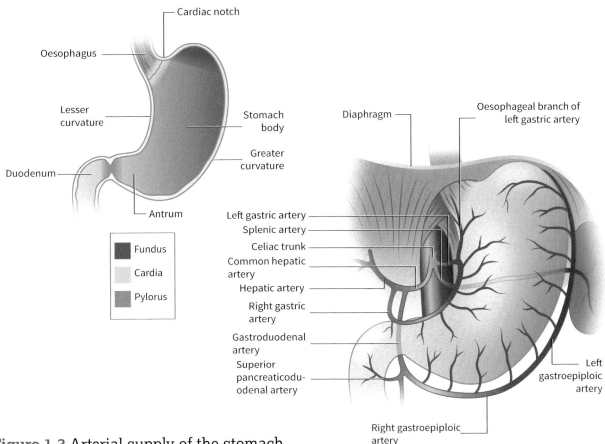

Figure 1.3 Arterial supply of the stomach

STEP-BY-STEP OPERATION

Anaesthesia: general.

Position: reverse Trendelenburg.

1   Three laparoscopic ports are required: midline camera port 15 cm below the xiphisternum, right and left upper quadrant working ports in the mid-clavicular line. A fourth port may be required below the left lateral costal margin.

2   A liver retractor is inserted through an incision below the xiphisternum to retract the left lobe of the liver.

3   The lesser omentum is incised, avoiding the hepatic branch of the anterior vagus nerve, and dissection is continued towards the right crus.

4   The phreno-oesophageal ligament is divided, and the oesophagus and superior stomach are dissected to free them from surrounding structures.

5   The right and left crura of the diaphragm are defined.

6   The oesophagus is mobilised to ensure that a 5 cm length is intra-abdominal (special attention being paid to preserve all branches of the vagus nerve).

7   Non-absorbable sutures are placed into the crura to close the oesophageal hiatus around the oesophagus.

8   Proximal short gastric vessels are identified and divided, freeing the fundus of the stomach.

9   The mobile fundus is pulled around the oesophagus at the level of the gastro- oesophageal junction to create a loose fundoplication, approximately 2 cm in length.

10   The instruments are removed. The 10 mm ports and the skin incisions are closed.

UPPER GASTROINTESTINAL

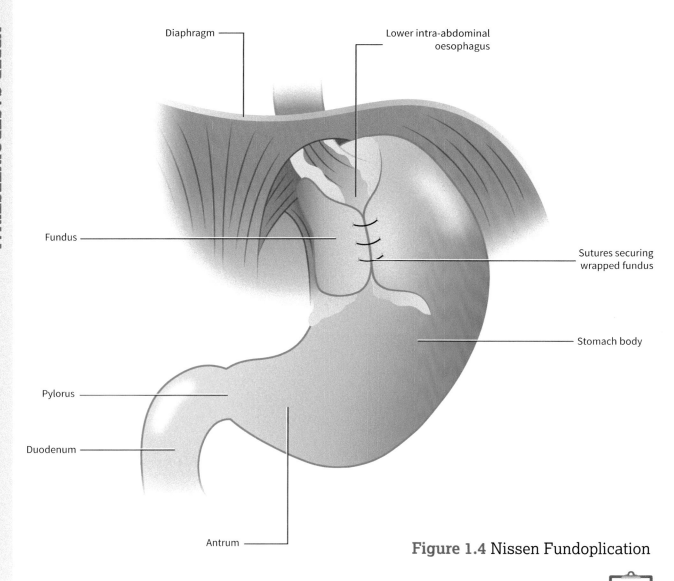

Figure 1.4 Nissen Fundoplication

COMPLICATIONS

Early

▸ Pneumo- or capnothorax caused by inadvertent opening of the pleura during the dissection whilst insufflating CO_2 (5–8%).

▸ Gastric or oesophageal perforation (<1%).

▸ Bleeding from the short gastric vessels, liver, or spleen.

Intermediate and late

▸ Bloating—early postoperative bloating is common and occurs with 30% of patients. Long-term "gas bloat" can occur due to difficulty belching.

▸ Dysphagia—caused by oedema from operative trauma, it normally resolves spontaneously over the first few weeks following surgery. Patients are advised to take a very soft diet for 6 weeks. A small proportion of patients have persistent dysphagia.

▸ Inadvertent vagal injury can cause widespread gastrointestinal dysfunction.

▸ Failure or recurrence of symptoms

▸ "Slipped Nissen"—the stomach can herniate upwards inside the fundoplication. This needs urgent attention, as it can lead to necrosis and perforation.

POSTOPERATIVE CARE

Inpatient

▸ Anti-reflux surgery can be performed as a day-case procedure, but large hiatal hernia will require admission.

▸ A very soft diet is advised for 6 weeks.

▸ Avoid heavy lifting for 6 weeks.

Outpatient

▸ Outpatient clinic follow-up 6–8 weeks postoperatively to ensure normal diet is returned and no postoperative complications.

SURGEON'S FAVOURITE QUESTION

What structure is in danger during posterior repair of the crura?

The aorta.

GASTRECTOMY

Lisa Grundy and Yashashwi Sinha

DEFINITION

Excision of the entire stomach (total) or a distal part of the stomach (partial or subtotal).

✓ INDICATIONS

- Malignant tumours:
  - › Adenocarcinoma.
  - › Carcinoid (Type III).
  - › Prophylactic gastrectomy in hereditary gastric cancer.
- Benign conditions:
  - › Perforated or bleeding peptic ulcers, having failed conservative medical or endoscopic treatment.

- › Refractory benign ulcers that fail to heal or cause pain, anaemia, or features of gastric outlet obstruction.
- › Caustic perforation.
- › Intractable reflux.

✗ CONTRAINDICATIONS

Relative

- Malnourishment—surgery can be delayed to allow for nutritional supplementation.

ANATOMY

Gross anatomy

- The angle of His, also known as the cardiac notch, is the acute angle between the cardia and the oesophagus. It is formed by the fibres of the collar sling and the circular muscles surrounding the gastro-oesophageal junction. It contributes to the physiological prevention of reflux.
- The stomach has two curvatures (lesser and greater) and five parts (cardia, fundus, body, antrum, and pylorus).
- The stomach is attached to structures by a series of ligaments:
  - › The gastrocolic ligament—part of the greater omentum; connects the greater curvature of the stomach and the transverse colon.
  - › The gastrosplenic ligament—connects the greater curvature of the stomach and the hilum of the spleen.
  - › The gastrophrenic ligament—connects the fundus of the stomach to the diaphragm.
  - › The hepatogastric ligament—connects the liver to the lesser curve of the stomach; forms part of the lesser omentum.
- The greater and lesser omenta are structures made of two layers of peritoneum folded on itself. The greater omentum hangs from the greater curvature of the stomach, whereas the lesser omentum attaches the stomach and duodenum to the liver.

- The omenta divide the abdominal cavity into the greater and lesser sacs, which communicate via the epiploic foramen.

Neurovasculature

- The parasympathetic nerve supply to the stomach is derived from the anterior and posterior vagus nerves.
- The sympathetic innervation is via the coeliac plexus (T6–T9).
- The blood supply is derived from the coeliac trunk, which branches from the abdominal aorta at T12.
- The left gastric artery (LGA), a direct branch of the coeliac trunk, supplies the superior lesser curvature of the stomach, whereas the right gastric artery (RGA), a branch of the common hepatic artery, supplies the inferior portion.
- The right gastro-epiploic (RGE) artery arises from the gastroduodenal artery and runs along the greater curvature from the distal aspect of the stomach.
- At the hilum of the spleen, the splenic artery divides into the short gastric arteries, which supply the fundus, and the left gastro-epiploic (LGE) artery, which supplies the proximal greater curvature.
- Gastric lymphatics run along the curvatures with the respective arteries and drain into the regional nodes.

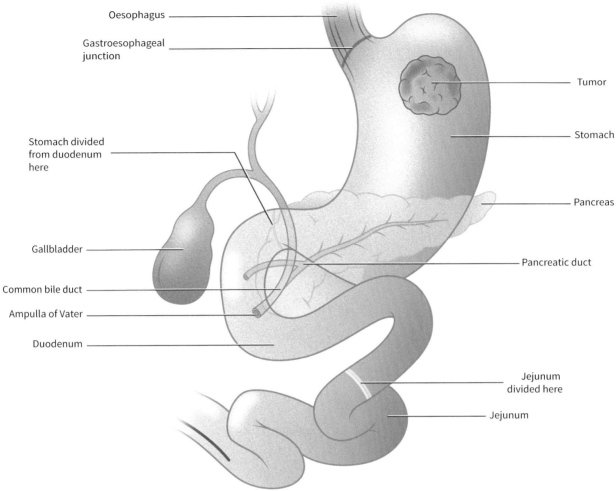

Figure 1.5 Gastrectomy
points of resection

Labels: Oesophagus, Gastroesophageal junction, Stomach divided from duodenum here, Gallbladder, Common bile duct, Ampulla of Vater, Duodenum, Tumor, Stomach, Pancreas, Pancreatic duct, Jejunum divided here, Jejunum

STEP-BY-STEP OPERATION

Anaesthesia: general.

Position: supine.

Considerations: Total gastrectomy requires Roux-en-Y reconstruction (described here); after partial gastrectomy, the proximal stomach may be anastomosed to the duodenum (Bilroth I), to a loop of jejunum (Polya) or Roux-en-Y (Bilroth II). Where appropriate, partial gastrectomy is preferred to total gastrectomy due to lower postoperative complications and superior quality of life.

1 Abdominal access is established (this can be either via a midline or rooftop incision, or laparoscopically).

2 Once the abdominal cavity is entered, an intraoperative assessment of resectability is performed, with the liver, the peritoneum, and the rest of the peritoneal cavity being examined for metastases.

3 Next, the greater omentum is dissected from the transverse colon, and the lesser sac is entered.

4 The greater curvature of the stomach is mobilised up to the level of the diaphragm, and the short gastric vessels are divided.

5 The lesser omentum is divided, and the RGE artery and vein and the RGA are identified, ligated, and divided.

6 The duodenum is mobilised and divided distal to the pylorus.

7 The coeliac axis is identified by finding the plane between the superior border of the pancreas and the left gastric vessels. The left gastric (or coronary) vein and the LGA are ligated and divided. The accompanying lymph nodes are removed.

8 The dissection is continued from the ligated LGA to the oesophageal hiatus of the diaphragm. The oesophagus is mobilised and divided, and the stomach is removed. Additional resection of the lymph nodes, spleen, distal pancreas, and transverse colon are sometimes required for oncological clearance.

9 Creating a Roux-en-Y loop: The jejunum is divided approximately 20 cm distal to the duodenojejunal flexure. The distal end of the jejunum (c) is anastomosed to the oesophagus (a), forming an oesphago-jejunostomy, and the proximal end of the divided jejunum (b) is anastomosed approximately 50 cm below the oesophago-jejunostomy to the jejunum (d) (jejunojejunostomy). The aim is to prevent bile reflux.

10 Drains around the duodenal stump and the oesophago/gastrojejunal anastomosis are left. The abdominal incision or port sites are closed.

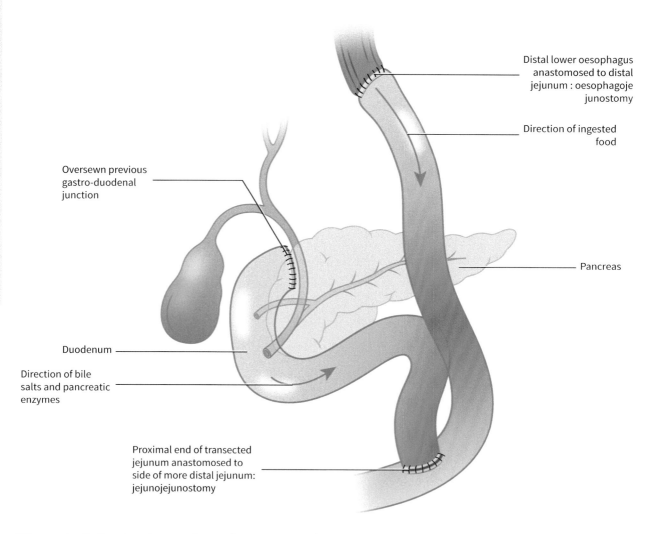

Distal lower oesophagus anastomosed to distal jejunum : oesophagoje junostomy

Direction of ingested food

Pancreas

Oversewn previous gastro-duodenal junction

Duodenum

Direction of bile salts and pancreatic enzymes

Proximal end of transected jejunum anastomosed to side of more distal jejunum: jejunojejunostomy

Figure 1.6 Gastrectomy sites of anastamosis

COMPLICATIONS

Early

▸ Bleeding from the splenic capsule—sometimes requires a splenectomy if this was not performed as part of the oncological excision.
▸ Anastomotic leak.
▸ Duodenal stump leakage.
▸ Pancreatitis or pancreatic fistula.
▸ Wound infection.
▸ Obstruction.

Intermediate and late

▸ Dumping syndrome (20%), when hyperosmolar carbohydrate-rich food enters the small bowel too quickly, causing nausea, vomiting, pain, and vasomotor symptoms such as palpitation and flushing.
▸ Anastomotic stricture.
▸ Nutritional problems—anaemia (vitamin B12 deficiency following total gastrectomy due to removal of intrinsic factor-producing parietal cells within the stomach).
▸ Adhesional small bowel obstruction.
▸ Rapid or slow transit, causing diarrhoea or vomiting.
▸ Marginal ulcer.
▸ Hernia.

POSTOPERATIVE CARE

Inpatient

▸ Nutritional support through total parenteral nutrition or via a jejunostomy tube if placed.
▸ Drains removed when output is minimal.
▸ Water-soluble contrast swallow may be performed on day 5–7 postoperatively to assess for anastomotic leak. Oral intake can then be built up if intact; liquids initially, then light diet. Meals will always be smaller after total gastrectomy but should return to normal size after partial gastrectomy.

▸ Vitamin and mineral supplementation.
▸ Patient discharged home once mobile and maintaining adequate nutritional intake.

Outpatient

▸ Dietician will be involved to help maintain nutrition.
▸ Follow-up depends upon the indication for surgery.

SURGEON'S FAVOURITE QUESTION

What vessel will supply the gastric remnant in a subtotal gastrectomy?

Short gastric vessels.

OMENTAL PATCH REPAIR OF A PERFORATED DUODENAL ULCER

Abhishek Chitnis

DEFINITION

The repair of a perforated duodenal ulcer using a pedicle of omentum.

✓ INDICATIONS

> To treat perforated peptic ulcers—prevent the leak of duodenal contents into the peritoneal cavity.
> Laparoscopic repair can be performed in haemodynamically stable patients with history of <24 hrs of acute symptoms.
> Open repair is more appropriate in patients with generalised peritonitis, those who are haemodynamically unstable, and those who have had signs of perforation for >24 hrs.

✗ CONTRAINDICATIONS

Relative

> Generalised abdominal infection.
> Duration of symptoms >24 hrs.

Absolute

> Severe cardio-respiratory insufficiency.
> Haemodynamic instability.
> Major coagulopathy.

ANATOMY

Gross anatomy

> The duodenum is divided into four sections:
> > The first (superior part) is intraperitoneal and lies at the level of L1. It extends from the pylorus of the stomach and ends at the superior duodenal flexure (SDF). Perforated duodenal ulcers typically occur in the first part of the duodenum, on the anterior superior surface.
> > The second (descending) part is a retroperitoneal structure that runs from the SDF down to the level of L3 to end at the corner of the inferior duodenal flexure (IDF). The pancreas and common bile duct enter the second part of the duodenum through the major duodenal papilla containing the sphincter of Oddi. This point demarcates the embryological transition from foregut to midgut.
> > The third (transverse) part runs from the IDF and across the midline.
> > The fourth (ascending) part joins with the jejunum at the duodenojejunal flexure marked by the ligament of Treitz.
> The omentum:
> > The greater omentum originates from the greater curvature of the stomach and descends anterior to the abdominal viscera to then fold back over itself to insert into the transverse colon.

Neurovasculature

> The duodenum:
> > Nervous supply derives from the vagus nerve and the greater and lesser splanchnic nerves.
> > The major duodenal papilla acts as a land mark between two adjacent blood supplies:
> > > Proximally—the arterial supply is from the gastroduodenal artery and its branch, the superior pancreaticoduodenal artery.
> > > Distally—the arterial supply is from the superior mesenteric artery and its branch, the inferior pancreaticoduodenal artery.
> > The venous drainage is into the superior pancreaticoduodenal vein (drains into the hepatic portal vein) and the inferior pancreaticoduodenal vein (drains into the superior mesenteric vein).
> The omentum:
> > The arterial supply is from the left and right gastro-epiploic arteries.
> > The venous drainage is into the left and right gastro-epiploic veins. The left gastro-epiploic vein drains into the splenic vein, whilst the right gastro-epiploic vein drains into the superior mesenteric vein.

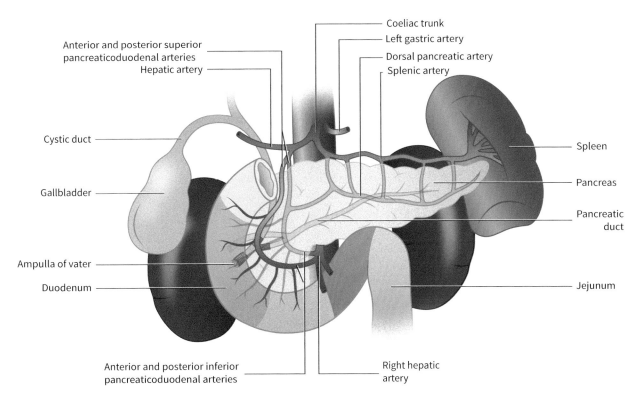

Figure 1.7 Vasculature of the duodenum and pancreas

STEP-BY-STEP OPERATION

Anaesthesia: general.

Position: supine with reverse Trendelenburg.

Considerations: This procedure can be performed via a laparotomy or laparoscopically. A nasogastric (NG) tube is required if not already in place.

1 An upper middle incision is made, which can be extended inferiorly.

2 The skin and fascia are dissected until the stomach and duodenum are identified.

3 Gastric contents are suctioned out of the peritoneal cavity, which is then irrigated with warm saline and the perforation is identified (most commonly located on the bulbous, first part of the duodenum).

4 If the perforation is not immediately identifiable, then the stomach and the first part of the duodenum should be mobilised to allow for full inspection.

5 Once the perforation has been identified, swabs are inserted around the perforation to prevent further leakage of gastric contents.

6 Three interrupted non-absorbable sutures are inserted across the site of the perforation.

7 A pedicle of omentum is mobilised without tension and is positioned across the perforation.

8 The previous interrupted sutures are then tied to secure the omentum in position, sealing the perforation (it is important that the sutures are strong enough to seal the perforation but not so strong that they compromise the omental blood supply).

9 The peritoneal cavity is then washed out with warm saline and the skin and fascial layers are closed. A drain may be placed for 24 hours.

10 For the laparoscopic procedure, three or four ports are required: supraumbilical, right mid-clavicular line, left mid-clavicular line, and an epigastric port if a liver retractor is necessary.

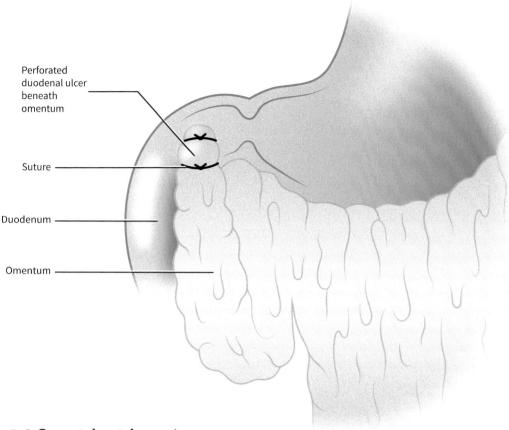

Perforated
duodenal ulcer
beneath
omentum

Suture

Duodenum

Omentum

Figure 1.8 Omental patch repair

COMPLICATIONS

Early

> Stenosis of the duodenal lumen resulting in gastric outlet obstruction (15%).
> Visceral injury.
> Death (5.5%).

Intermediate and late

> Strangulation of the omentum.
> Omental patch leak and fistula formation.
> Duodenal ulcer recurrence—in patients with no supplementary treatment (60%) and in patients with additional H. pylori eradication therapy (<5%).

POSTOPERATIVE CARE

Inpatient

> Analgesia.
> Nil by mouth and NG tube on free drainage for 24–48 hrs, after which commence oral fluids and slowly progress to a normal diet.
> Patients are usually discharged after 5–7 days, slightly sooner for laparoscopic procedures.

Outpatient

> H. pylori eradication therapy with proton pump inhibitors and antibiotics as 90% of cases are infected with H. pylori.

SURGEON'S FAVOURITE QUESTION

How do you identify the transition of the stomach to the duodenum?

Thickening of the pylorus, which underlies the pre-pyloric vein of Mayo.

OMENTAL PATCH REPAIR OF A PERFORATED DUODENAL ULCER

17

GASTRIC BYPASS

Yashashwi Sinha

DEFINITION

The creation of a small gastric reservoir and bypassing of the proximal small intestine using a Roux-en-Y technique.

✓ INDICATIONS

Patient must fulfil all:

- Obesity with or without comorbidities, defined as:
    - BMI ≥40.
    - BMI of 35–40 with a significant obesity-related comorbidity, including hypertension or diabetes.
    - BMI >30 with uncontrolled type 2 diabetes mellitus or metabolic syndrome.
- All non-surgical measures unsuccessful.
- Multidisciplinary management in a specialist obesity service.
- Fit for anaesthesia and the surgery, and self-motivated to adhere to follow-up.

✗ CONTRAINDICATIONS

- Inability or unwillingness to follow postoperative dietary recommendations.
- Stomach or intestinal disorders:
    - Severe reflux.
    - Chronic pancreatitis.
    - Oesophageal or gastric varices.
    - Portal hypertension.
- Pregnancy.
- Uncontrolled/untreated psychiatric disorder and/or suicide attempt in last 18 months or several in past five years.

ANATOMY

Gross anatomy

- The stomach has two curvatures (lesser and greater) and five parts (cardia, fundus, body, antrum, and pylorus).
- The acute angle between the cardia and oesophagus is known as the cardiac notch or angle of His. It is formed by the fibres of the collar sling and the circular muscles surrounding the gastro-oesophageal junction. It forms a sphincter to prevent reflux.
- The stomach is attached to other structures by a series of ligaments:
    - Gastrocolic ligament—part of the greater omentum, connects the greater curvature of the stomach and the transverse colon.
    - Gastrosplenic ligament—connects the greater curvature of the stomach and the hilum of the spleen.
    - Gastrophrenic ligament—connects the fundus of the stomach to the diaphragm.
    - Hepatogastric ligament—connects the liver to the lesser curve of the stomach; forms part of the lesser omentum.

Neurovasculature

- The parasympathetic nerve supply to the stomach is via the vagus nerves.
- The sympathetic innervation is derived from segments T6–T9 of the spinal cord via the coeliac plexus.
- The blood supply for the stomach is derived from the coeliac trunk, which branches from the abdominal aorta (T12).
- The left gastric artery (LGA), a direct branch of the coeliac trunk, supplies the superior lesser curvature of the stomach, whereas the right gastric artery (RGA), a branch of the common hepatic artery, supplies the inferior portion of the lesser curvatures.
- The right gastro-epiploic (RGE) artery arises from the gastroduodenal artery and runs along the greater curvature from the distal aspect of the stomach.
- At the hilum of the spleen, the splenic artery divides into the short gastric arteries, which supply the fundus, and the left gastro-epiploic (LGE) artery, which supplies the proximal greater curvature of the stomach.
- Gastric lymphatics run along the curvatures with the respective arteries and drain into the regional nodes.

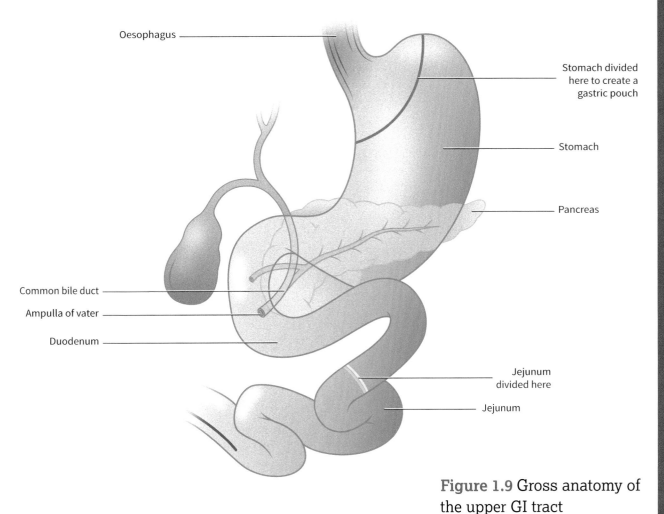

Oesophagus

Stomach divided here to create a gastric pouch

Stomach

Pancreas

Common bile duct

Ampulla of vater

Duodenum

Jejunum divided here

Jejunum

Figure 1.9 Gross anatomy of the upper GI tract

STEP-BY-STEP OPERATION

Anaesthesia: general.

Position: supine or lithotomy.

1. Access to the abdominal cavity is gained via five ports.
2. A window is created in the lesser sac.
3. A small gastric pouch is then created by dividing the cardia from the remainder of the stomach. This is performed using a stapler.
4. A Roux-en-Y loop is created by dividing the jejunum approximately 20 cm distal to the duodenojejunal flexure. The distal end of the jejunum is anastomosed to the gastric pouch, forming a gastro-jejunostomy.
5. The proximal end of the divided jejunum is anastomosed to the more distal jejunum to create a common channel that is approximately 100–150 cm long. The more distal the placement of this enteroenterostomy (i.e., the closer to the ileocaecal junction), the greater the degree of malabsorption experienced by the patient.
6. Mesenteric defects are sutured close to prevent internal herniation. Surgical drains may be placed.
7. Intraoperative leak testing can be done with methylene blue dye or endoscopically.
8. The peritoneal cavity is deflated, ports are removed, and the incisions are closed.

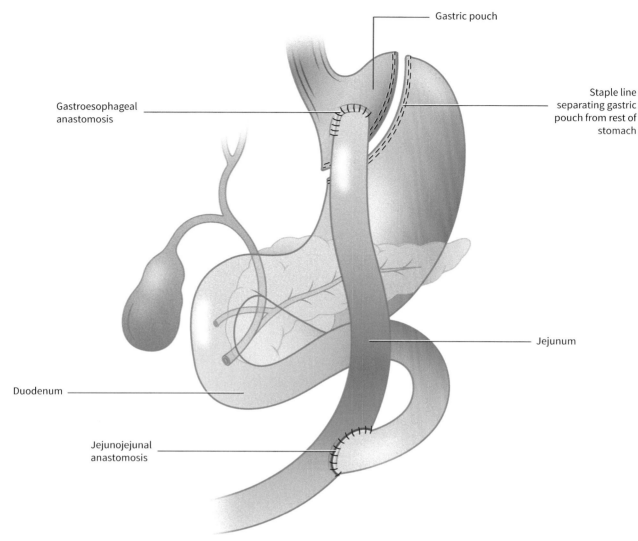

Gastric pouch

Staple line separating gastric pouch from rest of stomach

Gastroesophageal anastomosis

Jejunum

Duodenum

Jejunojejunal anastomosis

Figure 1.10 Gastric bypass sites of anastomosis

COMPLICATIONS

Early

- Anastomotic leak.
- Haemorrhage.
- Iatrogenic bowel perforation.
- Wound infection.
- Internal hernia causing obstruction.
- Anastomotic leakage.

Intermediate and late

- Gastric remnant distension—can be fatal if ruptures and causes peritonitis.
- Stomal stenosis—may require endoscopic balloon dilation.

- Marginal ulcers.
- Bowel obstruction due to internal herniation.
- Dumping syndrome when hyperosmolar carbohydrate-rich food enters the small bowel too quickly, causing nausea, vomiting, pain, and vasomotor symptoms such as palpitation and flushing.
- Gallstones secondary to malabsorption.
- Gastrogastric fistula.
- Incisional hernia.
- Short bowel syndrome.
- Metabolic and nutritional derangements.

POSTOPERATIVE CARE

Inpatient

▸ If intraoperative leak test was negative, the patient can slowly build up oral intake (e.g., water, clear liquid, full liquid diet).

▸ IV proton pump inhibitor should be administered until oral intake is established.

▸ Drains, if placed, are removed when output is minimal.

▸ Vitamin and mineral supplementation as soon as oral intake is established (e.g., multivitamin, iron, calcium citrate).

▸ Patient discharged home once mobile and maintaining adequate nutritional intake.

Outpatient

▸ Regular dietician support to ensure adequate nutrition and supplementation.

▸ Outpatient review at 4–6 weeks.

▸ Oral proton pump inhibitors for 1–3 months postoperatively.

▸ Depending upon weight loss, patients may develop gallstones requiring cholecystectomy.

💬 SURGEON'S FAVOURITE QUESTION

What should you do if a patient with gastric bypass is admitted with abdominal pain?

After a full history and examination, the patient will most likely need an urgent CT. Due to the long biliopancreatic limb and the number of mesenteric defects, the patient can develop internal hernias and bowel obstruction. Obstruction of the biliopancreatic limb will not result in vomiting or constipation, as food does not pass down this limb (i.e., it is harder to diagnose, and CT will help to diagnose this).

GASTRIC BAND

Nick Leaver

DEFINITION

Reducing the functional size of the stomach by placement of an adjustable silicone device at the gastric cardia to aid weight loss.

✓ INDICATIONS

Patient must fulfil all:

▸ BMI ≥40 or a BMI of 35–40 and a significant health condition (e.g., hypertension or diabetes).
▸ All non-surgical measures unsuccessful.
▸ Multidisciplinary management in a specialist obesity service.
▸ Fit for anaesthesia and the surgery, and self-motivated to adhere to follow-up.

✗ CONTRAINDICATIONS

▸ Inability or unwillingness to follow postoperative dietary recommendations.
▸ Stomach or intestinal disorders:
  › Reflux.
  › Chronic pancreatitis.
  › Oesophageal or gastric varices.
  › Portal hypertension.
▸ Pregnancy.
▸ Uncontrolled/untreated psychiatric disorder and/or suicide attempt in last 18 months or several in past five years.

ANATOMY

Gross anatomy

▸ The stomach has two curvatures (lesser and greater) and five parts (cardia, fundus, body, antrum, and pylorus).
▸ The acute angle between the cardia and oesophagus is known as the cardiac notch or angle of His. It is formed by the fibres of the collar sling and the circular muscles surrounding the gastro-oesophageal junction. It forms a sphincter to prevent reflux.
▸ The stomach is attached to other structures by a series of ligaments:
  › Gastrocolic ligament—part of the greater omentum; connects the greater curvature of the stomach and the transverse colon.
  › Gastrosplenic ligament—connects the greater curvature of the stomach and the hilum of the spleen.
  › Gastrophrenic ligament—connects the fundus of the stomach to the diaphragm.
  › Hepatogastric ligament—connects the liver to the lesser curve of the stomach; forms part of the lesser omentum.

Neurovasculature

▸ The parasympathetic nerve supply to the stomach is via the vagus nerves.
▸ The sympathetic innervation is derived from segments T6–T9 of the spinal cord via the coeliac plexus.
▸ The blood supply for the stomach is derived from the coeliac trunk, which branches from the abdominal aorta (T12).
▸ The left gastric artery (LGA), a direct branch of the coeliac trunk, supplies the superior lesser curvature of the stomach, whereas the right gastric artery (RGA), a branch of the common hepatic artery, supplies the inferior portion of the lesser curvatures.
▸ The right gastro-epiploic (RGE) artery arises from the gastroduodenal artery and runs along the greater curvature from the distal aspect of the stomach.
▸ At the hilum of the spleen, the splenic artery divides into the short gastric arteries, which supply the fundus, and the left gastro-epiploic (LGE) artery, which supplies the proximal greater curvature of the stomach.
▸ Gastric lymphatics run along the curvatures with the respective arteries and drain into the regional nodes.

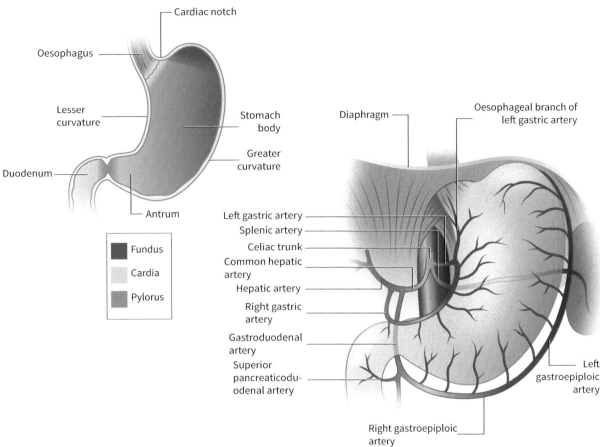

Figure 1.11 Arterial supply of the stomach

STEP-BY-STEP OPERATION

Anaesthesia: general.

Position: reverse Trendelenburg.

Considerations: A low-calorie diet a week prior to surgery is advocated to reduce fat around the stomach and in the liver.

1 The port positions are dependent on the approach used by the surgeon. One port is typically placed just below the left costal margin. Another is used to hold a liver retractor, and up to four more ports are placed in the epigastric, umbilical, and left hypochondriac regions.

2 A window is created in the lesser omentum, and fat is retracted to reveal the right crus of the diaphragm.

3 A window is created through the gastrophrenic ligament to reveal the stomach.

4 The band is washed in saline and tested. It is then inserted through the largest port.

5 The band is wrapped around the fundus to create a small pouch at the top of the stomach.

6 The band may be adjusted via a port that is placed subcutaneously in the epigastric or left hypochondriac regions. The band can be tightened or loosened by injecting or removing saline from the bubble in the adjustment port. The tubing for adjusting the band is inserted and connected to the device.

7 The adjustment port is placed under the skin by clearing a 2 cm area, inserting the port, and suturing it to the underlying muscle/fascia.

8 The system is tested and adjusted.

9 The wounds are injected with local anaesthetic and closed. Further adjustments can be made to the band at follow-up appointments.

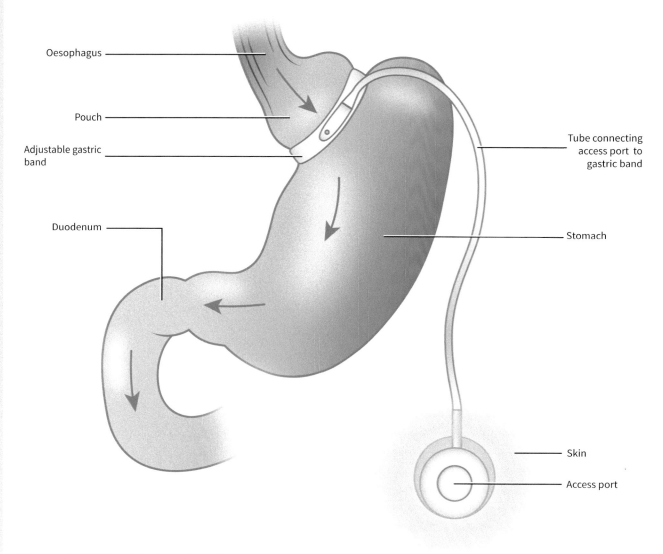

Figure 1.12 Gastric band and access port

COMPLICATIONS

Early

> Dysphagia.

> Bleeding.

> Infection of the band or port.

> Perforation.

> Acute stomal obstruction.

Intermediate and late

> Pouch or oesophageal dilation.

> Band slippage and gastric prolapse—distal stomach herniates upwards through the band; can be a surgical emergency, as it can cause gastric necrosis and leakage.

> Band failure (patient continues to eat soft foods through the band, and weight loss is negligible).

> Band erosion (band erodes into the stomach).

> Port tubing malfunction.

> Reflux.

> Almost 50% of patients will need surgical revision or removal of the band for the above complications.

POSTOPERATIVE CARE

Inpatient

▸ Most gastric bands are done as day cases, with patients being discharged once recovered from anaesthetic and eating safely.

Outpatient

▸ A liquid diet is recommended for the first 2 weeks postoperatively, and then purees and soft solids.

▸ Band adjustments can be made at regular intervals (e.g., every 3 months) if required.

 SURGEON'S FAVOURITE QUESTION

What is the normal postoperative X-ray appearance of a gastric band?

The band should lie at an approximately 30- to 45-degree angle. It should not lie in the horizontal plane—this suggests slippage. You should also not be able to see the open-face 'O' of the ring; if this is seen, it may indicate displacement.

CHOLECYSTECTOMY

Abhishek Chitnis

DEFINITION
Removal of the gallbladder.

✓ INDICATIONS

- Symptomatic gallstones (cholelithiasis) with or without complications:
  - Biliary colic.
  - Acute or chronic cholecystitis.
  - Gallstone pancreatitis.
  - Choledocholithiasis (bile duct stones), which may be removed by Endoscopic Retrograde Cholangiopancreatography (ERCP) prior to cholecystectomy or removed during the procedure via common bile duct exploration at the time of cholecystectomy.
  - Gallbladder polyps or porcelain gallbladder—due to potential for malignancy.
- Gallbladder carcinoma (may also require liver resection)—open approach favoured over laparoscopic.
- As part of a larger hepatobiliary resection (Whipple's procedure).

✗ CONTRAINDICATIONS

Relative

- Cholecystitis of more than 48-72 hours duration, indicating an interval cholecystectomy (typically at 6 weeks) after inflammation has subsided
- Previous upper abdominal adhesions.
- Significant comorbidities—these patients may be suitable for less invasive alternatives such as cholecystostomy or spinal anaesthesia + laparoscopic technique.

Absolute

- Cirrhosis of the liver with portal hypertension.

ANATOMY

Gross anatomy

- The gallbladder is divided into the fundus, body, and neck, which follow into a narrow infundibulum and the cystic duct.
- Bile drains through the left and right hepatic ducts, which unite to form the common hepatic duct. The cystic duct joins the common hepatic duct to form the common bile duct (CBD). The CBD is joined by the pancreatic duct to form the ampulla of Vater, which drains into the duodenum through the sphincter of Oddi.
- Calot's triangle is an anatomical space relevant for cholecystectomy. It is considered to be bordered by the cystic duct inferiorly, the lower border of the liver superiorly, and the common hepatic duct medially. The cystic artery crosses this triangle. When Calot's triangle was originally described in the 19th century, it was defined as bordered by the common hepatic duct medially, the cystic duct laterally and the cystic artery superiorly.

Neurovasculature

- Sympathetic nervous supply is via the coeliac nerve plexus (T7–T9).
- Parasympathetic nervous supply is from the right vagus nerve.
- Arterial supply is via the superficial and deep branches of the cystic artery, a branch of the right hepatic artery. Multiple cystic veins drain the neck and the cystic duct. These enter the liver directly or drain through the hepatic portal vein to the liver.
- The veins from the fundus and the body drain directly into the hepatic sinusoids.
- Lymphatic drainage is via the lymph node of Lund (also called Mascagni's lymph node) found at the neck of the gallbladder.

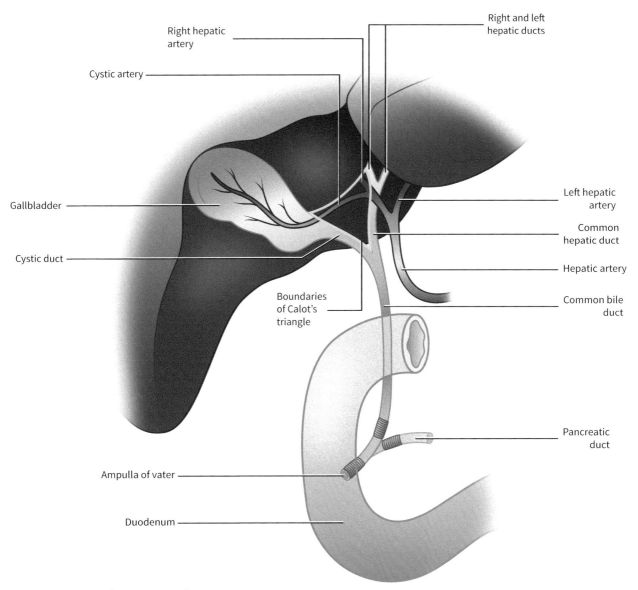

Figure 1.13 Calot's triangle

STEP-BY-STEP OPERATION

Anaesthesia: general.

Position: supine.

Considerations: Laparoscopic cholecystectomy (described here) is the gold standard treatment, but open cholecystectomy may be indicated in complex pathology or suspected gallbladder cancer. Conversion to open cholecystectomy is required for significant bleeding, concern about anatomy, or injury to other structures.

1. Three ports are placed—umbilical, right mid-clavicular line, and epigastrium—and pneumoperitoneum is established via the Hassan method. A fourth port in the right anterior axillary line is frequently added. A camera and instruments are inserted into the abdomen.

2. The tissue surrounding the biliary structures is dissected so that the cystic artery and cystic duct can be identified. In difficult cases, a "fundus first" retrograde dissection approach can be used instead.

3. Prior to clipping the cystic duct and the cystic artery, a large window is created behind each of these structures. This establishes the "critical view of safety" and minimises the risk of bile duct injury.

4. The cystic artery is clipped and divided.

5 On-table cholangiography can be performed if common bile duct stones are suspected (abnormal liver function tests or common bile duct dilatation on ultrasound scans) or to clarify the anatomy to prevent injury to the CBD. The cystic duct is clipped distally, cannulated, and injected with contrast to perform cholangiography. This displays the anatomy of the biliary ductal system, identifies ductal stones, and ensures that the contrast passes freely into the duodenum.

6 The cystic duct is then clipped and divided, ensuring that the CBD is identified to avoid injury.

7 The gallbladder is then dissected from the liver bed using diathermy and removed via a retrieval bag.

8 The peritoneal cavity is deflated, the ports are removed, and port sites are closed. For larger port sites, the fascial layer is closed in addition to the skin.

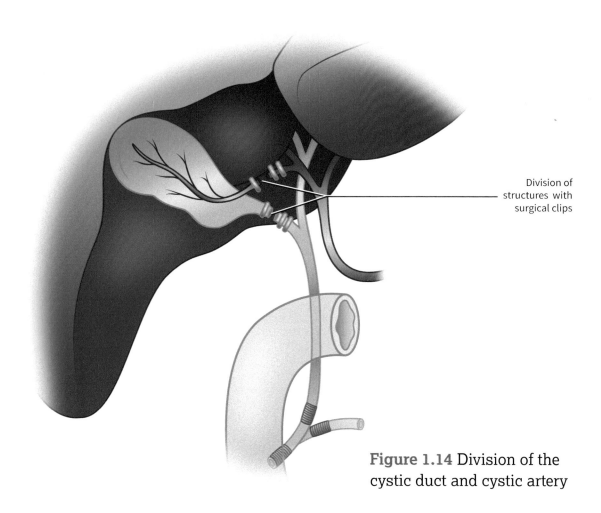

Division of structures with surgical clips

Figure 1.14 Division of the cystic duct and cystic artery

COMPLICATIONS

Early

- Laparoscopic conversion to open (2%).
- Bleeding from the cystic artery or liver bed.
- Infection—wound, intra-abdominal abscess, pneumonia, and urinary tract infection.
- Bile leak (1%) resulting in biliary peritonitis, usually from the cystic duct or the duct of Luska (accessory small bile duct).
- CBD injury (0.1%).

- Retained stone in the CBD.
- Damage to surrounding structures.

Intermediate and late

- Incisional hernia (rare in laparoscopic surgery).
- Adhesional small bowel obstruction.
- Post-cholecystectomy syndrome—persistence of presenting symptoms postoperatively.
- Increased frequency and looser stool passage.

POSTOPERATIVE CARE

Inpatient

- Eat and drink as tolerated.
- After laparoscopic cholecystectomy, patients are normally discharged the same day and normal activity is resumed within 2 weeks.
- After open cholecystectomy, patients are usually discharged after 2–4 days and normal activity is resumed within 4 weeks.

Outpatient

- No routine outpatient review.

 SURGEON'S FAVOURITE QUESTION

What is the name of the lymph node in Calot's triangle?

Lymph node of Lund.

WHIPPLE'S PROCEDURE (PANCREATICODUODENECTOMY)

Sasha Shoba Devi Thrumurthy

DEFINITION

The removal of the following structures *en bloc*:

> Head of pancreas.

> Stomach antrum and pylorus.

> Duodenum.

> Proximal jejunum.

> Common bile duct (CBD).

> Gallbladder.

✔ INDICATIONS

Malignancy of the head of the pancreas, ampulla of Vater, duodenum, or distal CBD in the absence of metastasis and/or vascular involvement.

> Chronic pancreatitis causing severe pain that is refractory to medical therapy.

✘ CONTRAINDICATIONS

> Metastatic disease.

> Nodal involvement out of the field of dissection.

> Involvement of the following structures: aorta, inferior vena cava (IVC), coeliac trunk, superior mesenteric artery (SMA), or superior mesenteric vein (SMV).

ANATOMY

Gross anatomy

> The pancreas is a retroperitoneal organ that lies within and is fixed to the curve of the first three parts of the duodenum.

> There are five components of the pancreas: head, uncinate process, neck, body, and tail.

> The pancreas drains via the pancreatic duct of Wirsung, which unites with the CBD to form the ampulla of Vater, which drains through the sphincter of Oddi into the second part of the duodenum.

Arterial supply

> The pancreas is primarily supplied by the coeliac trunk and the SMA.

> The head and uncinate process are supplied by the anterior and posterior divisions of the superior pancreaticoduodenal artery (SPA), which stems from the gastroduodenal artery (a branch of the common hepatic artery (CHA)). The anterior and posterior branches of the SPA run inferiorly to anastomose with

the anterior and posterior divisions of the inferior pancreaticoduodenal artery (branch of the SMA).

> The tail and body of the pancreas are supplied by the splenic artery.

Venous drainage

> The venous drainage of the pancreas parallels the arterial supply and drains into the portal vein

> The head of the pancreas drains into the SMV, while the body and tail of the pancreas drain into the splenic vein.

Lymphatic drainage and innervation

> Lymph drains via the peripancreatic and retroperitoneal nodes and into the thoracic duct, coeliac nodes, and superior mesenteric nodes.

> The pancreas is supplied by both the sympathetic system (the greater thoracic splanchnic nerves, coeliac plexus, and superior mesenteric plexus) and the parasympathetic system (the vagus nerve).

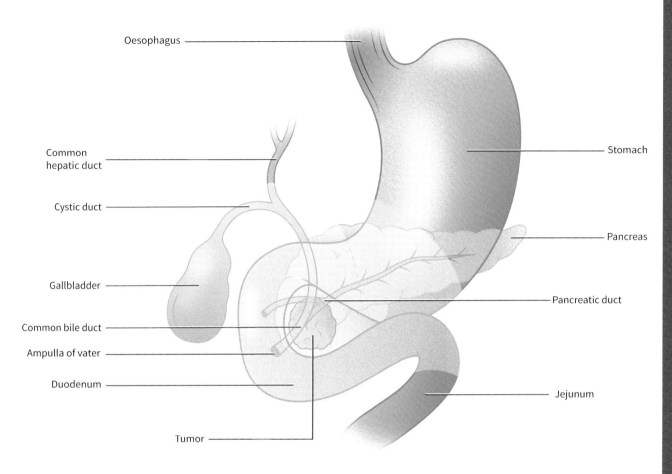

Structures removed

Figure 1.15 Structures removed en bloc in a Whipple's procedure

STEP-BY-STEP OPERATION

Anaesthetic: general.

Position: supine.

Considerations: The operation can be divided into three stages: assessment of resectability, resection, and reconstruction.

1 A vertical midline incision is made in the abdomen.

2 Assessment of resectability: the duodenum and pancreas are mobilised to ensure the absence of metastasis to either the aorta or the IVC. The SMV and neck of pancreas are inspected for the absence of tumour involvement between the two structures.

3 Resection:

  a A cholecystectomy is performed, and the CBD is divided superior to the insertion of the cystic duct.

  b The portal vein is dissected from its surrounding peritoneum, and the gastroduodenal artery is ligated and divided. The CHA is identified, and the surrounding lymph nodes are resected. The right gastro-epiploic vessels are then ligated and divided.

  c The antrum and pylorus of the stomach, together with the neck of the pancreas, are subsequently excised.

  d The duodenojejunal (DJ) flexure is mobilised, and 15 cm of the jejunum that is immediately distal to the DJ flexure is excised.

  e The uncinate process is dissected from the SMA and SMV, and all the small branches are ligated. The duodenum is then removed along with the head of the pancreas.

4 Reconstruction (consists of three main anastomosis):

  a Pancreaticojejunostomy: the proximal part of the jejunal loop is anastomosed to the end of the pancreatic remnant.

b Hepaticojejunostomy: the middle of the jejunal loop is anastomosed to the end of the common hepatic duct.

c Gastrojejunostomy: the distal side of the jejunal loop is anastomosed to the end of the gastric remnant.

5 Drainage and closure: two percutaneous silicone drains are inserted with one placed inferior

to the left lobe of the liver and anterior to the pancreaticojejunostomy. The second drain is placed into the hepatorenal space inferior to the hepaticojejunostomy. The abdomen is irrigated with warm saline and closed in layers.

Figure 1.16 Whipple's post-resection sites of anastomosis

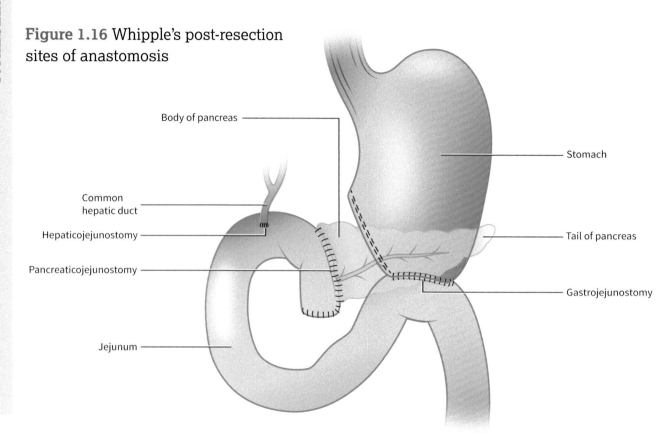

COMPLICATIONS

Early

› Haemorrhage.
› Delayed gastric emptying.
› Anastomotic leakage.
› Intra-abdominal infection.
› Paralytic ileus.

Intermediate and Late

› Intra-abdominal abscess—predominantly due to fistulae and/or anastomotic leaks.
› Acute pancreatitis of the remnant pancreas.
› Chyle leak.
› Pancreatic fistula.
› Dumping syndrome—loss of gastric reservoir and accelerated gastric emptying of osmotic contents;

presents with diarrhoea, vomiting, and/or abdominal pain ~30 min after a meal.
› Pseudoaneurysm (e.g., of the gastroduodenal artery) and secondary haemorrhage (intra-abdominal or gastrointestinal)—due to a ruptured pseudoaneurysm in relation to pancreatic leak, anastomotic leak, peptic ulceration, and/or sepsis.
› Pancreatic endocrine insufficiency—may cause brittle diabetes.
› Pancreatic exocrine insufficiency—may cause fat malabsorption.
› Tumour recurrence.

POSTOPERATIVE CARE

Inpatient

‣ Average length of hospital stay: 10–14 days with the first 24–48 hrs on High Dependency Unit (HDU).

‣ IV proton pump inhibitor should be administered.

‣ Octreotide may be administered to reduce pancreatic secretions.

‣ Amylase level from abdominal drains may be checked postoperatively.

Outpatient

‣ Patients should be reviewed regularly.

‣ Multidisciplinary team (MDT) involvement, including dietetic and psychosocial input, is vital.

 SURGEON'S FAVOURITE QUESTION

What structures are removed in a Whipple's operation?

• **Head of pancreas.**

• **Stomach antrum and pylorus.**

• **Duodenum.**

• **Proximal jejunum.**

• **Common bile duct (CBD).**

• **Gall bladder.**

LIVER RESECTION

James Brooks

DEFINITION
Surgical removal of part of the liver.

✓ INDICATIONS

- Removal of a primary liver cancer (e.g., hepatocellular carcinoma (HCC)).
- Removal of an isolated metastasis—most commonly secondary to colorectal cancer.
- Removal of locally spreading tumours from the gallbladder and the bile duct.
- Removal of benign symptomatic lesions such as tumours or cysts.

✗ CONTRAINDICATIONS

- Underlying disease of the liver parenchyma can prevent vital postoperative regeneration of the liver. Patients with HCC or cirrhosis should be carefully evaluated for risk of postoperative liver failure.
- Care should be taken in patients with severe lung disease, as they have a higher risk of pleural effusions due to the high abdominal incision.

ANATOMY

Gross anatomy

- The liver can be divided into four anatomical lobes: the larger left and right lobes and the smaller caudate and quadrate lobes.
- The liver can also be divided into two functional lobes (left and right), with each lobe being supplied by its own hepatic portal vein and hepatic artery.
- Anatomically, the divide between the left and right functional lobes is from the fundus of the gallbladder to the inferior vena cava (IVC).
- For surgical purposes, the liver is divided into eight segments, with each segment being supplied by a secondary or tertiary branch of the portal triad.
- The round ligament (ligamentum teres) is found on the inferior border of the liver and is a remnant of the umbilical vein.
- On the anterior surface, the falciform ligament divides the subphrenic recess into left and right.
- The liver is attached to the diaphragm by several peritoneal reflections (ligaments):
  - The coronary ligament surrounds the bare area of the liver (not covered in peritoneum).
  - Bilaterally, the anterior and posterior layers of the coronary ligament converge to form the right and left triangular ligaments.
- The lesser omentum (formed by the hepatogastric and hepatoduodenal ligaments) attaches the liver to the stomach and duodenum.

Neurovasculature

- The hepatic portal vein provides 75% of the liver's blood supply and is formed from the superior mesenteric and splenic veins. It carries venous blood, rich in nutrients absorbed from the intestines, for "first pass" metabolism. This blood has a lower oxygen content and supplies approximately half of the liver's oxygen requirements.
- The hepatic artery proper originates from the coeliac trunk and provides 25% of the liver's blood supply. This artery supplies the liver with oxygenated blood from the general arterial circulation, accounting for the other half of the liver's oxygen requirements.
- Blood drains from the liver via the right, left, and intermediate (middle) hepatic veins directly into the IVC.
- The portal triad consists of the hepatic portal vein, the hepatic artery proper, and the common bile duct. The portal triad enters the liver at the porta hepatis and is bounded by a fibrous capsule called Glisson's capsule.

Figure 1.17 Segmental anatomy of the liver

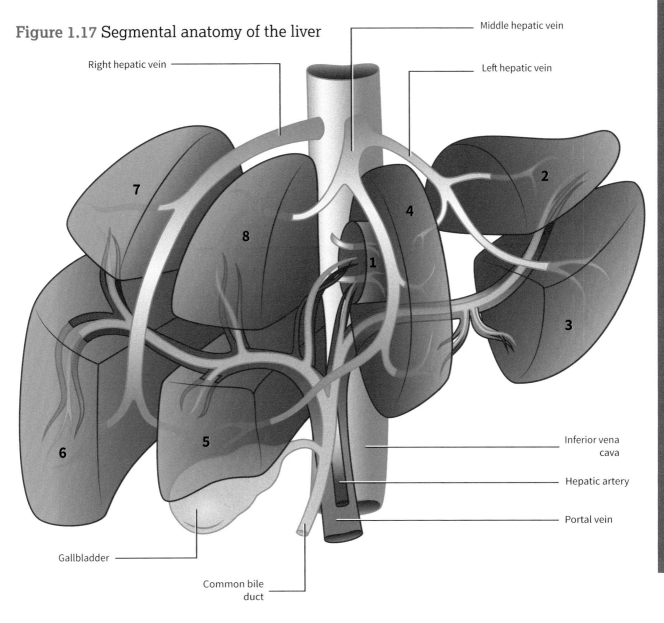

Middle hepatic vein

Right hepatic vein

Left hepatic vein

Inferior vena cava

Hepatic artery

Portal vein

Gallbladder

Common bile duct

Right posterior section   **Right anterior section**   **Left medial section**   **Left lateral section**

STEP-BY-STEP OPERATION

Anaesthesia: general.

Position: supine.

1   Four to five access ports are placed, and pneumoperitoneum is established using the Hassan method.

2   Visual exploration of the liver and laparoscopic staging of the cancer are performed.

3   The round ligament, falciform ligament, and left triangular ligament are divided.

4   The arteries and the portal vein supplying the relevant segments are dissected and clipped. The segments now appear darker in colour than the rest of the liver.

5   The transection line is marked on the liver with diathermy. The parenchyma is transversely resected 1 cm to the left of the falciform ligament as far as the Glissonian sheath surrounding the portal triad.

6 The bile duct is dissected and clipped. Deeper transection is now completed, and the liver is placed in a specimen bag.

7 The remaining surface of the liver is inspected for bleeding and biliary leaks. A fibrin sealant may be sprayed on the surface.

8 A large drain is placed near the surface.

9 The specimen bag is delivered through a port and the incisions.

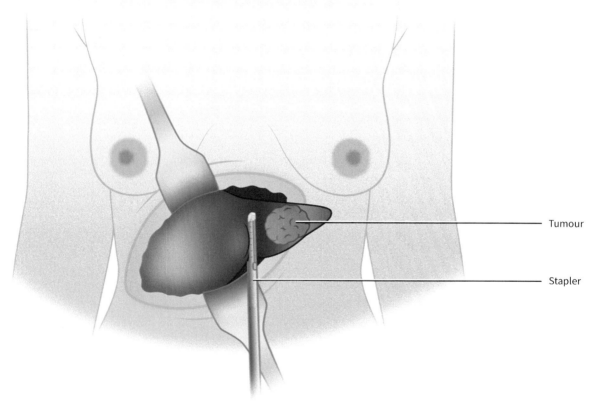

Tumour

Stapler

Figure 1.18 Liver resection

COMPLICATIONS

Early

> Bleeding—due to the immense vascularity of the liver.
> Biliary leak.
> Gas embolism—damage to the IVC can allow CO_2 into the circulatory system.

Intermediate and late

> Wound or deep intra-abdominal infection.
> Hypophosphataemia—thought to be due to the uptake of phosphate by the remaining hepatocytes.
> Coagulopathy—derangement of the INR is common and usually self-limiting.
> Encephalopathy.

POSTOPERATIVE CARE

Inpatient

▸ Initial postoperative management is usually in a High Dependency Unit (HDU)/Intensive Treatment Unit (ITU) setting with careful monitoring of vitals.

▸ Liver function is monitored using Liver Function Tests (LFTs) and INR.

▸ Drains are removed at 48 hours or when output is minimal.

▸ The patient is usually discharged 4–5 days postoperatively.

Outpatient

▸ Routine follow-up appointment at 2–3 weeks and from then on according to original indication/MDT outcome.

 SURGEON'S FAVOURITE QUESTION

What are the causes of hepatomegaly?

Infections (viral hepatitis, EBV, CMV, malaria), tumours (primary or secondary), metabolic (haemochromatosis and Wilson's disease), toxins (alcoholic hepatitis and alcoholic fatty liver).

SPLENECTOMY

James Brooks

DEFINITION
Removal of the spleen.

✔ INDICATIONS

Emergency
› Splenic trauma (blunt, penetrating, or iatrogenic) resulting in uncontrolled bleeding.

Elective (although often clinically urgent)
› Haematological disease—idiopathic thrombocytopenic purpura, hereditary spherocytosis, autoimmune haemolytic anaemia, thrombotic thrombocytopenic purpura.
› Oncological—Hodgkin and non-Hodgkin lymphoma, chronic lymphocytic leukaemia, hairy cell leukaemia, or part of a tumour debulking or eradicating procedure (e.g., gastric carcinoma excision).

› Portal hypertension.
› Felty's syndrome—a triad of rheumatoid arthritis, splenomegaly, and neutropaenia.
› Cyst or abscess.
› Tuberculosis infection.
› Sarcoidosis.

✘ CONTRAINDICATIONS

▸ Young age—splenectomy for haematological indications should ideally be done after age 6 (and not before age 3); this decreases the risk of overwhelming post-splenectomy sepsis.
▸ Untreated coagulopathy.

ANATOMY

▸ The spleen is located in the left upper quadrant of the abdomen. It is approximately 12 cm in length and 7 cm in width and is covered in visceral peritoneum.
▸ The splenic artery originates from the coeliac trunk and enters the spleen at the splenic hilum. It has multiple branches:
  › Short gastric arteries—five to seven short gastric arteries arise from the terminal branches of the splenic artery and supply the fundus and upper body of the stomach.
  › Left gastroepiploic artery—supplies the lateral aspect of the greater curvature of the stomach and part of the greater omentum

  › Pancreatic branches—throughout its course, the splenic artery travels superiorly to the pancreas and supplies the neck, body, and tail of the pancreas through multiple small pancreatic branches.
▸ The splenic vein drains from the splenic hilum and joins the superior mesenteric vein to form the hepatic portal vein at the level of L1 behind the neck of the pancreas.
▸ There are two important attachments to other organs: the gastrosplenic ligament, which attaches the spleen to the greater curvature of the stomach, and the splenorenal ligament, which attaches the spleen to the left kidney. The tail of the pancreas is often found in contact with the splenic hilum but is not attached.

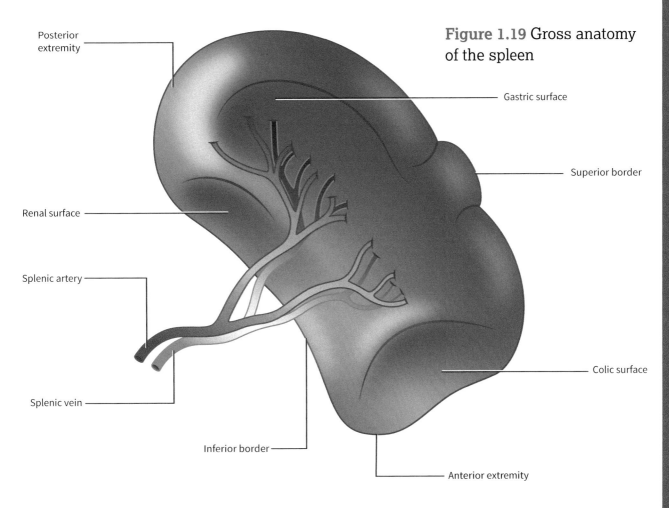

Figure 1.19 Gross anatomy of the spleen

Posterior extremity

Gastric surface

Superior border

Renal surface

Splenic artery

Splenic vein

Colic surface

Inferior border

Anterior extremity

STEP-BY-STEP OPERATION

Anaesthesia: general.

Position: right lateral decubitus position.

Considerations: Splenectomy can be either open or laparoscopic (described here). Open is preferred in trauma and in gross splenomegaly (larger than 1000 g). In the elective setting, the patient is immunised against haemophilus influenza, pneumococcus, and meningococcus at least 2 weeks before surgery.

1 Laparoscopic ports are inserted according to patient size, position, and spleen size: generally, four ports are introduced.

2 The inferior attachments of the spleen (splenocolic ligament) are dissected.

3 The lateral attachments (splenorenal ligament) and retroperitoneal attachments (vessels) are dissected.

4 The medial aspect of the spleen is now in view. The gastrosplenic ligament is divided, and then the lower short gastric vessels are divided.

5 The tail of the pancreas is identified to avoid injury.

6 The splenic artery and vein are ligated (ligature or vascular stapler) and divided at the upper border of the pancreas.

7 The remaining short gastric vessels are then divided, freeing the spleen.

8 The spleen is placed into a specimen retrieval bag, which is removed through the abdominal wall, usually through a Pfannenstiel incision.

9 A drain is inserted into the intra-abdominal cavity, haemostasis is ensured, and the incisions are closed with absorbable sutures.

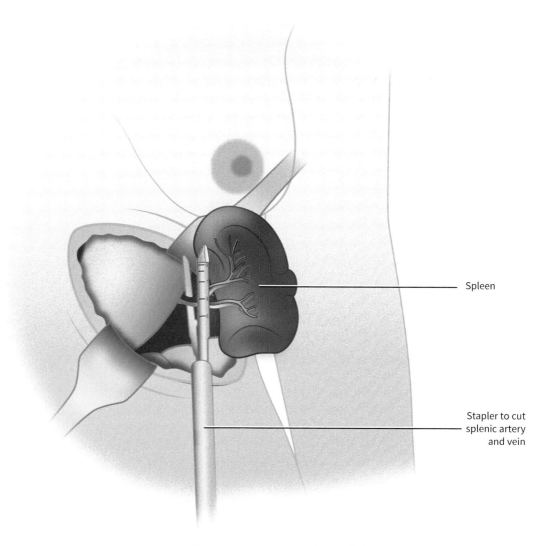

Spleen

Stapler to cut splenic artery and vein

Figure 1.20 Ligation of the splenic artery and vein

COMPLICATIONS

Early:

▸ Bleeding—if significant, requires transfusion and urgent conversion to laparotomy

▸ Damage to surrounding structures, particularly the tail of the pancreas with formation of pancreatic fistula.

▸ Infection—wound, intra-abdominal abscess (particularly sub-phrenic), pneumonia, and urinary tract infection.

Immediate and late:

▸ Left-sided atelectasis due to diaphragmatic splintage.

▸ Portal or splenic vein thrombosis.

▸ Gastric dilatation due to gastric ileus.

▸ Ischaemia of the greater curvature of the stomach.

▸ Thrombocytosis, increasing the risk of venous thrombosis.

▸ Sepsis from encapsulated bacteria—most cases occur within 2 years and are due to haemophilus influenza, pneumococcus, or meningococcus. The risk of this occurring in a patient's lifetime is 5% with a high mortality.

POSTOPERATIVE CARE

Inpatient

- If drains are left in situ, they are removed once output is significantly reduced.
- In the elective setting, patients may be discharged after 2–3 days. In the emergency setting, this depends on the status of other injuries.

Outpatient

- To prevent sepsis from encapsulated organisms:
  - The patient is immunised against haemophilus influenza, pneumococcus, and meningococcus (if not done preoperatively).
  - The patient is discharged on prophylactic antibiotics (often penicillin) for a minimum of 2 years.
  - Annual influenza vaccination is recommended, as well as pneumococcal boosters.
- Outpatient follow-up depends upon the indication—e.g., patients with thrombocytosis are discharged on antiplatelet therapy (such as aspirin).

❓ SURGEON'S FAVOURITE QUESTION

How do you differentiate between a spleen and a kidney on clinical examination?

A kidney is dull to percussion, can be balloted, you can get above it, and it is not notched.

HELLER MYOTOMY

Sameena Mohamedally

DEFINITION
Incision of the muscle of the cardia of the stomach and lower oesophageal sphincter for the treatment of achalasia.

✓ INDICATIONS

- Type 2 (intermittent pan-oesophageal pressurisation) achalasia.
- Recurrent achalasia with dysphagia.
- Failure of pneumatic dilatation.
- Young patients with achalasia who otherwise may need recurrent dilatations.
- Patients at risk of perforation with dilatation.

✗ CONTRAINDICATIONS

- None.

ANATOMY

Gross anatomy

- The oesophagus is a muscular tube (~ 25 cm long) that allows food to pass from the pharynx to the stomach.
- There are three major constrictions made by structures around the oesophagus:
    1. The cervical stricture at the pharyngo-oesophageal junction, known as the upper oesophageal sphincter.
    2. The thoracic constriction, occurring due to the impressions of the arch of the aorta and the left main bronchus.
    3. The diaphragmatic constriction (lower oesophageal sphincter), where the oesophagus passes through the diaphragm at the oesophageal hiatus in the right crus of the diaphragm (T10).
- The oesophagus is attached to the diaphragm by the phrenoesophageal ligament and a layer of epiphrenic fat.
- The anterior surface of the oesophagus is covered by peritoneum. The left vagus nerve runs along the anterior surface of the oesophagus, and the right vagus nerve lies posteromedially. Oesophageal branches of the left gastric artery provide the arterial supply.

Histology

- Histologically, the oesophagus is made up of four main layers:
    1. The innermost is the mucosa, which contains the epithelial lining.
    2. The submucosa is a layer of connective tissue with blood vessels and lymphatics embedded in it.
    3. The muscularis externa is made up of two layers of muscle: an inner circular layer and an outer longitudinal layer that changes from striated to smooth muscle as it reaches the lower third of the oesophagus.
    4. The last layer is the adventitia. There is no serosa.
- Histologically, the stomach is composed of similar layers; however, the muscularis externa has a third layer of muscle, known as the oblique layer, that sits between the longitudinal and circular layers.

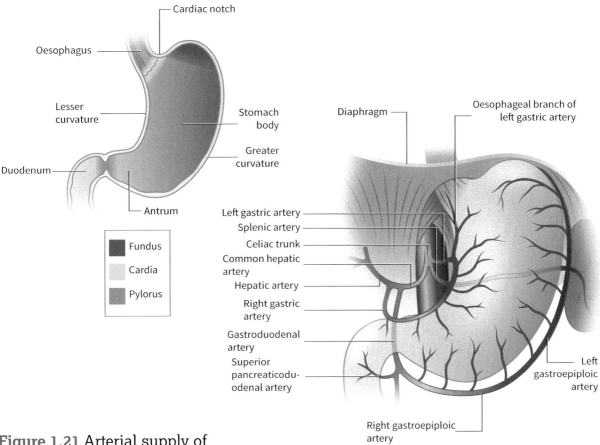

Figure 1.21 Arterial supply of the stomach

STEP-BY-STEP OPERATION

Anaesthesia: general.

Position: reverse Trendelenburg; the surgeon stands between the legs.

Considerations: Heller Myotomy is usually performed laparoscopically, but laparotomy is required occasionally. Thoracotomy is rarely required, except when a very long myotomy is indicated. A nasogastric (NG) tube is inserted.

1 Three laparoscopic ports are required: a midline camera port 15 cm below the xiphisternum, and right and left upper quadrant working ports in the mid-clavicular lines.

2 A liver retractor is inserted through an incision below the xiphisternum to retract the left hemi-liver.

3 The anterior vagus nerve is identified, and the lesser omentum is dissected in the direction of the right crus of the diaphragm.

4 The oesophagus and superior stomach are dissected to free them from surrounding structures.

5 The vagus nerve is identified on the anterior surface of the oesophagus for the full length of the myotomy.

6 An incision is made through the longitudinal and circular muscle across the gastro-oesophageal junction extending 4 cm proximally onto the oesophagus and 2 cm distally.

7 In this incision, both layers of muscle fibres of the muscular externa are dissected laterally until the plane of the submucosa is reached. The innermost layer, the mucosa, is left intact.

8 A careful inspection is made for inadvertent mucosal perforation. Air insufflation into the submerged oesophagus or intraoperative endoscopy may be helpful. Any mucosal perforations can be repaired with 4/0 absorbable sutures.

9 This procedure is usually combined with a Dor or Toupet partial fundoplication to prevent postoperative reflux.

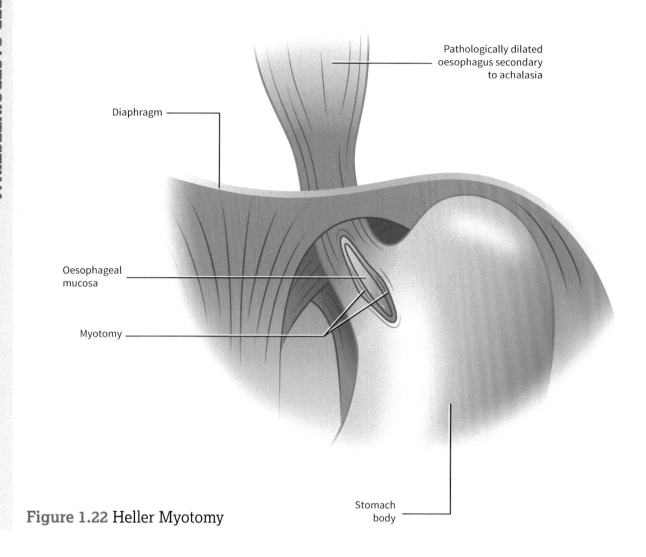

Figure 1.22 Heller Myotomy

COMPLICATIONS

Early

‣ Gastrointestinal perforation (20%).
‣ Pneumothorax (7%).

Intermediate and late

‣ Gastro-oesophageal reflux disease—most common complication; most institutes combine a Heller

Myotomy with a partial fundoplication as a preventative measure.

‣ Dysphagia—as with any fundoplication, swallowing will improve over the first 8–12 weeks.
‣ Respiratory complication (4%)—patients are at higher risk of aspiration pneumonia from anaesthesia.
‣ Recurrent achalasia requiring further procedure (20%).

POSTOPERATIVE CARE

Inpatient

- Admit overnight to monitor for undetected perforation.
- Start free fluids as tolerated after operation but leave NG tube on free drainage overnight.
- Soft diet from day 1 and progress as tolerated. Avoid bony fish and tablets for first 2 weeks.

Outpatient

- The patient is discharged with liquid oral analgesics and proton pump inhibitor (sublingual) for 2 weeks.
- The patient can resume normal activities within 7–14 days.
- Outpatient follow-up at 4–6 weeks.
- An annual outpatient follow-up to assess symptoms.

💬 SURGEON'S FAVOURITE QUESTION

What other forms of treatment can be considered for achalasia?

Nifedipine, endoscopic botulinum toxin injection into the lower oesophageal sphincter, per-oral endoscopic myotomy (POEM).

ENDOSCOPIC RETROGRADE CHOLANGIOPANCREATOGRAPHY (ERCP)

Nimeshi Jayakody

DEFINITION

An endoscopic procedure carried out to diagnose and treat biliary and pancreatic duct conditions. It involves cannulation of the common bile duct (CBD) via a side viewing endoscope with injection of contrast media to delineate the duct.

✓ INDICATIONS

- ERCP and sphincterotomy with stone removal:
  - Choledocholithiasis with jaundice.
  - Choledocholithiasis with dilated CBD.
  - Choledocholithiasis with acute pancreatitis.
  - Choledocholithiasis with cholangitis.
- Biliary strictures causing biliary obstruction—require stent insertion (e.g., malignant compression).
- To obtain tissue sampling through biopsy/brushings for histological diagnosis (e.g., suspected pancreatic, biliary, or ampullary cancers).
- Type 1 sphincter of Oddi dysfunction secondary to papillary stenosis.

✗ CONTRAINDICATIONS

- Untreated coagulopathies—INR must be <1.5 to proceed.
- Structural abnormalities (e.g., previous Roux-en-Y procedure).
- Low likelihood of biliary stone or stricture.
- As a diagnostic/evaluation method of abdominal pain—MRI cholangiopancreatography or endoscopic ultrasound are preferred, as they are less invasive.

ANATOMY

Embryology

- The duodenum comprises four parts. The first and second parts develop from the foregut and are supplied by the anterior and posterior superior pancreaticoduodenal arteries, which branch from the gastroduodenal artery.
- The third and fourth parts are midgut in origin and are supplied by the anterior and posterior inferior pancreatoduodenal arteries, which branch from the superior mesenteric artery.

Gross anatomy

- Bile is drained from the liver by the right and left hepatic ducts. They join to form the common hepatic duct. This is joined by the cystic duct to form the CBD. The CBD joins the pancreatic duct(s) at the ampulla of Vater, which opens into the duodenum at the sphincter of Oddi. There is a visible protrusion where these

structures enter the duodenum, termed the duodenal papilla.
- The second and third parts of the duodenum are retroperitoneal.

Neurovasculature

- The pancreatic blood supply is from the superior and inferior pancreaticoduodenal arteries and the dorsal pancreatic artery (a branch of the splenic artery). The bile ducts and the gallbladder are supplied by the cystic artery.
- The pancreas is drained by the splenic vein and the superior and inferior pancreaticoduodenal veins. The biliary system drains into the hepatic portal vein from tributaries.
- The lymphatic drainage of the pancreas and the bile ducts drains into nodes along the hepatic, splenic, and mesenteric arteries to eventually drain into the coeliac, superior mesenteric, and para-aortic lymph nodes.

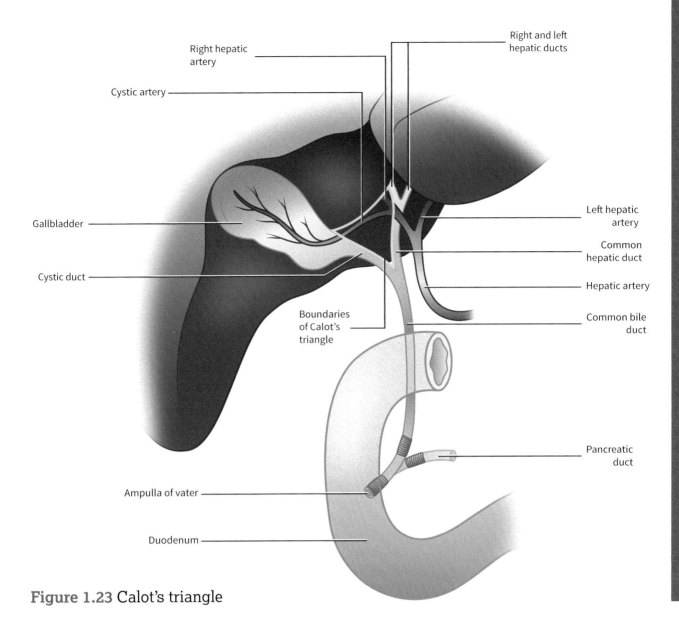

Right hepatic artery

Right and left hepatic ducts

Cystic artery

Gallbladder

Cystic duct

Boundaries of Calot's triangle

Left hepatic artery

Common hepatic duct

Hepatic artery

Common bile duct

Pancreatic duct

Ampulla of vater

Duodenum

Figure 1.23 Calot's triangle

STEP-BY-STEP OPERATION

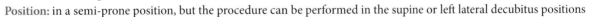

Anaesthesia: under sedation with local anaesthetic spray to the throat; may be carried out under general anaesthesia in complex cases.

Position: in a semi-prone position, but the procedure can be performed in the supine or left lateral decubitus positions

1 The endoscope is passed through the oral cavity and pharynx into the oesophagus.
2 The endoscope is carefully manoeuvred through the oesophagus and passes through the gastro-oesophageal junction. The endoscope is then angled so that the fundus can be seen before following along the greater curvature of the stomach.
3 The pylorus is then identified in the 6 o'clock position.

4 The endoscope is inserted into the first part of the duodenum (due to the position of the second part of the duodenum, careful manoeuvring is required).
5 The major duodenal papilla is identified (as it protrudes into the duodenum). To enter the biliary system, a wire is inserted through the Ampulla of Vater, through which a cannula is inserted. Sometimes, a sphincterotomy (a division of the sphincter of Oddi) is required at the duodenal papilla to gain access.

6 Contrast medium is injected to view the biliary system, and fluoroscopic images of the biliary tree are taken, termed a 'cholangiogram'.

7 Once clear images of the biliary tree have been obtained, interventions may be performed (e.g., brushings for cytology, balloon or basket retrieval of stones, stenting of strictures). Stents may be permanent (metallic) or temporary (plastic), depending on the indication for the procedure.

8 After the procedure, the endoscope is removed under direct visualisation.

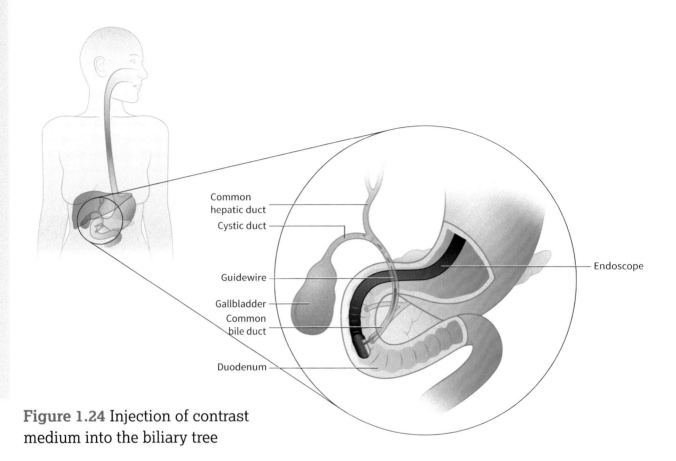

Figure 1.24 Injection of contrast medium into the biliary tree

COMPLICATIONS

Early

▸ Post-ERCP pancreatitis (1%).
▸ Bleeding (particularly after sphincterotomy).
▸ Infection (cholangitis).
▸ Duodenal perforation.
▸ Aspiration pneumonia.
▸ Contrast allergy anaphylaxis.

Intermediate and late

▸ Complications relating to therapeutic interventions and underlying pathology, e.g.:
  › Stent migration.
  › Recurrence of strictures.
  › Recurrence of impacted calculi.
  › Recurrent ascending cholangitis following sphincterotomy.

POSTOPERATIVE CARE

Inpatient

- Commonly performed as a day case procedure in simple cases, with patients being discharged home provided they are pain free and the effect of sedation has worn off.
- In more complex cases, patients return to the ward and continue with previous treatment.
- Mobilisation and adequate analgesia are critical.
- Serum amylase is measured in some centres post-procedure for early detection of pancreatitis.

Outpatient

- Patients are reviewed in clinic within 2–3 weeks if indicated; further management is dictated by underlying pathology.
- Most patients with choledocholithiasis will require cholecystectomy to prevent recurrence of ductal stones, though therapeutic ERCP may be all that is required in elderly patients with comorbidities.

SURGEON'S FAVOURITE QUESTION

What procedure may be carried out during an ERCP in the case of a patient with pancreatic cancer and obstructive jaundice?

Stenting of the common bile duct to treat biliary obstruction.

ALISON BRADLEY

SMALL BOWEL RESECTION

Sasha Shoba Devi Thrumurthy

DEFINITION
Removal of part of the small intestine.

✓ INDICATIONS

- Ischaemia from an incarcerated hernia, small bowel volvulus, adhesive small bowel obstruction, or embolism.
- Neoplasm—either primary small bowel tumour (rare) or small bowel stuck to a secondary e.g. colorectal or peritoneal malignancy.
- Perforation.
- Inflammation secondary to Crohn's disease following failure of medical management.
- Strictures.
- Meckel's diverticulitis.
- Irreducible intussusception.
- Trauma.

✗ CONTRAINDICATIONS

Relative

- Extensive Crohn's disease—extensive resection can lead to short gut syndrome; medical management is preferred if possible.
- Unresectable tumours—may be preferable to create a side-to-side anastomosis of uninvolved bowel proximal and distal to obstruction in order to bypass the obstruction whilst leaving the tumour in situ.

ANATOMY

Gross anatomy

- The 1st and 2nd part of the duodenum originate from the foregut, the rest of the small bowel, the 3rd and 4th part of duodenum, the jejunum and ileum originate from the midgut embryologically. From here, the term "small bowel" will exclude the duodenum. .
- The small bowel is intraperitoneal and is suspended on its mesentery—a double layer of peritoneum.
- The mesentery contains the arteries, veins, lymphatics, and nerve supply to the small bowel.
- The mesenteric border is the concave margin of the small bowel facing towards the root of the mesentery, and the antimesenteric border is the convex margin of the small bowel facing away from the root of the mesentery.

- The root of the mesentery runs from the duodenojejunal flexure to the caecum.

Neurovasculature

- Innervation is by the sympathetic system (via the superior mesenteric plexus) and the parasympathetic system (via the vagus nerve).
- Arterial supply is from the superior mesenteric artery (SMA). Jejunal and ileal branches of the SMA form arcades within the mesentery.
- Venous drainage occurs via the superior mesenteric vein (SMV), which drains into the hepatic portal vein.
- Lymphatic drainage is via the superior mesenteric nodes.

Figure 2.1 Small bowel anatomy with arterial supply

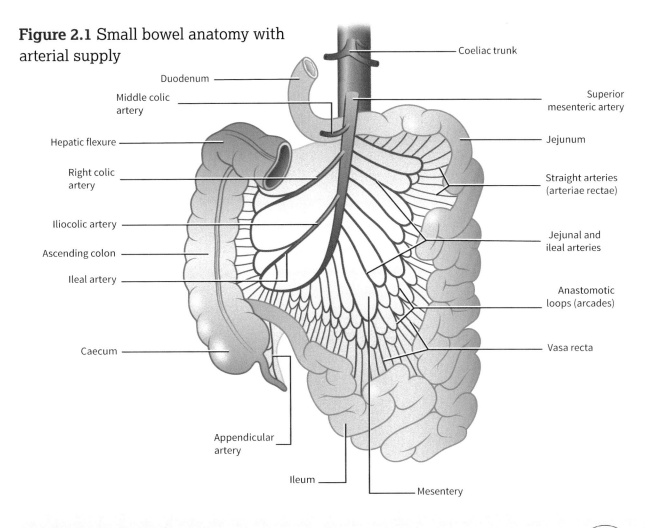

STEP-BY-STEP OPERATION

Anaesthesia: general.

Position: supine.

Considerations: In small bowel obstruction, a urinary catheter and a nasogastric (NG) tube are inserted.

1 A midline laparotomy is performed. An initial inspection of the bowel is done to assess for what needs to be done. If a hernia is seen, the bowel is removed and assessed for viability.

2 The bowel is wrapped in a warm, saline soaked swab (unless there is a perforation) and left for 5 minutes, after which the small bowel is assessed for signs of non-viability (these include poor colour, absence of peristalsis, and no pulsation in mesenteric artery).

3 The margins of proximal and distal resection are identified and clamped off.

4 Non-crushing bowel clamps are placed proximal (afferent loop) and distal (efferent loop) to the section of bowel to be resected. This technique avoids large enteric content contamination when the bowel is divided.

5 The mesentery is then divided between the resection margins, and the mesenteric vessels are ligated and divided.

a For benign disease, a small section of mesentery adjacent to the bowel is removed.

b For malignant disease, a deep V-shaped wedge is removed.

6 Straight crushing clamps are applied across the bowel, angled slightly towards the mesenteric border.

7 The bowel is cut flush against the outer aspect of each crushing clamp. Care must be taken not to contaminate the abdominal cavity with bowel contents.

8 The bowel ends are anastomosed, either hand sewn or stapled end-to-end anastomosis.

9 The mesenteric defect is closed, avoiding damage to the vasculature. The bowel is inspected for bleeding and leaks, and patency is assessed by palpation.

10 The midline laparotomy is repaired; firstly mass closure of the midline abdominal wall and then the skin separately

LOWER GASTROINTESTINAL

Figure 2.2 Resection of small bowel tumour

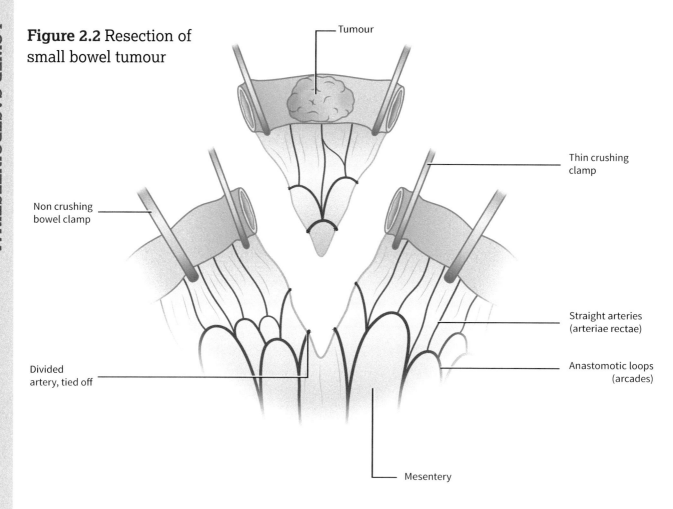

Tumour

Thin crushing clamp

Non crushing bowel clamp

Straight arteries (arteriae rectae)

Divided artery, tied off

Anastomotic loops (arcades)

Mesentery

COMPLICATIONS

Early

> Bleeding.
> Paralytic ileus.

Intermediate and late

> Deep Vein Thrombisis (DVT) and Pulmonary Embolism (PE).
> Infection—wound, intra-abdominal abscess, pneumonia, and urinary tract infection.
> Anastomotic leak (typically 5–7 days postoperatively).

> Wound dehiscence.
> Adhesive bowel obstruction.
> Incisional hernia.
> Gallstones (after ileal resections—formation of cholesterol-rich stones is facilitated by a combination of gallbladder hypomotility and decreased bile salt concentration as a result of depletion of the body's pool of bile salts).
> Short bowel syndrome—occurs if more than 50% of small bowel is lost.

POSTOPERATIVE CARE

Inpatient

> If the bowel was obstructed preoperatively, the NG tube is left on free drainage and fluids permitted. Once evidence of absorption is noted; decreased NG tube returns, and bowel activity resumes, then the tube can be removed and diet introduced.

> If resection is done for a non obstructing lesion then normal diet can be commenced post op. Intravenous fluids are maintained until the patient has adequate oral intake to maintain hydration.

> If there is a prolonged period of bowel inactivity, parenteral nutrition must be considered.

> Early sitting up and ambulation are encouraged with input from physiotherapy.

> Urinary catheters are removed within 48 hours of surgery to prevent infection.

> If drains are left in situ, they are removed once output is significantly reduced.

Outpatient

> Patients are reviewed 2–6 weeks postoperatively with the results of pathology.

> In cases of small bowel malignancy, further treatment is decided upon by a multidisciplinary team (MDT) and depends on the results of pathology and the patient's comorbid state.

💬 SURGEON'S FAVOURITE QUESTION

What three factors are required for an anastomosis to successfully heal?

An adequate blood supply, minimal tension, and mucosal apposition.

LAPAROSCOPIC APPENDICECTOMY

Shiying Wu

DEFINITION
An elective or emergency surgical procedure to resect the vermiform appendix.

✓ INDICATIONS

- Acute appendicitis.
- Suspected malignancy of the appendix.

✗ CONTRAINDICATIONS

- Contraindications to laparoscopy (laparotomy preferred):
  - Severe cardiopulmonary disease where establishing pneumoperitoneum would put too much pressure on the cardiovascular system.
  - Extensive adhesions.
  - Patients too unstable to tolerate pneumoperitoneum.
  - Extensive contamination
- Relative;
  - Pregnancy

ANATOMY

Gross anatomy

- The vermiform appendix is 2–20 cm long (average 9 cm), arising embryonically from the midgut.
- The three taeniae coli of the caecum converge at the caecal pole, which marks the base of the appendix.
- The position of the appendix is variable:
  - Two-thirds are retrocaecal.
  - One-third are pelvic.
  - The remainder are paracaecal, subcaecal, preileal, postileal, or subileal.

Neurovasculature

- The appendix is supplied by the appendicular artery within the mesoappendix (a branch of the ileocolic artery, in turn a branch of the superior mesenteric artery).
- Venous drainage is via small appendicular veins leading to the posterior caecal or ileocolic vein, which drain into the superior mesenteric vein.
- Lymphatic tissue drains to ileocolic lymph nodes and then to superior mesenteric nodes.

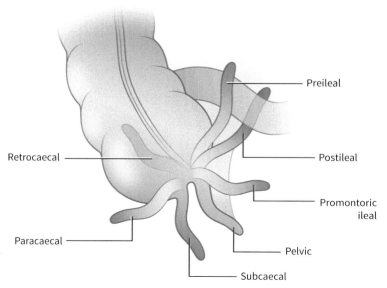

Figure 2.3 Potential anatomical locations of the appendix

STEP-BY-STEP OPERATION

Anaesthesia: general.

Position: supine and trendelenburg.

Considerations: A urinary catheter can be inserted, and prophylactic antibiotics are administered.

1   Pneumoperitoneum is achieved using the Hasson technique by inserting a port at:
    a   the umbilicus,
    b   the suprapubic region (inserted under direct vision), and
    c   the left iliac fossa (inserted under direct vision).

2   A diagnostic laparoscopy is performed (inspecting all four quadrants of the abdomen to exclude alternative diagnosis). If purulent material is present, a sample is sent to microbiology.

3   The patient is placed in the Trendelenburg position with their right side tilted up to allow the small bowel to move out of the pelvis and right iliac fossa.

4   Adherent bowel loops or omentum are brushed away with forceps.

5   The appendix is grasped at its tip, and adhesions to the lateral wall are divided with diathermy, mobilising the appendix towards the appendicular base.

6   Using diathermy, a window is created in the mesoappendix near the appendicular base.

7   The mesoappendix is dissected away from the appendix, and the appendicular artery is clipped and then divided.

8   The base of the appendix is secured with nooses of pre-tied sutures (two sutures are placed at the base of the appendix, and a third suture is placed slightly distally on the appendix). The appendix is then divided between the second and third sutures.

9   The appendix is removed in a specimen bag through the umbilical port.

10 The abdomen is washed out, ports are removed, and the incisions are closed.

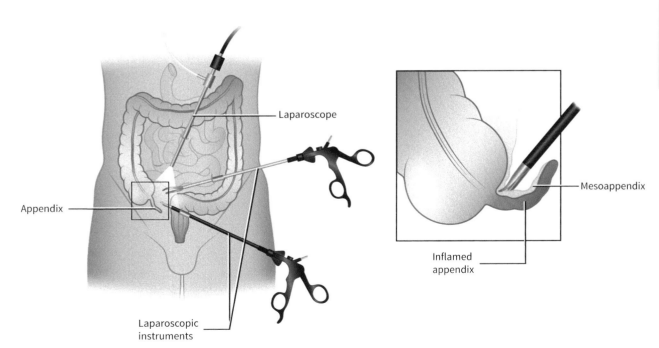

Figure 2.4 Laparosopic appendicectomy

COMPLICATIONS

Early

> Bleeding.
> Enteric injury.
> Paralytic ileus.

Intermediate and late

> Infection—wound, intra-abdominal collection, abscess, pneumonia, and urinary tract infection.
> Wound dehiscence.
> Stump appendicitis.
> Adhesions.
> Incisional hernia.

POSTOPERATIVE CARE

Inpatient

> Patients are discharged within 24–48 hours, provided they are mobile, able to void, and pain is adequately controlled.
> In perforated appendicitis, antibiotics are continued 5 days postoperatively.

Outpatient

> Routine follow-up is not required.
> Patients may be reviewed 6 weeks postoperatively with pathology results (occasionally, unexpected pathology such as carcinoid tumours are encountered).

SURGEON'S FAVOURITE QUESTION

Where is McBurney's Point?

The point two-thirds of the way along an imaginary line drawn from the umbilicus to the anterior superior iliac spine, marking the base of the appendix.

RIGHT HEMICOLECTOMY

Shiying Wu

DEFINITION

Removal of the terminal ileum and right colon, including the caecum, appendix, ascending colon, hepatic flexure, and a portion of the transverse colon. An extended right hemicolectomy includes removal of the transverse colon, the splenic flexure and proximal descending colon.

✓ INDICATIONS

- Tumours or inflammatory conditions of the right colon or terminal ileum, transverse colon or splenic flexure.
- Large adenomatous polyps.
- Inflammatory bowel disease.
- Diverticular disease involving the right colon.
- Caecal volvulus.

✗ CONTRAINDICATIONS

Contraindications to laparoscopic right hemicolectomy

- Bowel obstruction or ileus leading to severe abdominal distension with poor operative view.
- Multiple previous abdominal surgeries.
- Dense adhesions.

ANATOMY

Gross anatomy

- Embryonically, the ascending colon to the proximal two thirds of the transverse colon originates from the midgut. The distal one third of the transverse colon to the sigmoid colon originates from the hindgut.
- The transverse colon and caecum are peritoneal structures.
- The ascending colon is retroperitoneal.

Neurovasculature

- Parasympathetic nerve supply is from the vagus nerve.
- Sympathetic nerve supply is from the thoracic splanchnic nerves via the coeliac and superior mesenteric ganglia and the superior mesenteric plexus.
- The arterial supply to the right colon comes from branches of the superior mesenteric artery (SMA):

  › Ileocolic artery—supplies the terminal ileum, appendix and caecum.
  › Right colic artery (only present in 20% of people)—supplies the ascending colon. Where absent the ascending colon is supplied by the ileocolic artery and right branch of middle colic artery.
  › Middle colic artery—supplies the proximal two-thirds of the transverse colon.
- Venous drainage is from the ileocolic, right colic, and middle colic veins, which correspond to the arterial anatomical distribution and drain into the superior mesenteric vein, which drains into the portal circulation.
- Ileocolic, right colic, and middle colic lymph nodes drain into the superior mesenteric nodes, which are located at the origin of the superior mesenteric artery.

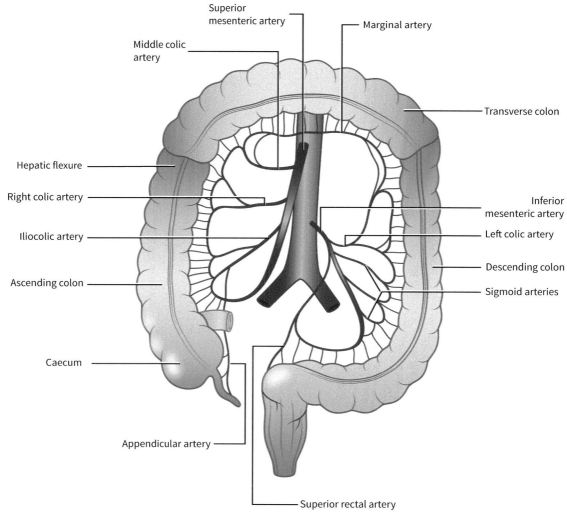

Figure 2.5 Large bowel anatomy with arterial supply

STEP-BY-STEP OPERATION

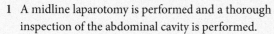

Anaesthesia: general.

Position: supine.

Considerations: A urinary catheter is inserted and, in cases of obstruction, a nasogastric (NG) tube is inserted. Prophylactic antibiotics are administered.

1 A midline laparotomy is performed and a thorough inspection of the abdominal cavity is performed.

2 In cases of malignancy, the abdominal cavity and viscera are assessed for tumour spread.

3 Dissection is commenced by dividing the peritoneum lateral to the right colon. The ascending colon and caecum are mobilised and retracted medially (care must be taken to identify and not injure the duodenum, right ureter, and right gonadal vessels).

4 The mesentery is palpated and inspected to identify the position of the ileocolic and the right branch of the middle colic artery, which are then ligated and divided near their origin.

5 In an extended right hemicolectomy (for tumours of the transverse colon or splenic flexure), dissection is continued to the splenic flexure or beyond as determined by the site of the lesion.

6 Dissection is continued until the bowel can be held freely, from terminal ileum to mid-transverse colon.

7 Non-crushing bowel clamps are placed on the margins of resection, one on the ileum and one one-third of the way along the transverse colon. A crushing bowel clamp is placed on the side of the bowel to be resected, and the bowel is divided at each end between the crushing and non-crushing clamps. The resected bowel is then removed and sent for histology.

8 The remaining bowel ends are inspected for viability, and an ileocolic anastomosis is fashioned, either hand sewn or with a stapling device. Alternatively an end ileostomy is performed if required.

9 The midline laparotomy is repaired; firstly mass closure of the midline abdominal wall and then the skin separately.

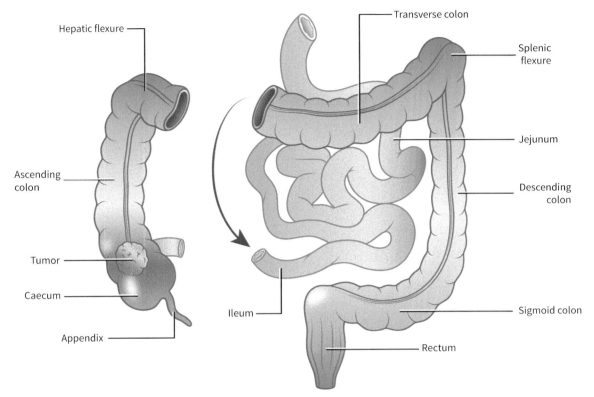

Figure 2.6 Resection of caecal tumour

COMPLICATIONS

Early

- Damage to surrounding structures—right ureter, gonadal vessels, duodenum.
- Paralytic ileus.
- Atelectasis.
- Anastomotic leak.

Intermediate and late

- Infection—wound, intra-abdominal abscess, pneumonia, and urinary tract infection.
- Incisional hernia.
- Deep Vein Thrombosis (DVT) or Pulmonary Embolism (PE).
- Adhesive bowel obstruction.
- Anastomotic stricture.
- Change in bowel habit.
- Mortality.

POSTOPERATIVE CARE

Inpatient

> If the bowel was obstructed preoperatively, the NG tube is kept in until bowel activity resumes.
> If there was evidence of perforation or sepsis, antibiotics are continued postoperatively.
> Diet is gradually built up as bowel activity resumes; in prolonged ileus, parenteral nutrition must be considered.
> Early ambulation with input from physiotherapy.
> Urinary catheters are removed within 48 hours to prevent infection.

> If drains are left in situ, they are removed once output is minimal.
> DVT prophylaxis is given in-hospital and continued for 28 days for colorectal cancer patients.

Outpatient

> Patients are reviewed 2–6 weeks postoperatively.
> In cases of malignancy, further treatment is decided upon by a multidisciplinary team (MDT) and depends on the results of pathology and the patient's comorbid state.

❓ SURGEON'S FAVOURITE QUESTION

Describe the course of the ureter

Ureters begin at the ureteropelvic junction (L2), posterior to the renal artery and vein, and descend anterior to the psoas as a retroperitoneal structure, coursing under the gonadal vessels at the inferior pole of the kidney. They continue medially to the sacroiliac joint. They run lateral in the pelvis, crossing anterior to the iliac vessels at the bifurcation of the common iliac artery, then medially to penetrate the base of the bladder.

LEFT HEMICOLECTOMY

Yasoda Dupaguntla

DEFINITION

Resection of the descending left colon.

✓ INDICATIONS

> Tumours of the colon in the region supplied by the inferior mesenteric artery.
> Diverticular strictures.
> Large adenomatous polyps that cannot be resected using a colonoscope.
> Segmental Crohn's colitis.
> Trauma and ischaemic injury.

✗ CONTRAINDICATIONS

Contraindications to laparoscopic left hemicolectomy

> Bowel obstruction or ileus leading to severe abdominal distension with poor operative view.
> Multiple previous abdominal surgeries.
> Dense adhesions.

ANATOMY

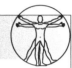

Gross anatomy

> The embryological hindgut develops into the distal third of the transverse colon, splenic flexure, descending and sigmoid colons, and upper rectum.
> The transverse and sigmoid colon are intraperitoneal and mobile on their mesenteries.
> The descending colon and upper rectum are retroperitoneal and fixed.

Neurovasculature

> Parasympathetic nerve supply comes from the pelvic splanchnic nerves (S2–4), and sympathetic from the inferior mesenteric plexus.
> The inferior mesenteric artery (IMA) branches off the descending aorta at the level of L3 and supplies the hindgut.

> Branches of the IMA:
>> Left colic artery—supplies the descending colon.
>> Sigmoid arteries (2–4)—supply the sigmoid colon.
>> Superior rectal artery—supplies the upper rectum.
> Venous drainage is from the left colic, sigmoid, and superior rectal veins, which correspond to the arterial anatomical distribution. The inferior mesenteric vein (IMV) ultimately drains into the portal venous system and terminates when it joins the splenic vein. The splenic vein joins the superior mesenteric vein to form the portal vein.
> Lymphatic drainage of the sigmoid and the upper rectum is to the para-aortic lymph nodes.

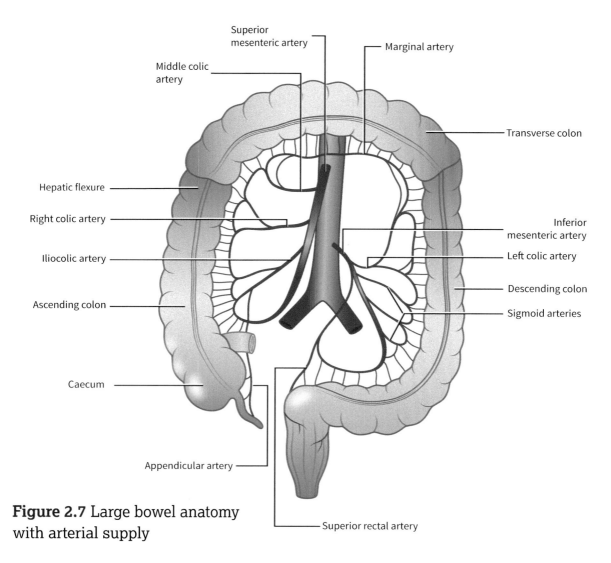

Figure 2.7 Large bowel anatomy with arterial supply

STEP-BY-STEP OPERATION

Anaesthesia: general.

Position: supine or Lloyd-Davies.

Considerations: Prophylactic antibiotics are administered. An enema can be given to clear the left colon. This procedure can be performed as a laparotomy or laparoscopically.

1 A midline laparotomy and a thorough inspection of the abdominal cavity is performed.

2 In cases of malignancy, the abdominal cavity is assessed for tumour spread, including palpation of the liver.

3 Dissection is commenced by dividing the peritoneum lateral to the left colon. Care is taken to identify and preserve the left ureter and gonadal vessels.

4 The origin of the IMA and IMV are identified with palpation; they are then ligated and divided.

5 Once the transverse colon, splenic flexure and descending colon are completely mobilised, the proximal and distal points of transection are identified (5 cm resection margin of healthy bowel should be left on either side of the diseased area).

6 The bowel is divided proximally and distally, either between bowel clamps or with a linear cutting stapler.

7 The diseased segment is removed and sent for pathology.

8 The proximal and distal segments are brought together, and an end-to-end anastomosis is fashioned using staples or sutures.

9 The anastomosis is checked for any leakage before closing. This is done by submerging the anastomosis in water and inflating the colon with gas.

10 The midline laparotomy is repaired; firstly mass closure of the midline abdominal wall and then the skin separately.

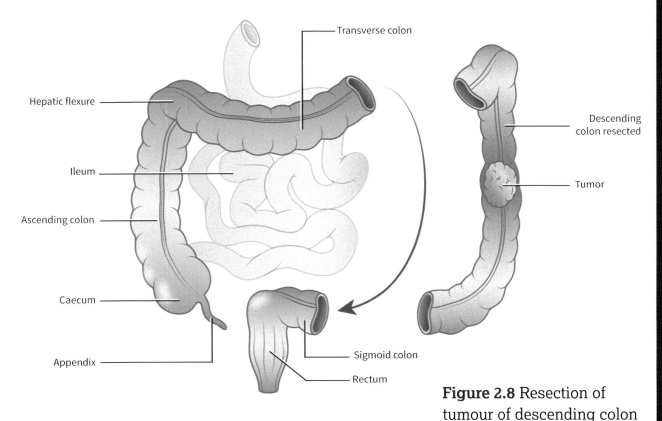

Transverse colon

Hepatic flexure

Ileum

Ascending colon

Caecum

Appendix

Descending colon resected

Tumor

Sigmoid colon

Rectum

Figure 2.8 Resection of tumour of descending colon

COMPLICATIONS

Early

› Bleeding.
› Splenic or left ureter injury.
› Anastomotic leak.
› Ileus.

Intermediate and late

› Infection—chest, urinary, and intra-abdominal collection.

› Deep Vein Thrombosis (DVT) or Pulmonary Embolism (PE).
› Enteric fistula formation.
› Adhesive bowel obstruction.
› Incisional hernia.
› Anastomotic stricture.
› Change in bowel habit.
› Mortality.

POSTOPERATIVE CARE

Inpatient

› If the bowel was obstructed preoperatively, the NG tube is kept in until bowel activity resumes.
› In cases of perforation or sepsis, antibiotics are continued postoperatively.
› Diet is gradually built up as bowel activity resumes; in prolonged ileus, parenteral nutrition must be considered.
› Urinary catheters are removed within 48 hours to prevent infection.
› If drains are left in situ, they are removed once output is minimal.

› DVT prophylaxis is given in-hospital and continued for 28 days for colorectal cancer patients.

Outpatient

› Patients are reviewed 2–6 weeks postoperatively.
› In cases of malignancy, further treatment is decided upon by a multidisciplinary team (MDT), and depends on the results of pathology and the patient's comorbid state.

LOWER GASTROINTESTINAL

 SURGEON'S FAVOURITE QUESTION

What is the difference between a Hartmann's procedure and a left hemicolectomy?

In a Hartmann's procedure, an end-colostomy is fashioned, and a rectal stump is left in the pelvis; in a left hemicolectomy, a primary anastomosis is formed.

HARTMANN'S PROCEDURE

Joon Park

DEFINITION

An emergency procedure to remove the sigmoid colon and upper rectum, resulting in an end colostomy (colonic stoma) and an over-sewn rectal stump.

✓ INDICATIONS

- Diverticular disease of the sigmoid colon with perforation, abscess, and/or peritonitis.
- Rectosigmoid cancer causing obstruction or perforation.
- Unresolved sigmoid volvulus.
- Other sigmoid pathology where a primary anastomosis would be at significant risk of breakdown:
  - Anastomotic dehiscence.
  - Ischaemia.

✗ CONTRAINDICATIONS

- The Hartmann's procedure is usually conducted as an emergency procedure due to bowel perforation. Patient comorbidities should be considered prior to surgery, with some comorbid patients opting for palliation.

ANATOMY

Gross anatomy

- The embryological hindgut develops into the distal third of the transverse colon, splenic flexure, descending colon, sigmoid colon, and upper rectum.
- The transverse and sigmoid colon are intraperitoneal and mobile on their mesenteries.
- The descending colon and upper rectum are retroperitoneal and fixed.

Neurovasculature

- Parasympathetic nerve supply comes from the pelvic splanchnic nerves (S2–4), and sympathetic from the inferior mesenteric plexus.
- The inferior mesenteric artery (IMA) branches off the descending aorta at the level of L3 and supplies the hindgut.

- Branches of the IMA:
  - Left colic artery–supplies the descending colon.
  - Sigmoid arteries (2–4)—supply the sigmoid colon.
  - Superior rectal artery—supplies the upper rectum.
- Venous drainage is from the left colic, sigmoid, and superior rectal veins, which correspond to the arterial anatomical distribution. The inferior mesenteric vein (IMV) ultimately drains into the portal venous system and terminates when it joins the splenic vein. The splenic vein joins the superior mesenteric vein to form the portal vein.
- Lymphatic drainage of the sigmoid and the upper rectum is to the para-aortic lymph nodes.

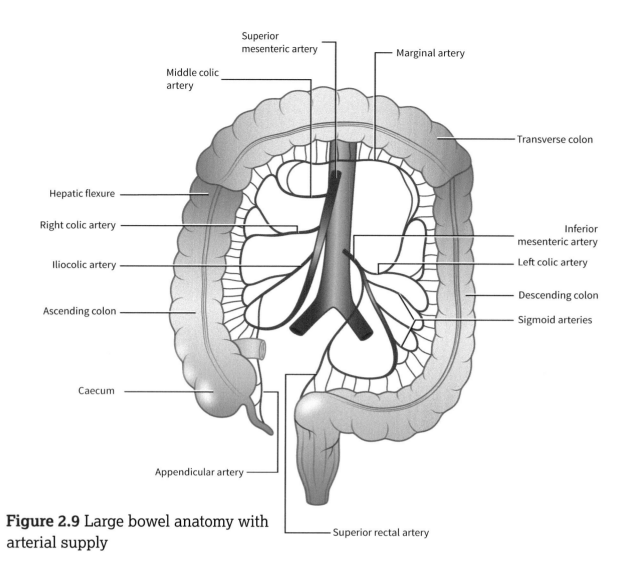

Figure 2.9 Large bowel anatomy with arterial supply

STEP-BY-STEP OPERATION

Anaesthesia: general.

Position: Lloyd-Davies position.

Considerations: A urinary catheter is inserted. In cases of obstruction, a nasogastric (NG) tube is inserted, and prophylactic antibiotics are given. The stoma site is marked on the left lower quadrant.

1 A midline laparotomy is performed.
2 The abdominal cavity is inspected, and any free fluid is sent to microbiology.
3 Dissection is commenced by dividing the peritoneum lateral to the left colon. Care is taken to identify and preserve the left ureter throughout its length.
4 The sigmoid vessels are identified within the mesentery and divided.
5 Once the sigmoid and descending colon are completely mobilised, the proximal and distal points of transection are identified.
6 The bowel is divided proximally and distally, either between bowel clamps or with a linear cutting stapler.

Peritoneal lavage is performed using warm saline (water if a cancer case), and drains are inserted.
7 The rectal stump (either stapled or sewn-over by hand) is left in situ.
8 A circular incision is made over the site of the previously marked stoma site, and the abdominal cavity is entered. The proximal colon is brought out of the abdomen and through the incision, ensuring it is not under tension.
9 The midline laparotomy is repaired; firstly mass closure of the midline abdominal wall and then the skin separately.
10 The protruding bowel is then fashioned into a stoma, and a bag is placed over the stoma (colostomy).

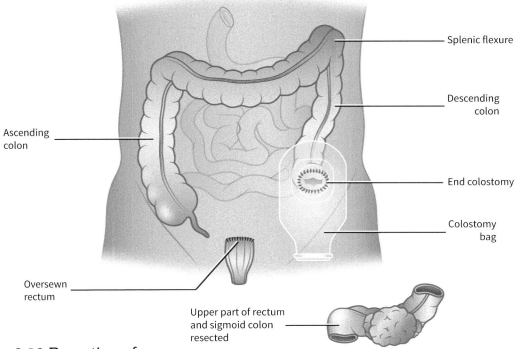

Splenic flexure

Descending colon

Ascending colon

End colostomy

Colostomy bag

Oversewn rectum

Upper part of rectum and sigmoid colon resected

Figure 2.10 Resection of tumour of sigmoid colon

COMPLICATIONS

Early

▸ Iatrogenic damage to surrounding structures—ureters and gonadal vessels.
▸ Paralytic ileus.
▸ Atelectasis.
▸ Stoma—retraction or ischaemia.

Intermediate and late

▸ Infection—wound, intra-abdominal abscess, pneumonia, and urinary tract infection.
▸ Deep Vein Thrombosis (DVT) or Pulmonary Embolism (PE).
▸ Incisional hernia.
▸ Adhesive bowel obstruction.
▸ Stoma—stenosis, prolapse, or para-stomal hernia.

POSTOPERATIVE CARE

Inpatient

▸ Initial postoperative care in an Intensive Treatment Unit (ITU)/High Dependency Unit (HDU) environment.
▸ Antibiotics are continued for 5–7 days postoperatively.
▸ Full and normal diet is encouraged immediately post op; in prolonged ileus, parenteral nutrition must be considered.
▸ Urinary catheters are removed within 48 hours to prevent infection.
▸ If drains are left in situ, they are removed once output is minimal.
▸ DVT prophylaxis is given in-hospital and continued for 28 days for colorectal cancer patients.

▸ The patient is instructed in stoma care and must be confident with the stoma management before discharge.

Outpatient

▸ Patients are reviewed 2–6 weeks postoperatively.
▸ Stoma reversal is considered once the patient has fully recovered, usually after 6 months.
▸ In cases of malignancy, further treatment is decided upon by a multidisciplinary team (MDT) and depends on the results of pathology and the patient's comorbid state.

LOWER GASTROINTESTINAL

 SURGEON'S FAVOURITE QUESTION

How do you differentiate between a colostomy and an ileostomy?

A colostomy tends to be flush with the skin, and an ileostomy is spouted. Do not simply rely on the position when attempting to differentiate between the two.

ANTERIOR RESECTION OF THE RECTUM

Stephen Ali

DEFINITION

Excision of the rectum, mesorectum, and regional lymphatics via the anterior abdominal wall.

✓ INDICATIONS

Rectal cancers without invasion of the anal sphincter complex.

✗ CONTRAINDICATIONS

Relative

› Localised, superficial, T1 rectal cancers—may be endoscopically treated with local excision.

Absolute

› Rectal cancers very close to or involving the sphincters—managed by abdominoperineal resection.

ANATOMY

Gross anatomy

› The rectum arises embryologically from the hindgut.
› The upper rectum is intra-peritoneal, the middle third is lined by peritoneum anteriorly only, and the lower third, below the pelvic peritoneal reflection, is extra-peritoneal.
› In males, the rectovesical pouch, base of bladder, seminal vesicles, and prostate lie anterior to the rectum, with Denonvilliers' fascia separating it from the prostate.
› In females, the posterior vaginal wall, rectovaginal septum, and bladder lie anteriorly.
› For both sexes, the sacrum, coccyx, lower sacral nerves, and middle sacral artery all lie posterior to the rectum.
› The levator ani and coccygeus muscles lie lateral and inferior to the peritoneal reflection.

Neurovasculature

› Nerve supply arises from the pelvic plexus (hypogastric nerves) and splanchnic nerves (S2–S4).
› Blood supply is from the superior rectal artery (branch of the inferior mesenteric artery) and the middle and inferior rectal arteries (branches of the pudendal arteries).
› Venous drainage is via the superior rectal vein to the inferior mesenteric vein, draining to the hepatic portal circulation.
› Lymphatic drainage is to the mesorectum, then the inferior mesenteric lymph nodes. Total mesorectal excision (TME)—removal of mesorectal fat and lymph nodes—is crucial in an oncological anterior resection.

71

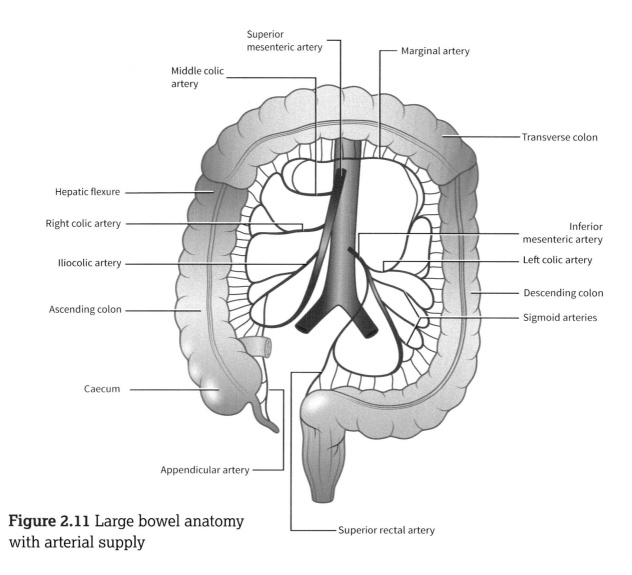

Superior mesenteric artery

Marginal artery

Middle colic artery

Transverse colon

Hepatic flexure

Right colic artery

Inferior mesenteric artery

Iliocolic artery

Left colic artery

Descending colon

Ascending colon

Sigmoid arteries

Caecum

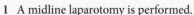

Appendicular artery

Superior rectal artery

Figure 2.11 Large bowel anatomy with arterial supply

STEP-BY-STEP OPERATION

Anaesthesia: general

Position: Lloyd-Davies

Considerations: A urinary catheter is inserted. Bowel preparation can be considered.

1 A midline laparotomy is performed.

2 The abdominal cavity is assessed for tumour spread, including palpation of the liver.

3 Dissection is commenced by dividing the peritoneum lateral to the left colon. Care is taken to identify and preserve the left ureter throughout its length.

4 The origin of the inferior mesenteric artery (IMA) and inferior mesenteric vein (IMV) are identified with palpation. They are then ligated and divided.

5 Once the splenic flexure, descending colon, sigmoid and rectum are completely mobilised, the proximal and distal points of transection are identified.

6 Total mesorectal excision (TME) is then performed. Anteriorly, the dissection commences by opening

the peritoneum at the rectovesical pouch in men, and between the anterior mesorectum and posterior vaginal wall in women. Dissection is then continued towards the pelvic floor, laterally and posteriorly (anterior to the coccyx).

7 After mobilisation and TME, the bowel is divided at its proximal and distal resection margins, either between bowel clamps or with a linear cutting stapler device. The specimen is sent to pathology.

8 An end-to-end anastomosis is formed between the descending colon and the rectal stump, using either a circular stapling device or by hand-sewing. The anastomosis is checked for any leakage before closing. This is done by submerging the anastomosis in saline

(water if a cancer case) and inflating the rectum with gas. There should be no leak of bubbles from the staple line.

9 A defunctioning loop ileostomy may be formed to divert faeces away from a healing anastomosis if within 6cm of the anal verge. Defunctioning loop ileostomy should also be considered at other times if there have

been technical difficulties during construction of the anastomosis. This is placed in the right iliac fossa and can be reversed 3–6 months later.

10 The midline laparotomy is repaired; firstly mass closure of the midline abdominal wall and then the skin separately.

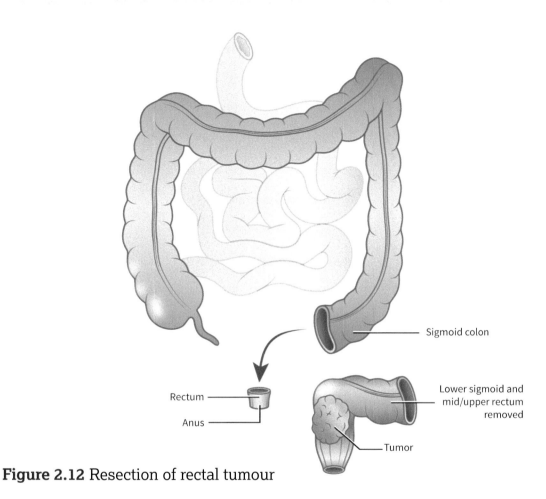

Figure 2.12 Resection of rectal tumour

COMPLICATIONS

Early

> Damage to surrounding structures—the ureter and gonadal vessels.
> Anastomotic leak.
> Paralytic ileus.
> Atelectasis.
> Stoma retraction and ischaemia.

Intermediate and late

> Infection—wound, intra-abdominal abscess, pneumonia, and urinary tract infection.
> Anastomotic stricture.
> Bladder and sexual dysfunction.
> Deep Vein Thrombosis (DVT) or Pulmonary Embolism (PE).
> Incisional hernia.
> Adhesive bowel obstruction.
> Stoma stenosis, prolapse, or para-stomal hernia.
> Mortality.

POSTOPERATIVE CARE

Inpatient

➤ Diet is gradually built up as bowel activity resumes; in prolonged ileus, parenteral nutrition must be considered.

➤ Early ambulation with input from physiotherapy.

➤ Urinary catheters removed within 48 hours—attention must be paid to voiding, as bladder tone may be lost postoperatively.

➤ If drains are left in situ, they are removed once output is minimal.

➤ DVT prophylaxis is given in-hospital and continued for 28 days.

➤ If a loop ileostomy is formed, the patient is instructed in stoma care and must be confident with stoma management before discharge.

Outpatient

➤ Patients are reviewed 2–6 weeks postoperatively.

➤ Further treatment is decided upon by a multidisciplinary team (MDT) depending on the results of pathology and the patient's comorbid state.

❓ SURGEON'S FAVOURITE QUESTION

In what circumstances may a patient end up with an intestinal stoma after an anterior resection?

1. Anastomosis too low- they are likely to have a defunctioning loop ileostomy which may subsequently be reversed.

2. Not technically possible - insufficient length of vascularised bowel (commonest reason), or not sensible to do so e.g. gross examination by the naked eye shows tumour present at the resection margin or blood supply too poor, an end colostomy is performed, which would usually be permanent.

3. Anastomotic leak - the patient will likely need emergency surgery and take down of the anastomosis into an end colostomy.

ABDOMINOPERINEAL RESECTION (APR)

Jane Lim

DEFINITION
Removal of the sigmoid colon, rectum, and anus with the creation of a permanent end-colostomy.

✓ INDICATIONS

> Anal cancer with failed neoadjuvant therapy.
> Recurrent anal cancer.
> Low-lying rectal cancer with involvement of the anal sphincter.

✗ CONTRAINDICATIONS

> Patients with significant morbidity may be deemed unsuitable to undergo major colorectal resection.

ANATOMY

Gross anatomy

> The anal canal is extra-peritoneal and measures 2–4 cm.
> The anal canal is embryologically part hindgut and part proctoderm. The dentate line divides the anal canal based on this:
>> The proximal two-thirds of the anal canal lie above the dentate line. This section is hindgut in origin and is lined with columnar mucosa.
>> The distal third lies below the dentate line—this section is proctoderm in origin and is lined with squamous epithelium.

Neurovasculature

> Above the dentate line:
>> Innervated by the inferior hypogastric plexus.
>> Arterial supply is from the superior rectal artery (a branch of the IMA) and the middle rectal artery (a branch of the inferior vesicular artery).
>> Venous drainage is via the internal haemorrhoidal plexus to the superior rectal vein.
> Below the dentate line:
>> Innervated by the inferior rectal nerve, a branch of the pudendal nerve from the sacral plexus.
>> Arterial supply is via the inferior rectal arteries from the pudendal artery.
>> Venous drainage is via the external haemorrhoidal plexus to the inferior and middle rectal veins.

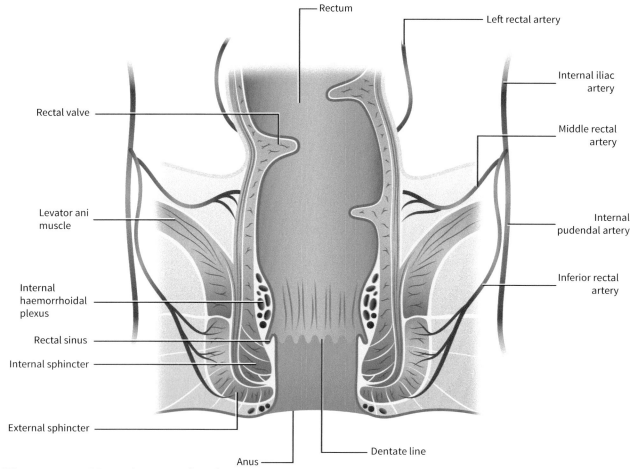

Figure 2.13 Vascular supply of rectum

STEP-BY-STEP OPERATION

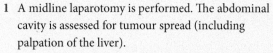

Anaesthesia: general.

Position: supine and Lloyd-Davies.

Considerations: A urinary catheter is inserted. The abdominal and perineal components of the operation can be done concurrently if there are two surgeons.

1 A midline laparotomy is performed. The abdominal cavity is assessed for tumour spread (including palpation of the liver).

2 The small bowel and sigmoid colon are retracted to the patient's right-hand side. The parietal peritoneum is dissected, starting from the junction between the sigmoid colon and the retroperitoneal descending colon. Care is taken to identify and preserve the left ureter and the left common iliac artery.

3 The inferior mesenteric artery and vein are ligated and then the left peritoneal dissection is carried down into the total mesorectal excision plane. The peritoneum on the right is then divided and the two sides joined below the level of the bifurcation of the aorta. This allows mobilisation of the rectum and sigmoid colon.

4 The superior rectal artery is ligated. The descending colon is divided at its proximal resection margin,

either between bowel clamps or with a linear cutting stapler device.

5 The proximal end of the colon is brought out through the abdominal wall and an end-colostomy is fashioned.

6 Next, the perineal resection is commenced. The patient may be repositioned prone or Lloyd-Davis for this part of the procedure. An elliptical perineal incision is made from the perineal body to a point midway between the anus and coccyx.

7 The rectum is mobilised from the prostate/vagina and surrounding tissues. The inferior rectal vessels are ligated, and the rectum, sigmoid colon, and anus are removed.

8 The levator muscles are reapproximated with sutures. A mesh may be used to add extra support.

9 The perineal wound is closed in layers.

10 The midline laparotomy is repaired; firstly mass closure of the midline abdominal wall and then the skin separately.

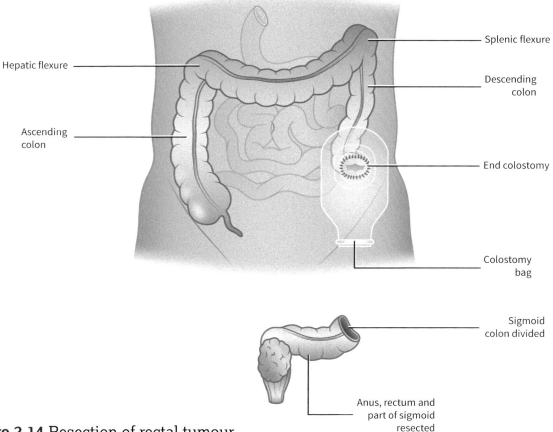

Hepatic flexure

Ascending colon

Splenic flexure

Descending colon

End colostomy

Colostomy bag

Sigmoid colon divided

Anus, rectum and part of sigmoid resected

Figure 2.14 Resection of rectal tumour with formation of end colostomy

COMPLICATIONS

Early

> Damage to surrounding structures—the ureters and gonadal vessels.
> Paralytic ileus.
> Atelectasis.
> Stoma problems—retraction or ischaemia.

Intermediate and late

> Infection—wound, intra-abdominal abscess, pneumonia, and urinary tract infection.
> Deep Vein Thrombosis (DVT) or Pulmonary Embolism (PE).

> Wound dehiscence.
> Persistent perineal sinus (perineal wound that has not healed 6 months postoperatively).
> Bladder and sexual dysfunction.
> Incisional hernia.
> Perineal hernia.
> Adhesive bowel obstruction.
> Stoma problems—stenosis, prolapse, or para-stomal hernia.

POSTOPERATIVE CARE

Inpatient

▸ Full and normal diet is encouraged immediately post op; in prolonged ileus, parenteral nutrition must be considered.

▸ Early ambulation with input from physiotherapy.

▸ Urinary catheters removed within 48 hours—attention must be paid to voiding, as bladder tone may be lost postoperatively.

▸ If drains are left in situ, they are removed once output is significantly reduced.

▸ DVT prophylaxis is given in-hospital and continued for 28 days in cases of malignancy.

▸ The patient is instructed in stoma care and must be confident with stoma management before discharge.

Outpatient

▸ Patients are reviewed 2–6 weeks postoperatively.

▸ Further treatment is decided upon by a multi disiplinary team (MDT) and depends on the results of pathology and the patient's comorbid state.

---

⑦ SURGEON'S FAVOURITE QUESTION

When perineal defects are too large for primary repair, what are the reconstructive options available for this area?

Reconstruction can be done with either a biological mesh or a myocutaneous flap. These include a pedicled gluteus maximus, gracilis, or rectus abdominis flap.

HERNIA REPAIR

Carly Bisset

DEFINITION

Repair of an inguinal hernia, which may be either indirect (through the deep inguinal ring) or direct (through Hesselbach's triangle).

✓ INDICATIONS

Elective
- Symptomatic inguinal hernia.

Emergency
- Incarcerated or strangulated hernia.

✗ CONTRAINDICATIONS

- Pregnancy—repair should be delayed unless there are signs of an acute incarceration, strangulation, or bowel obstruction.
- Small asymptomatic hernias- can undergo watchful waiting.

ANATOMY

Gross anatomy
- The deep and superficial inguinal rings are the internal and external openings of the inguinal canal.
- The inguinal canal contains the ilioinguinal nerve in both sexes, in females it contains the round ligament, in males the spermatic cord.
- The deep ring is found deep to the midpoint of the inguinal ligament, which lies halfway between the pubic tubercle and the anterior superior iliac spine (ASIS). The superficial inguinal ring is located ~ 1 cm superolateral to the pubic crest.
- The borders of the inguinal canal are:
  › Anterior—aponeurosis of external and internal oblique muscles.
  › Posterior—transversalis fascia and the conjoint tendon.
  › Superior—internal oblique and transverse abdominus.
  › Inferior—inguinal and lacunar ligaments.
- Hesselbach's triangle is demarcated by:
  › Medial—rectus abdominis.
  › Lateral—inferior epigastric vessels.
  › Inferior—inguinal ligament.

Pathology
- Direct inguinal hernias arise directly through the posterior wall of the inguinal canal, medial to the inferior epigastric vessels in Hesselbach's triangle.
- Indirect inguinal hernias arise through the deep ring with the spermatic cord, lateral to the inferior epigastric vessels. Indirect hernias traverse the inguinal canal to the superficial ring and may descend into the scrotum.

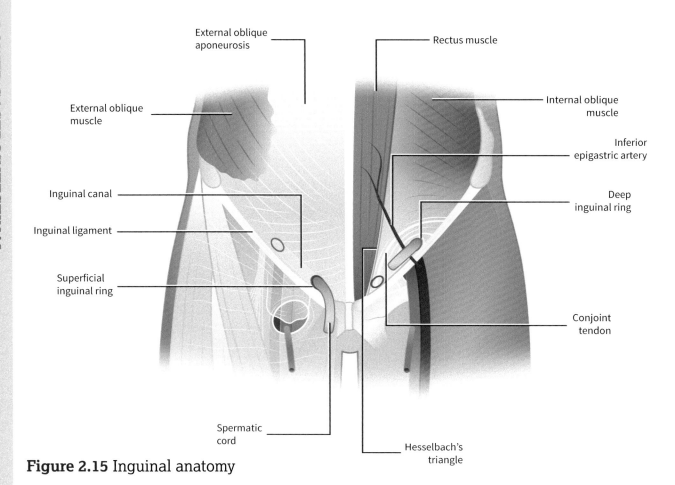

Figure 2.15 Inguinal anatomy

STEP-BY-STEP OPERATION

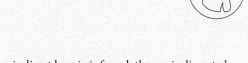

Anaesthesia: general, regional, or local.

Position: supine.

Considerations: A urinary catheter can be considered.

1 A skin crease incision is made in the groin, running superior to, but approximately in line with, the inguinal ligament, from the pubic tubercle to the level of the deep inguinal ring.

2 Dissection is continued until the external oblique aponeurosis is visible.

3 The external oblique fibres are split as far as the superficial inguinal ring (just superior to the pubic tubercle).

4 The ilioinguinal nerve is identified and protected.

5 The contents of the inguinal canal are identified and inspected. The sac is then dissected free from the cord structures, and a tape is passed around the spermatic cord.

6 Sac relocation:

   a If a direct hernia is found, the sac is pushed back into the extra-peritoneal space, and non-absorbable sutures are used to plicate the posterior wall over it.

   b If an indirect hernia is found, the sac is dissected to the deep ring and opened to determine its contents. Once emptied, it is then transfixed at its base.

7 The mesh is cut to the shape and size of the inguinal canal. The apex is sutured to the pubic tubercle with the suture being placed a short distance away from the apex ensuring some medial overlap. A slit made at the lateral end to create two 'tails'.

8 The inferior edge of the mesh is sutured along the inguinal ligament, and the superior edge is sutured onto the internal oblique muscle. The 'tail ends' of the mesh are sutured together around the spermatic cord lateral to the cord contents, recreating the deep inguinal ring.

9 The wound is closed in layers with absorbable sutures.

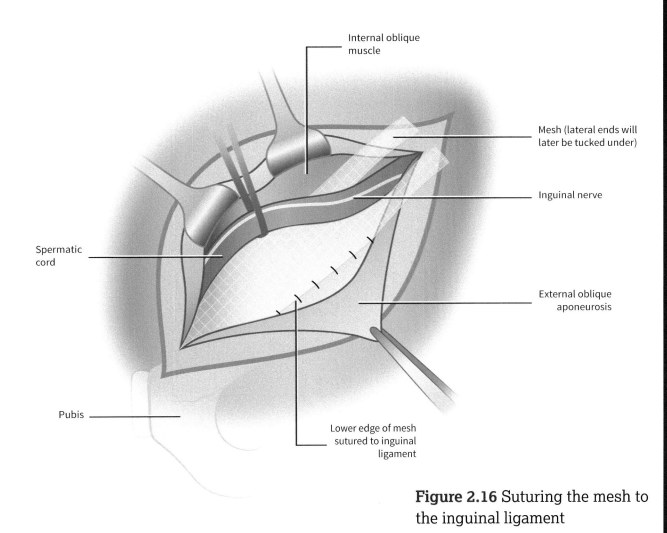

Internal oblique muscle

Mesh (lateral ends will later be tucked under)

Inguinal nerve

External oblique aponeurosis

Spermatic cord

Pubis

Lower edge of mesh sutured to inguinal ligament

Figure 2.16 Suturing the mesh to the inguinal ligament

COMPLICATIONS

Early

> Bleeding.
> Haematoma and seroma formation.
> Damage to vas deferens.
> Ischaemic orchitis or testicular atrophy.
> Ilioinguinal nerve damage.
> Femoral vessel damage.

Intermediate and late

> Infection—wound, mesh, intra-abdominal abscess, pneumonia, and urinary tract.
> Chronic inguinal pain secondary to ilioinguinal nerve damage.
> Recurrence (0–2%).
> Chronic mesh infection.

POSTOPERATIVE CARE

Inpatient

> Patients can be discharged the same day, provided there were no immediate complications.

Outpatient

> Avoid heavy lifting and straining for 4–6 weeks.

LOWER GASTROINTESTINAL

 SURGEON'S FAVOURITE QUESTION

How is the difference between an indirect and direct hernia identified intra-operatively?

An indirect hernia protrudes lateral to the inferior epigastric artery; a direct hernia protrudes medial to the inferior epigastric artery

FEMORAL HERNIA REPAIR

Joon Park

DEFINITION

Surgical closure of the femoral ring, with removal of pre-peritoneal fat or intestine from the femoral ring (if present).

✓ INDICATIONS

Elective

> Femoral hernias are associated with a high risk of strangulation; therefore, elective repair is recommended.

Acute

> Incarcerated or strangulated hernia.

✗ CONTRAINDICATIONS

> In patients with severe comorbidities, elective operative management may be deemed inappropriate in order to minimise risk.

ANATOMY

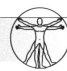

Gross anatomy

> The femoral ring forms the base of the femoral canal.
> Boundaries of the femoral canal:
> › Anterior—inguinal ligament.
> › Posterior—pectineal (Cooper's) ligament.
> › Medial—lacunar ligament.
> › Lateral—femoral vein.
> The femoral canal contains loose fatty connective tissues, lymphatic vessels, and lymph nodes.

Pathology

> A femoral hernia is the protrusion of pre-peritoneal fat or intestine into the femoral ring and canal.
> Femoral hernias arise inferolateral to the pubic tubercle in the anterior thigh.

Figure 2.17 Femoral anatomy

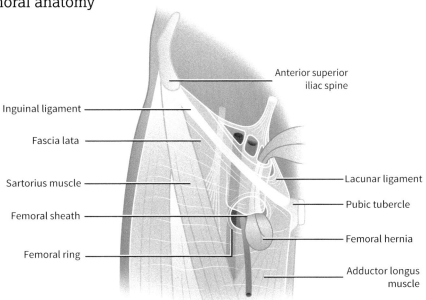

Anterior superior iliac spine

Inguinal ligament

Fascia lata

Sartorius muscle

Femoral sheath

Femoral ring

Lacunar ligament

Pubic tubercle

Femoral hernia

Adductor longus muscle

STEP-BY-STEP OPERATION

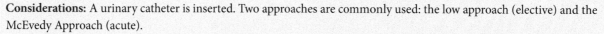

Anaesthesia: general.

Position: supine.

Considerations: A urinary catheter is inserted. Two approaches are commonly used: the low approach (elective) and the McEvedy Approach (acute).

Low approach:

1 An incision is made 1 cm below and parallel to the medial inguinal ligament. The subcutaneous fat is blunt dissected through to the level of the femoral hernia sac.

2 The hernia sac is dissected down to its neck, and the femoral and long saphenous veins are identified and preserved.

3 The sac is opened to assess contents and viability. The contents of the sac are then returned through the femoral ring to the peritoneum.

McEvedy Approach:

1 An 8–10 cm incision is made over the lower abdominal wall commencing at the pubic tubercle, running obliquely and laterally.

2 The rectus sheath is opened, and the rectus muscles are retracted. The preperitoneal fat and areolar tissue are dissected and then peritoneum is pulled up.

3 The hernia sac is identified and dissected down to its neck and then reduced upwards through the femoral ring.

4 The sac is then opened to assess contents and their viability; any non-viable bowel should be excised.

Both:

5 The neck of the sac is ligated as high as possible, and the femoral ring is closed with mesh sutures or interrupted non-absorbable sutures between the inguinal and pectineal ligaments.

6 The skin is closed with subcutaneous absorbable sutures.

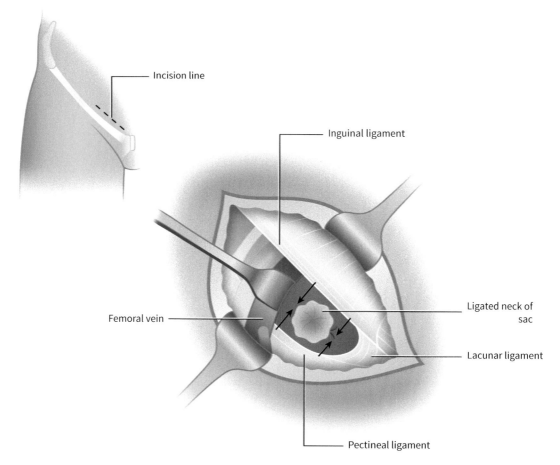

Figure 2.18 Ligation of the hernia sac and suture closure of the femoral ring.

COMPLICATIONS

Early

> Bleeding.
> Haematoma and seroma.
> Bowel injury.
> Femoral vein compression.

Intermediate and late

> Infection—wound, mesh (if used), intra-abdominal abscess, pneumonia, and urinary tract infection.
> Hernia recurrence.
> Stenotic stricture of the small bowel following strangulation (stenosis of Garré).
> Persistent groin pain.

POSTOPERATIVE CARE

Inpatient

> Elective patients can be discharged the same day.

Outpatient

> Patients are advised to avoid heavy lifting and straining for 4–6 weeks.

⚛ SURGEON'S FAVOURITE QUESTION

What are the borders of the femoral ring?

Anteriorly—inguinal ligament.

Posteriorly—pectineal ligament.

Medially—lacunar ligament.

Laterally—femoral vein.

HAEMORRHOIDECTOMY

Shiying Wu

DEFINITION

Surgical procedure to remove haemorrhoids (anorectal vascular cushions).

✓ INDICATIONS

External haemorrhoids

> Symptomatic haemorrhoids refractory to conservative management.
> Large or severely symptomatic external haemorrhoids.

Internal haemorrhoids

> Prolapsed internal haemorrhoids that can be manually reduced (Grade III).
> Prolapsed and incarcerated internal haemorrhoids (Grade IV).
> Symptomatic internal haemorrhoids refractory to conservative measures.
> Combined haemorrhoids.

✗ CONTRAINDICATIONS

Relative

> Previous operations involving the anal canal resulting in poor anal sphincter tone.
> Faecal incontinence.
> Portal hypertension with rectal varices.

Absolute

> Active disease in the anal canal or rectum, including Crohn's, colitis, and peri-anal abscess.

ANATOMY

Gross anatomy

> The anal canal is extra-peritoneal and measures 2–4 cm.
> The anal canal is embryologically part hindgut and part proctoderm. The dentate line divides the anal canal based on this:
> › The proximal two-thirds of the anal canal lie above the dentate line. This section is hindgut in origin and is lined with columnar mucosa.
> › The distal third lies below the dentate line. This section is proctoderm in origin and is lined with squamous epithelium.

Neurovasculature

> Above the dentate line
> › Innervated by the inferior hypogastric plexus.
> › Arterial supply is from the superior rectal artery (a branch of the IMA) and the middle rectal artery (a branch of the inferior vesicular artery).
> › Venous drainage is via the internal haemorrhoidal plexus to the superior rectal vein.
> Below the dentate line
> › Innervated by the inferior rectal nerve, a branch of the pudendal nerve from the sacral plexus.
> › Arterial supply is via the inferior rectal arteries from the pudendal artery.

> › Venous drainage is via the external haemorrhoidal plexus to the inferior and middle rectal veins.

Pathology

> Haemorrhoids are dilated anal vascular cushions and occur due to arterial inflow from branches of the superior rectal artery in the left lateral, right anterolateral, and right posterolateral positions.
> Haemorrhoids classically arise in the 3, 7, and 11 o'clock positions in lithotomy position.
> Haemorrhoids are termed depending on whether they arise from above or below the dentate line. Haemorrhoids proximal to the dentate line are classed as internal, distal as external, and mixed if they are both proximal and distal.
> Internal haemorrhoids are classified according to the degree from which they prolapse from the anal canal:
> › Grade I—bulge into the lumen but do not prolapse below the dentate line.
> › Grade II—prolapse out of the anal canal with defecation/straining but spontaneously reduce.
> › Grade III—prolapse out of the anal canal with defecation/straining and require manual reduction.
> › Grade IV—are irreducible and therefore have the potential to strangulate.

Figure 2.19 Internal and external haemorrhoidal locations

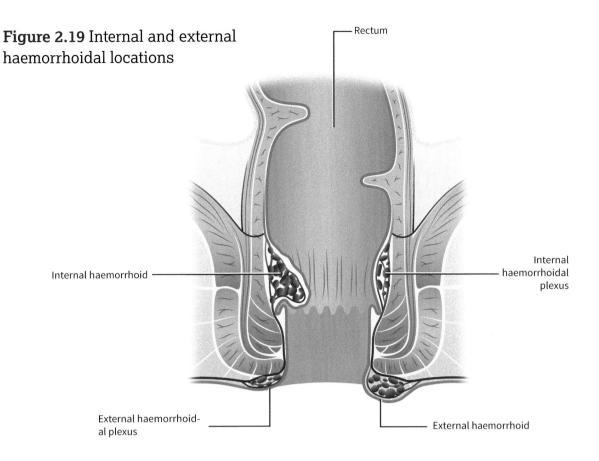

Rectum

Internal haemorrhoid

Internal haemorrhoidal plexus

External haemorrhoid-al plexus

External haemorrhoid

STEP-BY-STEP OPERATION

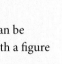

Anaesthesia: general.
Position: lithotomy.

Haemorrhoidectomy:

1 A digital rectal examination is performed, and an anal retractor is used to identify and examine the haemorrhoids.
2 A clip is applied to each haemorrhoid, and local anaesthetic is infiltrated into each.
3 The haemorrhoid and overlying skin are grasped and retracted. Diathermy is used to dissect the tissue off the internal anal sphincter until it remains on a pedicle.
4 The pedicle is transfixed, and the haemorrhoid is removed.
5 The skin at the anal verge can be closed or left to heal by secondary intention.

Haemorrhoidal Artery Ligation (HALO):

1 A probe containing bright LEDS with an integrated doppler ultrasound is inserted into the anus. This allows direct visualization of the mucosa of the anus and rectum by the surgeon whilst combining feedback on doppler flow and depth perception of arteries.
2 The probe is rotated slowly until an artery is detected, and its depth assessed; safe ligation can occur on arteries up to 8mm deep.
3 Through the window of the probe a suture can be placed to ligate the artery, double ligation with a figure of eight knot is often used.
4 The probe is then rotated until the next artery is detected and ligated. A whole turn of the probe is made then the probe is withdrawn 1.5cm and the process repeated. In general 5-7 arteries can be ligated but this can vary.
5 The series of suture ligations created reduce the arterial supply to the haemorrhoidal cushions which in time shrink over the next 6-8 weeks.

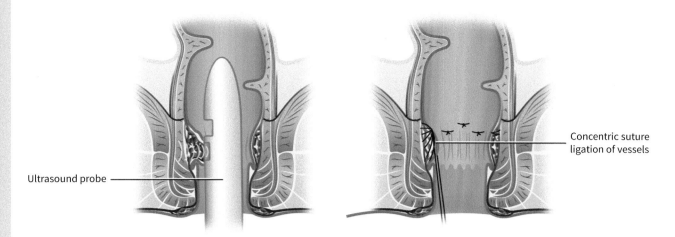

Ultrasound probe

Concentric suture ligation of vessels

Figure 2.20 Ultrasound probe insertion and circumferential suture ligations in the HALO (Haemorrhoidal Artery Ligation) technique

COMPLICATIONS

Early
> Pain.
> Bleeding.
> Urinary retention.

Intermediate and late
> Pelvic sepsis.
> Anal canal stenosis.
> Secondary haemorrhage 10–14 days after treatment (notorious in banding).
> Faecal incontinence.
> Rectovaginal fistula (if staples are used).
> Recurrence

POSTOPERATIVE CARE

Inpatient
> The patient is discharged on laxatives, analgesia, and anti-inflammatories.
> A course of oral metronidazole is prescribed postoperatively.

Outpatient
> Follow-up at outpatient clinic in 4 weeks.

SURGEON'S FAVOURITE QUESTION

What is the grading system used for internal haemorrhoids?

Grade I—no prolapse.

Grade II—prolapse upon bearing down but reduces spontaneously.

Grade III—prolapse upon bearing down and requires reduction manually.

Grade IV—prolapsed, cannot be reduced.

EXCISION OF PILONIDAL SINUS

Stephen Ali

DEFINITION

The surgical removal of a small hole or tunnel in the skin at the natal cleft.

✓ INDICATIONS

> A chronic or recurrently infected pilonidal sinus.

✗ CONTRAINDICATIONS

> Asymptomatic patients with a simple pilonidal sinus where there is a small pit or non-tender lump in the

natal cleft, which may have an emergent hair—these patients do not require treatment.

> Acutely infected pilonidal sinuses—these should be drained and later return for definitive excision.

ANATOMY

Gross anatomy

> A pilonidal sinus is a subcutaneous sinus in the natal cleft lined by squamous epithelium and containing hair.

> The natal cleft is the groove between the buttocks extending inferiorly from the sacrum to the anus.

Pathology

> An infected sinus is usually lined with purulent material and granulation tissue.

> The sinus may be part of a deeper tract extending along the midline or to one side.

> The sinus may have one or more openings.

> Less commonly, sinuses occur in the interdigital clefts, face, and axilla.

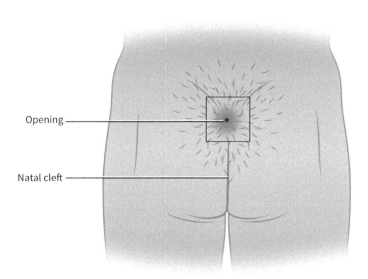

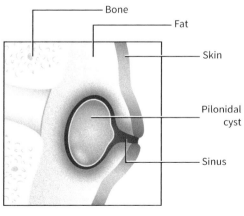

Figure 2.21 Pilonidal sinus with infected cyst

STEP-BY-STEP OPERATION

Anaesthesia: general or local.

Position: prone with elevated hips or lateral decubitus position.

Considerations: The buttocks are taped apart to expose the sinus, and the area is shaved.

1 The sinus is palpated, and probes are used to delineate the sinus tracts. If the sinus is difficult to palpate, methylene blue dye can be injected into the sinus tracts to delineate anatomy.

2 An elliptical incision is made around the cavity incorporating any lateral sinus tracts, an incision line lateral to the midline suture line is preferred.

3 The incision is made through the subcutaneous fat and extends down to the presacral fascia incorporating all the sinus tract and any secondary openings.

4 All of the sinus tract with a cuff of surrounding subcutaneous fat is included in the specimen

5 The cavity is then thoroughly irrigated with normal saline and local anaesthetic can be instilled.

6 A subcutaneous fat flap is then raised by undermining the subcutaneous layer so that it is roughly 1cm thick and 2cm deep to allow a two layered tension free closure.

7 The subcutaneous layer is closed with absorbable sutures.

8 The skin is then closed with the suture line being placed laterally to the midline. A vertical mattress suture with non-absorbable sutures is preferred superiorly with absorbable sutures in the inferior natal cleft.

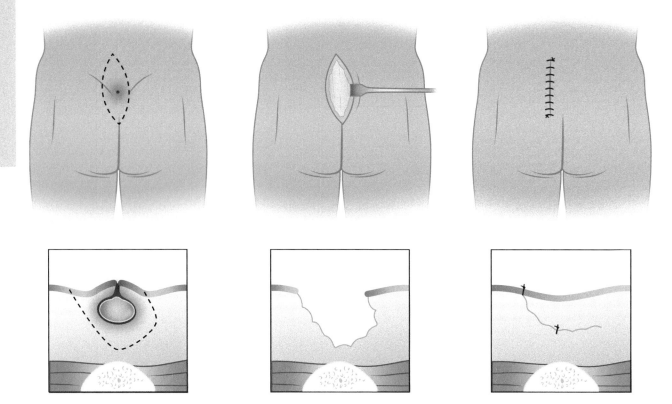

Figure 2.22 Pilonidal sinus surgery

COMPLICATIONS

Early
> Bleeding.

Intermediate and late
> Wound infection.
> Further recurrence of pilonidal sinus.

> Chronic wound and delayed wound healing.
> Scarring.
> Pain
> Paraesthesia

POSTOPERATIVE CARE

Inpatient
> Patients are discharged within 24–48 hrs, provided they are mobile, able to void, and pain is adequately controlled.

Outpatient
> If packed to heal by secondary intention, the patient is seen by the practice nurse for frequent (initially every 48 hrs) dressing changes. This involves removing the ribbon gauze and repacking the cavity to allow healing by secondary intention.
> Good hygiene to keep the area clean and dry and free from any loose hairs is essential.

SURGEON'S FAVOURITE QUESTION

What might you expect to find lining a pilonidal sinus or cavity?

Macroscopically: hair follicles, stratified squamous epithelium with slight cornification, chronic granulation tissue, epithelial debris, and young granulation tissue.

Microscopically: lymphocytes, plasma cells, and foreign body giant cells.

INCISION AND DRAINAGE OF PERIANAL ABSCESS

Christina Cheng

DEFINITION
The surgical washout of a localised collection of pus within the tissues situated around or near the anus.

✓ INDICATIONS

> Acute perianal abscess.

✗ CONTRAINDICATIONS

> Spontaneously ruptured perianal abscess.

ANATOMY
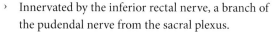

Gross anatomy
> The anal canal is extraperitoneal and measures 2–4 cm.
> The anal canal is embryologically part hindgut and part proctoderm. The dentate line divides the anal canal based on this:
>> The proximal two-thirds of the anal canal lie above the dentate line. This section is hindgut in origin and is lined with columnar mucosa.
>> The distal third lies below the dentate line. This section is proctoderm in origin and is lined with squamous epithelium.

Neurovasculature
> Above the dentate line:
>> Innervated by the inferior hypogastric plexus.
>> Arterial supply is from the superior rectal artery (a branch of the IMA) and the middle rectal artery (a branch of the inferior vesicular artery).
>> Venous drainage is via the internal haemorrhoidal plexus to the superior rectal vein.

> Below the dentate line:
>> Innervated by the inferior rectal nerve, a branch of the pudendal nerve from the sacral plexus.
>> Arterial supply is via the inferior rectal arteries from the pudendal artery.
>> Venous drainage is via the external haemorrhoidal plexus to the inferior and middle rectal veins.

Pathology
> Anorectal abscesses arise from infection of the anal intersphincteric glands.
> Anorectal abscesses are classified according to their anatomical location:
>> Perianal—around the anal orifice (60%).
>> Ischiorectal—in the ischiorectal fossa, a space between the anal canal and the levator ani muscles (30%).
>> Submucosal—deep to the anal canal mucosa (5%).
>> Pelvirectal—between the levator ani and the pelvic peritoneum (5%).

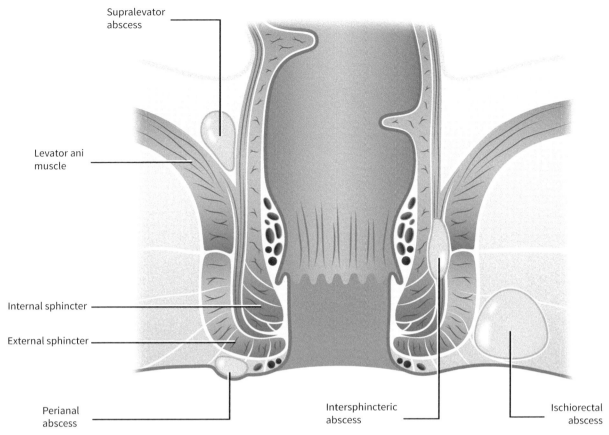

Supralevator abscess

Levator ani muscle

Internal sphincter

External sphincter

Perianal abscess

Intersphincteric abscess

Ischiorectal abscess

Figure 2.23 Perianal abscess locations

STEP-BY-STEP OPERATION

Anaesthesia: general.

Position: lateral, prone, or Lloyd-Davies position.

Considerations: If there is suspicion of anal fistula, a rectal examination is performed.

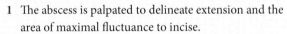

1 The abscess is palpated to delineate extension and the area of maximal fluctuance to incise.
2 An incision circumferential to the anus (not radial) is made over the abscess.
3 In large abscess some skin may need to be de-roofed in order to prevent early closure and reformation of the abscess
4 When the abscess cavity is entered, there should be an expulsion of purulent material.

5 A swab is taken for microbiology.
6 The purulent material is expelled, and the cavity is curetted.
7 A digit is inserted and swept around the cavity to break down loculations.
8 The cavity is thoroughly irrigated with normal saline.
9 The cavity is packed with absorbent ribbon and left to heal by secondary intention.
10 A pressure dressing is applied.

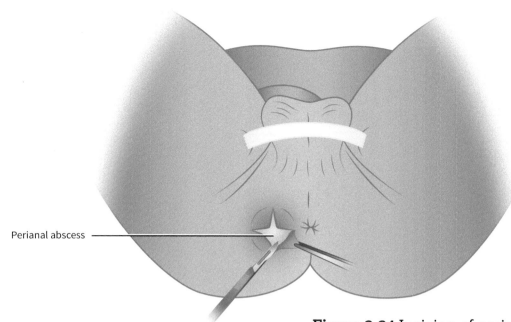

Perianal abscess

Figure 2.24 Incision of perianal abscess in the Lloyd-Davies position

COMPLICATIONS

Early

› Bleeding.

Intermediate/Late

› Wound infection.
› Recurring abscess requiring further surgical management.
› Chronic wound and delayed wound healing.
› Scarring.

POSTOPERATIVE CARE

Inpatient

› The dressing is removed after 24–48 hours.
› Patients are discharged within 24–48 hours, provided they are mobile, able to void, and pain is adequately controlled.
› If there is evidence of surrounding cellulitis, antibiotics are continued for 5 days postoperatively.

Outpatient

› The patient is seen by the practice nurse for frequent (initially every 48 hours) dressing changes. This involves removing the ribbon gauze and repacking the cavity to allow healing by secondary intention.
› Hygiene education—keeping the area clean, and dry.

 SURGEON'S FAVOURITE QUESTION

What is the difference between healing by primary and secondary intention?

Healing by primary intention occurs when wound edges are re-approximated and healing occurs with minimal tissue loss and scarring. Healing by secondary intention occurs when wound edges are left apart and healing occurs from the bottom of the wound upwards.

3 BREAST

KATRINA MASON

MASTECTOMY

Jane Lim

DEFINITION

- ▸ Simple or total mastectomy (SM)—removal of all breast tissue and the nipple.
- ▸ Radical mastectomy (RM)—a simple mastectomy + clearance of axillary lymph nodes + removal of pectoral muscles.
- ▸ Modified radical mastectomy (MRM)—simple mastectomy + clearance of axillary lymph nodes, but the pectoral muscles are spared.
- ▸ Skin-sparing mastectomy—a new technique used for patients having mastectomy and reconstruction where the skin envelope is preserved as much as possible for better cosmesis.

✓ INDICATIONS

- ▸ Breast cancer unsuitable for breast conserving therapy (BCT):
  - › Local recurrence after previous wide local excision (WLE) and radiotherapy.
  - › New primary tumour after previous BCT.
  - › Multifocal disease or extensive ductal carcinoma in situ (DCIS).
  - › Central tumour that involves the nipple and is not suitable for central WLE.
  - › Large tumour relative to breast size.
  - › Locally advanced disease with extensive skin changes.

- ▸ Patient preference for mastectomy over BCT.
- ▸ If BCT is inadequate and resection margins remain positive despite re-excision (generally, only one further re-excision is done).
- ▸ Prophylactic bilateral mastectomy for women with a strong family history of breast or ovarian cancer and with high-risk gene mutations (e.g., BRCA1 or BRCA2 mutation).

✗ CONTRAINDICATIONS

- ▸ Inoperable locally advanced breast cancer.

ANATOMY

Gross anatomy

- ▸ The breast normally extends from the second to the sixth ribs.
- ▸ The breast overlies:
  - › Pectoralis major.
  - › Serratus anterior.
  - › External oblique.
  - › The upper portion of the rectus abdominis muscle.
- ▸ Structurally, the breast parenchyma is made up of glandular tissue, arranged in lobes.
- ▸ Interspersed within the parenchyma is the fibrous stroma (Cooper's ligaments), which anchors the glandular lobes and the skin covering the breast to the pectoralis major.
- ▸ The fatty stroma makes up the rest of the breast tissue.

Neurovasculature

- ▸ The breast is innervated by the anterior and lateral cutaneous branches of the thoracic intercostal nerves (T3–T5). Sensory fibres provide innervation to the skin; autonomic fibres provide innervation to vessels and the smooth muscles of the nipple and areola.
- ▸ Arterial supply to the breast:
  1. Internal mammary artery (60%).
  2. Branches of axillary artery.
  3. Terminal branches of the intercostal arteries.
- ▸ The superficial veins of the breast drain into the internal thoracic vein, while the deep veins drain into the internal thoracic, intercostal, and axillary veins.
- ▸ 75% of the lymphatic drainage of the breast is into the axillary lymph nodes, with the rest to the internal mammary lymph nodes. Lymphatic vessels follow the blood supply.

Figure 3.1 Gross anatomy of the breast

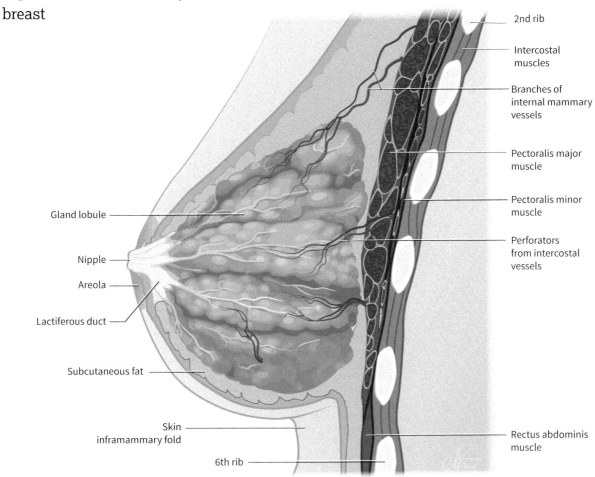

- 2nd rib
- Intercostal muscles
- Branches of internal mammary vessels
- Pectoralis major muscle
- Pectoralis minor muscle
- Perforators from intercostal vessels
- Rectus abdominis muscle

- Gland lobule
- Nipple
- Areola
- Lactiferous duct
- Subcutaneous fat
- Skin inframammary fold
- 6th rib

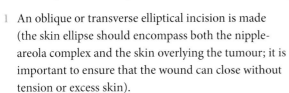

STEP-BY-STEP OPERATION

Anaesthesia: general.

Position: supine with the ipsilateral arm abducted ≤90° on padded arm boards away from the breast.

1. An oblique or transverse elliptical incision is made (the skin ellipse should encompass both the nipple-areola complex and the skin overlying the tumour; it is important to ensure that the wound can close without tension or excess skin).
2. The incision is deepened through the subcutaneous fatty tissue, generating a skin flap approximately 7–8 mm thick.
3. Using a combination of diathermy and scissors, the skin flap is extended medially to the lateral border of the sternum, laterally to the anterior border of the latissimus dorsi muscle, superiorly to the clavicle, and inferiorly to the uppermost part of the rectus sheath.
4. The breast tissue is dissected off the pectoralis major muscle.
5. The breast tissue sample is marked with a stitch in the axillary tail (orientation for the histopathologist).
6. Closed suction drains are inserted to prevent seroma or haematoma formation.
7. The skin is closed in two layers—an absorbable dermal layer to bring the wound edges together under minimal tension and a sub-cuticular suture for the skin.
8. Steri-Strips can be placed over the wound and a compression dressing of gauze and tape is applied.

BREAST

Figure 3.2 Dissection of breast tissue off pectoralis major

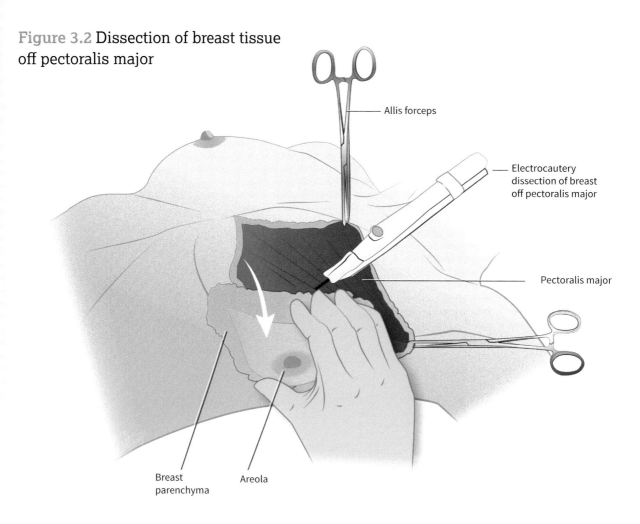

Allis forceps

Electrocautery dissection of breast off pectoralis major

Pectoralis major

Breast parenchyma

Areola

COMPLICATIONS

Early
> Haematoma.

Intermediate and late
> Skin flap necrosis (<10%).
> Nerve injuries causing:
  › Post-mastectomy pain syndrome (intercostobrachial nerve).
  › Phantom breast syndrome.
> Seroma
> Infection
> Pneumothorax—rare.

POSTOPERATIVE CARE

Inpatient

› Patients are typically discharged the next day.

Outpatient

› Breast nurse-led clinic within one week for wound check.

› Consultant-led clinic in 2 weeks after multidisciplinary team (MDT) review for results of histopathology and discussion of future treatment or reconstruction.

› Gentle arm and shoulder physiotherapy, starting from one day after the surgery, to prevent formation of significant scar tissue/fibrosis and to regain as much range of movement and shoulder function as possible.

 SURGEON'S FAVOURITE QUESTION

What is the difference between simple, radical, and modified radical mastectomy?

A radical mastectomy involves removal of the breast, axillary lymph nodes, and pectoralis muscles; modified radical is the same as radical but spares the pectoralis muscles; and simple mastectomy is removal of the breast only.

WIDE LOCAL EXCISION (WLE)

Jane Lim

BREAST

DEFINITION

The removal of a breast tumour with a clear margin of normal tissue.

✓ INDICATIONS

› WLE can offer a better cosmetic outcome without the need for mastectomy and reconstruction, but is only suitable in:
  › A single operable breast tumour that is small enough relative to the breast size to remove (e.g., <3 cm AND have no contraindications to further radiotherapy if required).
  › Paget's disease of the nipple (WLE of nipple-areolar complex).
  › Multifocal disease restricted to a single breast quadrant.

✗ CONTRAINDICATIONS

› Mastectomy +/- reconstruction is preferred over WLE in the following situations:
  › Multifocal breast cancer with ≥2 primary tumours in separate breast quadrants.
  › Diffuse malignant calcifications shown on breast mammogram.
  › If radiotherapy after WLE is contraindicated (e.g., in the first two trimesters of pregnancy, or connective tissue disease).
  › Positive resection margins after multiple re-excisions.

ANATOMY

Gross anatomy

› The breast normally extends from the second to the sixth ribs.
› The breast overlies:
  › Pectoralis major.
  › Serratus anterior.
  › External oblique.
  › The upper portion of the rectus abdominis muscle.
› Structurally, the breast parenchyma is made up of glandular tissues arranged in lobes.
› Interspersed within the parenchyma is the fibrous stroma (Cooper's ligaments), which anchors the glandular lobes and the skin covering the breast to the pectoralis major.
› The fatty stroma makes up the rest of the breast tissue.

Neurovasculature

› The breast is innervated by the anterior and lateral cutaneous branches of the thoracic intercostal nerves (T3–T5). Sensory fibres provide innervation to the skin; autonomic fibres provide innervation to vessels and the smooth muscles of the nipple and areola.
› Arterial supply to the breast:
  1 Internal mammary artery (60%).
  2 Branches of axillary artery.
  3 Terminal branches of the intercostal arteries.
› The superficial veins of the breast drain into the internal thoracic vein, whilst the deep veins drain into the internal thoracic, intercostal, and axillary veins.
› 75% of the lymphatic drainage of the breast is into the axillary lymph nodes, with the rest to the internal mammary lymph nodes. Lymphatic vessels follow the blood supply.

Figure 3.3 Gross anatomy of the breast

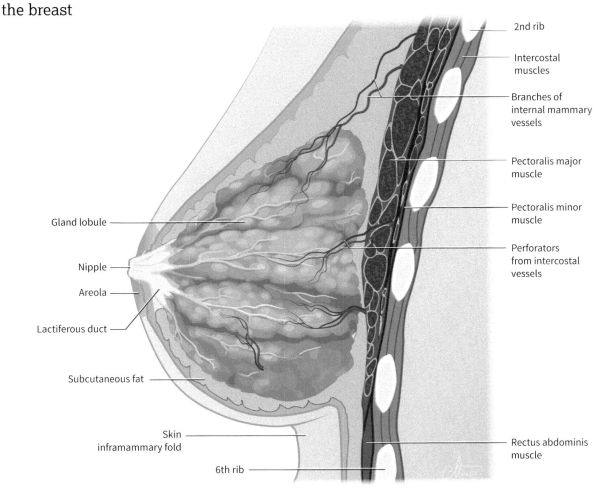

- 2nd rib
- Intercostal muscles
- Branches of internal mammary vessels
- Pectoralis major muscle
- Pectoralis minor muscle
- Perforators from intercostal vessels
- Rectus abdominis muscle

- Gland lobule
- Nipple
- Areola
- Lactiferous duct
- Subcutaneous fat
- Skin inframammary fold
- 6th rib

STEP-BY-STEP OPERATION

Anaesthesia: general, but can be performed under local anaesthetic with sedation.

Position: supine with the ipsilateral arm abducted ≤90° on padded arm boards away from the breast.

Considerations: Pre-operatively, whilst the patient is awake and upright, the breast lump is palpated and the incision marked; for non-palpable tumours, a breast radiologist will localise the tumour via guide wire insertion localisation. This involves a fine flexible wire inserted and tethered into the tumour so that the tip lies in the centre of the tumour.

1. An incision is made using oncoplastic principles (ensuring cancer clearance whilst preserving breast cosmesis), for example, using peri-areolar, infra-mammary, or round block technique incisions. Incisions should also try and include any previous open biopsy site scar).

2. The palpable tumour is excised using diathermy scissors or bipolar pen, with a 1–1.5 cm margin of surrounding macroscopically normal breast tissue (if a re-excision, a margin of similar thickness around the cavity of the previous excision is made).

3. For guide wire localised tumours, the surgeon dissects along the guide wire and resects a 2–3 cm margin around the wire tip.

4. The removed tissue is oriented for the histopathologist with sutures or surgical clips (e.g. long stich superior and short lateral).

5. Once the specimen is removed, an X-ray of the specimen is performed whilst the patient is still under anaesthesia to assess for adequate margins (calcifications within the specimen indicate the site of malignancy; if calcifications are too close to a margin, further cavity shavings are performed).

6 Haemostasis is achieved using diathermy.

7 Surgical metal clips are left in the site where the lump has been removed (assists in locating the site on later mammograms for administration of adjuvant radiotherapy and if re-excision of margins is required).

8 The cavity edges are closed with an absorbable suture, then the skin is closed with an absorbable subcuticular suture.

9 Steri-Strips can be applied across the wound edges, followed by a compression dressing with gauze and tape over the wound.

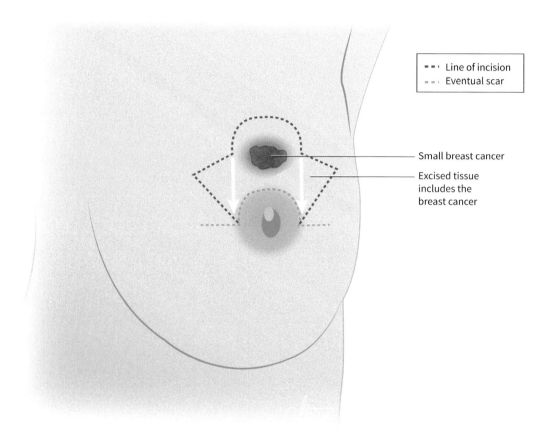

Line of incision
Eventual scar

Small breast cancer

Excised tissue includes the breast cancer

Figure 3.4 WLE lines of incision and closure

COMPLICATIONS

Early

▸ Haematoma (1%).

Intermediate and late

▸ Inadequate surgical margins (10%) requiring either further WLE or mastectomy.

▸ Infection.

▸ Seroma.

▸ Breast asymmetry and alteration of body image.

POSTOPERATIVE CARE

Inpatient

> WLE is usually day case surgery with discharge home the same day as long as there are no immediate postoperative complications.

Outpatient

> Review by the Breast Clinical Nurse Specialist (CNS) within a week of discharge to assess wound healing and monitor for seroma formation.

> Consultant-led follow-up clinic in 2 weeks after multidisciplinary team (MDT) review.

> Annual mammography for 5 years or until patient reaches NHS screening age. Frequency of further screening is in line with patient risk category.

 SURGEON'S FAVOURITE QUESTION

What are the types of breast cancer, and which is the commonest?

Breast cancers can be divided into 'invasive' or 'in situ'. 'In situ' carcinomas are the earliest form of cancer and are completely contained within the duct (DCIS—ductal carcinoma in situ) or lobule (LCIS—lobular carcinoma in situ) and have not invaded into surrounding tissues.

Invasive cancers have several histological subtypes:

Infiltrating ductal (75%).

Invasive lobular (8%).

Ductal/lobular (7%).

Mucinous, Tubular, Medullary, Papillary (all <2%).

AXILLARY NODE CLEARANCE (ANC)

Luke Conway

DEFINITION

Removal of axillary lymph nodes to treat invasive cancer.

✔ INDICATIONS

- ANC is used to treat local lymph node spread of cancer (breast or malignant melanoma) as proven by:
  - Sentinel node(s) positive for macro or micro metastases OR
  - A preoperative ultrasound-guided needle biopsy with histologically proven metastatic cancer.

✘ CONTRAINDICATIONS

Relative
- Pre-existing arm lymphoedema.

Absolute
- Known distant metastasis.
- Unknown lymph node status—should be offered sentinel lymph node biopsy (SLNB) first.
- Only isolated tumour cells in sentinel node biopsy samples (these patients are regarded as lymph node-negative).

ANATOMY

Gross anatomy
- The axilla is a quadrangular space with the following boundaries:
  - Superiorly—posterior border of clavicle, outer border of first rib and superior scapular border.
  - Medially—serratus anterior and the chest wall.
  - Laterally—intertubercular sulcus of the humerus.
  - Anteriorly—pectoralis major and minor.
  - Posteriorly—latissimus dorsi, teres major, and subscapularis.
  - Inferiorly—axillary skin.
- The axillary lymph nodes are divided into three surgical levels, corresponding to their anatomical location and path of drainage:
  - Level 1—up to the lateral border of the pectoralis minor.
  - Level 2—up to the medial border of the pectoralis minor.
  - Level 3—extend up to the apex of the axilla.

Neurovasculature
- The thoracodorsal nerve is approximately 2 cm medial to where the axillary vein crosses the latissimus dorsi and takes an inferior course along with the thoracodorsal vessels.
- The long thoracic nerve follows a similar course but is located in a more medial position, descending inferiorly close to the serratus anterior, which it supplies.
- The axillary vein and artery arise from the subclavian vessels, running from the lateral border of the first rib to the inferior border of the axilla.

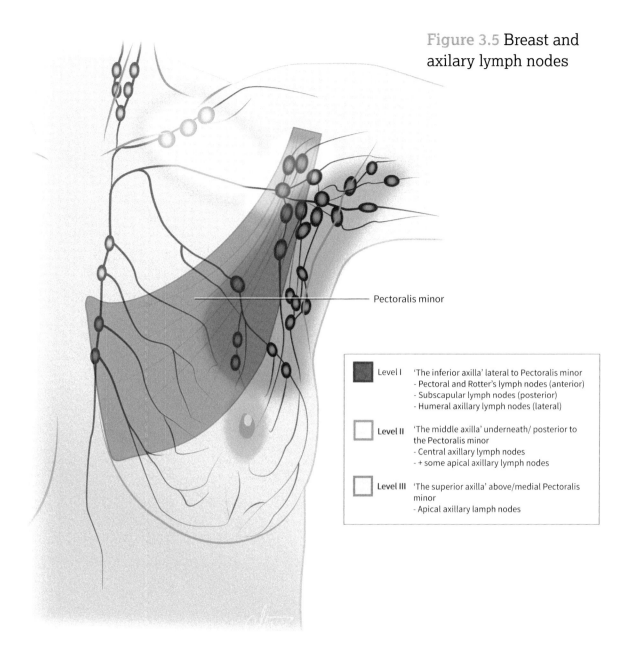

Figure 3.5 Breast and axilary lymph nodes

Pectoralis minor

	Level I	'The inferior axilla' lateral to Pectoralis minor - Pectoral and Rotter's lymph nodes (anterior) - Subscapular lymph nodes (posterior) - Humeral axillary lymph nodes (lateral)
	Level II	'The middle axilla' underneath/ posterior to the Pectoralis minor - Central axillary lymph nodes - + some apical axillary lymph nodes
	Level III	'The superior axilla' above/medial Pectoralis minor - Apical axillary lamph nodes

STEP-BY-STEP OPERATION

Anaesthesia: general.

Position: supine with arm abducted 90°–110° **on a padded arm board away from the breast.**

1 A 4–5 cm incision is made along the skin crease of the axilla between the borders of pectoralis major and latissimus dorsi.

2 Dissection is made into the axilla using a combination of diathermy, 'Mayo' scissors, and blunt dissection (e.g., 'peanut' swabs held in forceps).

3 The contents are visualised through the retraction of the pectoralis major and minor anteriorly and the latissimus dorsi posteriorly (as the axilla is deep and dark, the surgeon will often use a head-light and retractors with lights attached).

4 This axillary vein is dissected out and acts as the superior border of the axillary lymph node dissection (ALND).

5 Inferior branches of the axillary vein are clipped or ligated and cut.

6 The thoracodorsal pedicles are then identified and preserved via dissection inferior to the axillary vein following the posterior wall of the axilla.

7 The long thoracic nerve is dissected free from the contents of the axilla and preserved.

8 The axillary fat pad (containing level 1 lymph nodes) is retracted and removed.

9 Level 2 nodes are removed by medial retraction of the pectoralis minor and the removal of fatty nodal tissues.

Level 3 nodes are sometimes also removed. These are then sent to the laboratory with a stitch to orientate the pathologist.

10 A drain is inserted, and closure is performed with interrupted deep dermal sutures followed by a continuous subcuticular stitch.

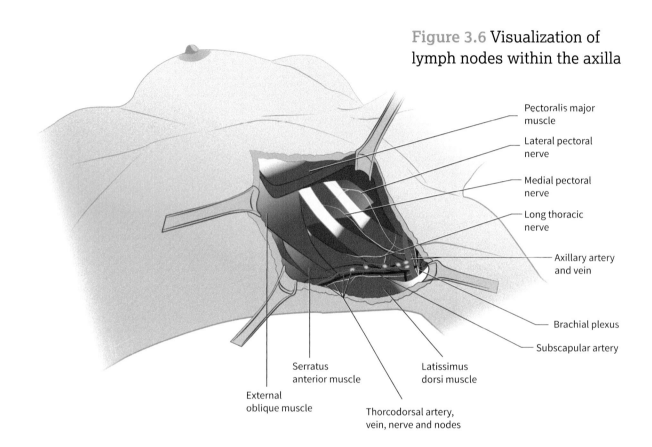

Figure 3.6 Visualization of lymph nodes within the axilla

Pectoralis major muscle

Lateral pectoral nerve

Medial pectoral nerve

Long thoracic nerve

Axillary artery and vein

Brachial plexus

Subscapular artery

Serratus anterior muscle

Latissimus dorsi muscle

External oblique muscle

Thorcodorsal artery, vein, nerve and nodes

COMPLICATIONS

Early
> Bleeding/haematoma (10%).

Intermediate and late
> Seroma.
> Temporary shoulder stiffness.
> Nerve injuries causing:
  › Numbness or paraesthesia of upper arm (medial cutaneous nerve and intercostobrachial nerve).
  › Post-mastectomy pain syndrome (intercostobrachial nerve).
  › Winged scapula (long thoracic nerve).
  › Immobility and loss of stabilisation of the shoulder (thoracodorsal and medial pectoral nerve).
> Lymphoedema of the arm (5%), increasing to up to 25% if level 3 nodes are cleared).
> Infection (5%).

POSTOPERATIVE CARE

Inpatient

› Drains removed at surgeon's discretion, usually when output <30ml/24hrs after mobilisation.

› Physiotherapy to reduce risk of lymphoedema and shoulder stiffness.

Outpatient

› Review by the Breast Clinical Nurse Specialist (CNS) within a week of discharge to assess wound healing and monitor for seroma formation.

› Consultant-led follow-up clinic in 4–6 weeks after multidisciplinary team (MDT) review.

 SURGEON'S FAVOURITE QUESTION

What complication is likely to have happened if a patient is found to have winged scapula after a mastectomy?

Injury and damage to the long thoracic nerve.

SENTINEL LYMPH NODE BIOPSY (SLNB)

Luke Conway

DEFINITION

Removal of sentinel nodes (first cancer-draining axillary lymph nodes) to identify local lymph node spread of breast cancer in order to stage disease.

✓ INDICATIONS

- Early invasive breast cancer with no evidence of lymph node involvement on preoperative ultrasound or following a negative ultrasound-guided needle biopsy. Axillary node spread is the most significant prognostic indicator and one of the major determinants of appropriate systemic adjuvant therapy.
- All patients having mastectomy for Ductal Carcinoma in Situ (DCIS).
- Patients having breast conserving surgery for:
  - High-grade DCIS.
  - DCIS + micro-invasion seen on core biopsy.
  - DCIS + mammography or ultrasound suggesting invasive disease.

✗ CONTRAINDICATIONS

Relative

- Allergy to radio-colloid or blue dye (an alternative is to have single technique—e.g., blue dye or radio isotope only).

Absolute

- Axillary lymph node positive at presentation—confirmed by core biopsy. These patients should have axillary lymph node clearance as first-line, without an SLNB.
- Inflammatory breast cancer.
- Previous axillary surgery or radiotherapy.

ANATOMY

Gross anatomy

- The axilla is a quadrangular space with the following boundaries:
  - Superiorly—posterior border of clavicle, outer border of first rib and superior scapular border.
  - Medially—serratus anterior and the chest wall.
  - Laterally—intertubercular sulcus of the humerus.
  - Anteriorly—pectoralis major and minor.
  - Posteriorly—latissimus dorsi, teres major, and subscapularis.
  - Inferiorly—axillary skin.
- The axillary lymph nodes are divided into three surgical levels, corresponding to their anatomical location and path of drainage:
  - Level 1—up to the lateral border of the pectoralis minor.
  - Level 2—up to the medial border of the pectoralis minor.
  - Level 3—extend up to the apex of the axilla.

Neurovasculature

- The thoracodorsal nerve is approximately 2 cm medial to where the axillary vein crosses the latissimus dorsi and takes an inferior course along with the thoracodorsal vessels.
- The long thoracic nerve follows a similar course but is located in a more medial position, descending inferiorly close to the serratus anterior, which it supplies.
- The axillary vein and artery arise from the subclavian vessels, running from the lateral border of the first rib to the inferior border of the axilla.

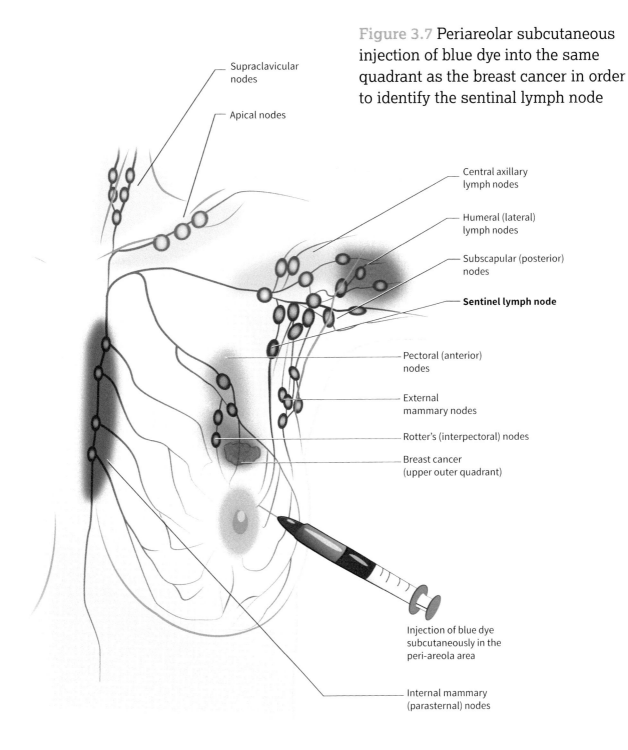

Figure 3.7 Periareolar subcutaneous injection of blue dye into the same quadrant as the breast cancer in order to identify the sentinal lymph node

Supraclavicular nodes

Apical nodes

Central axillary lymph nodes

Humeral (lateral) lymph nodes

Subscapular (posterior) nodes

Sentinel lymph node

Pectoral (anterior) nodes

External mammary nodes

Rotter's (interpectoral) nodes

Breast cancer (upper outer quadrant)

Injection of blue dye subcutaneously in the peri-areola area

Internal mammary (parasternal) nodes

STEP-BY-STEP OPERATION

Anaesthesia: general; can also be done under local anaesthetic.

Position: supine with arm abducted 90°–110° on padded arm board away from the breast.

Considerations: The day prior to, or morning of surgery, a peri-areolar injection of radioactive isotope is given.

BREAST

1 Once patient is under anaesthesia, a blue dye is injected subcutaneously next to the areola (both the radioactive isotope and blue dye travel through the lymphatic system of the breast and will be taken up by the sentinel node to allow for both visual (blue) and Geiger counter (radioactive) detection of the node, a 'dual technique').

2 A Geiger counter is used to detect the location of the sentinel node in axilla.

3 A small incision, approximately 2–3 cm in length, is made over the location of the sentinel lymph node.

4 Using forceps, scissors, or blunt dissection, the subcutaneous and axillary fat is dissected to visualise the sentinel lymph node (the Geiger counter and following a blue-dyed lymphatic channel can help locate the sentinel node).

5 Once visualised, the sentinel node is removed.

6 The axilla is then explored for further radioactive or blue nodes. If identified, these are removed and sent for analysis. The specific count on the Geiger counter is recorded on the histology form for each node (radioactive nodes are referred to as "hot" nodes and, if dyed, they are labelled as "blue." Nodes can be both, either, or none of these categories).

7 If available, one-step nucleic amplification testing (OSNA) is used to confirm malignancy in approximately 30 minutes. If OSNA shows the node(s) to be positive, then axillary node clearance can be performed whilst the patient is still anesthetised (and has appropriately consented).

8 The wound is then closed with subcuticular sutures.

9 A simple Steri-Strip dressing is applied to the skin.

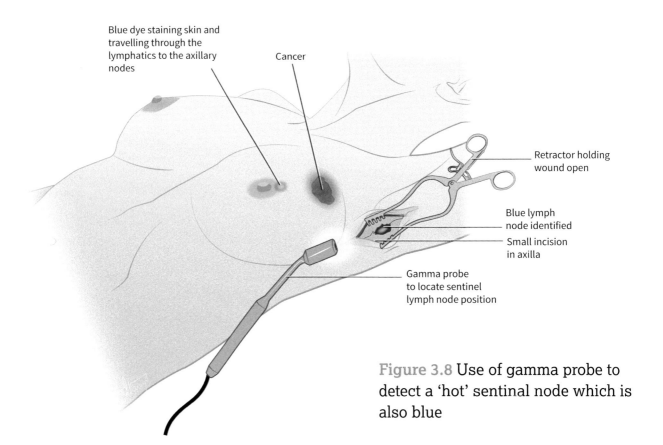

Blue dye staining skin and travelling through the lymphatics to the axillary nodes

Cancer

Retractor holding wound open

Blue lymph node identified

Small incision in axilla

Gamma probe to locate sentinel lymph node position

Figure 3.8 Use of gamma probe to detect a 'hot' sentinal node which is also blue

COMPLICATIONS

Early

- Anaphylaxis or allergic reaction to blue dye (0.2%).
- Blue-green discoloration of urine—resolves after a few days.
- Pain.
- Haematoma.

Intermediate and late

- Blue discolouration of the skin of the breast, which can last for months to years.
- Infection (5%).
- Seroma.

POSTOPERATIVE CARE

Inpatient

- SLNB is usually day-case surgery with discharge home the same day as long as there are no immediate postoperative complications.

Outpatient

- Node analysis takes approximately one week if OSNA is not available.
- Consultant-led clinic after multidisciplinary team (MDT) review in 4–6 weeks.

 ## SURGEON'S FAVOURITE QUESTION

Briefly outline the lymphatic drainage of the breast.

75% of lymphatic drainage is facilitated by the axillary nodes. The remainder occurs via the internal mammary/thoracic nodes. There are three axillary lymph node 'levels': levels 1, 2, and 3.

LATISSIMUS DORSI FLAP RECONSTRUCTION OF THE BREAST

Luke Conway

DEFINITION

Reconstruction of the breast using a pedicled latissimus dorsi (LD) flap.

✓ INDICATIONS

- Breast cancer reconstruction following mastectomy or wide local excision with significant defect can be done in conjunction with implant reconstruction.
- An alternative to other autologous tissue-based reconstruction (e.g., Deep Inferior Epigastric Perforator (DIEP) flap) if these donor sites are unsuitable.

✗ CONTRAINDICATIONS

Relative

- Active radiotherapy—should be completed before reconstructive surgery.
- Patient occupation greatly involves use of latissimus muscle (e.g., climbers and swimmers).

Absolute

- Previous surgery that has damaged the donor site or compromised its vascular supply.
- Extensive local and metastatic disease.

ANATOMY

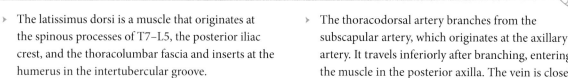

- The latissimus dorsi is a muscle that originates at the spinous processes of T7–L5, the posterior iliac crest, and the thoracolumbar fascia and inserts at the humerus in the intertubercular groove.
- It is responsible for extension, adduction, and internal rotation of the shoulder joint and has a synergistic role in lateral flexion and extension of the lumbar spine.
- It is vital in LD flap reconstruction to preserve the thoracodorsal pedicle, which comprises the thoracodorsal artery, vein, and nerve.

- The thoracodorsal artery branches from the subscapular artery, which originates at the axillary artery. It travels inferiorly after branching, entering the muscle in the posterior axilla. The vein is closely associated with the artery.
- The thoracodorsal nerve supplies the latissimus dorsi and is a branch of the posterior cord of the brachial plexus, from nerve roots C6–C8. It follows a similar inferior course to the artery.

Figure 3.9 The attachments and neurovasculature of latissimus dorsi

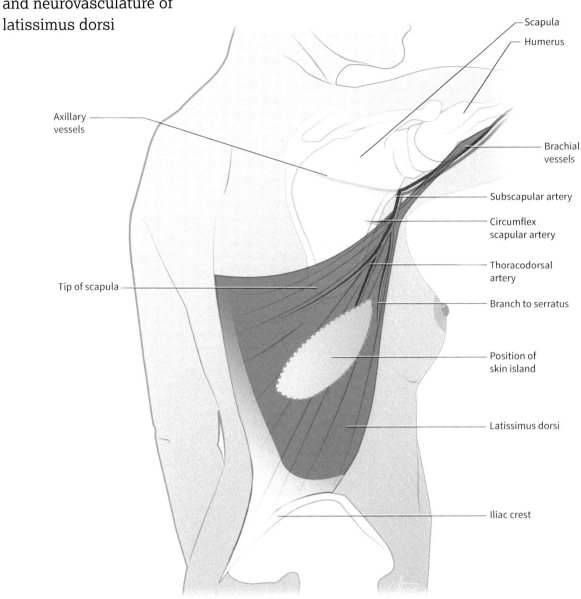

- Scapula
- Humerus
- Brachial vessels
- Subscapular artery
- Circumflex scapular artery
- Thoracodorsal artery
- Branch to serratus
- Position of skin island
- Latissimus dorsi
- Iliac crest
- Axillary vessels
- Tip of scapula

STEP-BY-STEP OPERATION

Anaesthesia: general.

Position: lateral decubitus position with the arm abducted; the patient lies on the contralateral side of the LD flap harvest and reconstruction site.

Considerations: LD flap reconstruction can be either immediate, at the same time as the mastectomy, or delayed once adjuvant therapy has been completed or at surgeon and patient preference. An LD flap is usually pedicled but can be a 'free flap' (lifted from the donor site and moved to a different anatomical location). When pedicled, the donor site is always ipsilateral to the recipient site.

1 The LD flap is marked out elliptically to give an "island" of skin and underlying muscle that is going to be positioned below the bra strap line.

2 The recipient site is then cleared and it's incision extended laterally, towards the axilla (if a delayed procedure, the old mastectomy is reopened).

3 The marked donor unit is then incised, and the underlying latissimus dorsi muscle is reflected by separating it from the serratus and the teres major, leaving an exposed thoracodorsal pedicle (nerve, artery, and vein).

4 A 'tunnel' is dissected through the subcutaneous tissues from the pedicle to the chest to allow the flap to be transferred to the anterior chest wall.

5 Minor branches of the thoracodorsal artery are clipped.

6 The thoracodorsal nerve is cut to stop nervous supply to the muscle.

7 The LD flap is then pulled anteriorly via the axillary tunnel to rest over the chest, creating a new breast mound or filling a breast defect (implants can be inserted at this point if it is a combined reconstructive procedure).

8 The LD flap is sutured to the chest wall with absorbable sutures and the skin island closed in two layers (deep and superficial) with buried sutures to distribute tension. The donor site is also closed.

9 Surgical drains are left in situ at both sites.

10 Simple dressings are applied to the wound; however, the skin of the LD flap must be accessible and visible for essential 'flap observations' postoperatively.

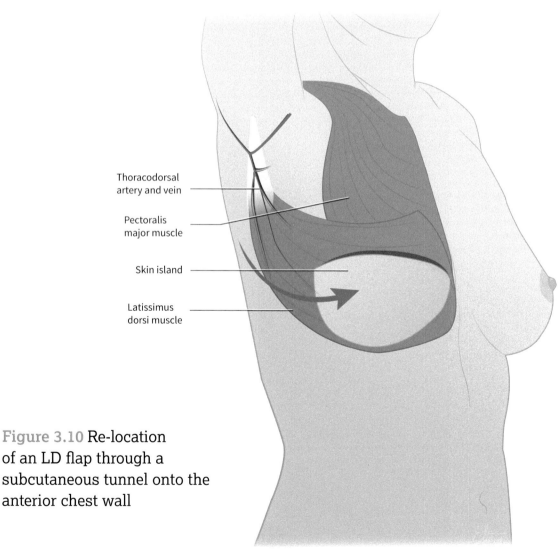

Thoracodorsal artery and vein

Pectoralis major muscle

Skin island

Latissimus dorsi muscle

Figure 3.10 Re-location of an LD flap through a subcutaneous tunnel onto the anterior chest wall

COMPLICATIONS

Early
› Haematoma (10%).
› Flap failure (1%).

Intermediate and late
› Necrosis of adipose tissue requiring further treatment (5%).

› Seroma.
› Infection.
› Asymmetry and alteration of body image.
› Reduced donor site function, particularly weakness of the latissimus dorsi muscles.

POSTOPERATIVE CARE

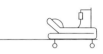

Inpatient
› Hourly 'flap observations' postoperatively, including blood pressure, urine output, and flap checks to assess for warmth, congestion, and turgor, all signs of vascular compromise of the flap. These are less important for pedicled versus 'free' LD flaps but are often still done.
› Surgical drains removed at surgeon's discretion, usually when output <30ml/24hrs after mobilisation.

Outpatient
› Review by the Breast Clinical Nurse Specialist (CNS) within a week of discharge to assess wound healing and monitor for seroma formation.
› Consultant-led follow-up clinic in 4–6 weeks.

 SURGEON'S FAVOURITE QUESTION

What is the difference between a flap and a graft?

A graft has no transferred blood supply and relies on the donor site, whilst a flap has an intact vascular supply.

ALEXANDER YAO, KATRINA MASON

TONSILLECTOMY

Maria Knöbel

DEFINITION
Surgical removal of the palatine tonsils from their fossae in the pharynx.

✓ INDICATIONS

- Recurrent tonsillitis.
- Scottish Intercollegiate Guidelines Network (SIGN) criteria:
    - 7 episodes in 1 year.
    - 5 episodes per year over 2 years.
    - 3 episodes per year over 3 years.
- Severely enlarged tonsils causing obstructive sleep apnoea (OSA) or dysphagia.
- Suspected malignancy.
- Peritonsillar abscess (quinsy).

✗ CONTRAINDICATIONS

Relative
- Severe bleeding diathesis.
- Acute tonsillitis—surgery should ideally be delayed.
- Patients at risk of atlanto-axial subluxation (e.g. Down's Syndrome, Achondroplasia)—often, modified positioning and spine stabilisation techniques can be employed.

ANATOMY

Gross anatomy

- Tonsils are glands of dense lymphoid tissue on the posterolateral walls of the oropharynx.
- Anatomical boundaries of the tonsils are:
    - Anterior—palatoglossus muscle.
    - Posterior—palatopharyngeus muscle.
    - Deep—superior constrictor muscle.
    - Superior—soft palate.
    - Inferior—lingual tonsil and tongue edge.
- Fibres of the palatopharyngeus and palatoglossus are found in the tonsil bed and attach to the capsule.

Neurovasculature

- Nerve supply is by the lesser palatine nerve (branch of maxillary division of the trigeminal nerve) and the glossopharyngeal nerve.
- Arterial supply:
    - Superior pole—tonsillar branches of the ascending pharyngeal artery, lesser palatine artery.
    - Inferior pole—branches of facial artery, dorsal lingual artery, and ascending palatine artery.
- Venous drainage is via the peritonsillar plexus, which drains into the lingual and pharyngeal veins, which then drain into the internal jugular vein.
- Lymphatic drainage is to the jugulodigastric nodes and deep cervical lymph nodes.

Figure 4.1 Blood supply to the tonsils

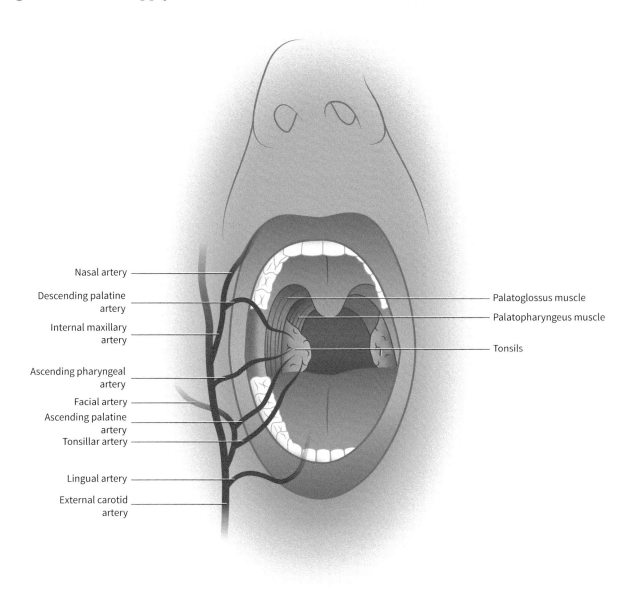

Nasal artery

Descending palatine artery

Internal maxillary artery

Ascending pharyngeal artery

Facial artery

Ascending palatine artery

Tonsillar artery

Lingual artery

External carotid artery

Palatoglossus muscle

Palatopharyngeus muscle

Tonsils

STEP-BY-STEP OPERATION

Anaesthesia: general; patients are often intubated to secure the 'shared airway'/protect from aspiration of blood. However, a laryngeal mask may be used.

Position: supine with a shoulder roll/sandbag under the shoulder blades to extend the neck and head.

1 A Boyle-Davis mouth gag with a mounted mouth guard is used to open the mouth, protect the teeth and expose the tonsils.

2 Forceps are used to grab hold of the tonsil, and traction is applied medially in order to assist dissection.

3 The following methods may be used to dissect the tonsils:

   a 'Cold steel' (dissectors and scissors).

   b Monopolar or bipolar cautery.

   c Radiofrequency ablation.

   d Coblation—where radiofrequency energy and saline are combined to create a plasma field at a relatively low temperature (preferred in young children, low weight, and complex comorbidities).

4 The tonsillar capsule is used as a plane of dissection, thereby 'shelling' the tonsil out from its fossa in a cranial-to-caudal direction.

5 Methods used in haemostasis include:
  a Pressure with gauze (can be soaked with adrenaline).
  b Silk ties around the bleeding vessel.
  c Bipolar diathermy cautery.
6 Once the tonsil has been dissected to the base of the tongue, it is often tied with silk ties and the remaining attachment cut with scissors.
7 The post-nasal space is suctioned for clots using a soft suction catheter passed through the nostril until it is seen in the oropharynx.

8 The mouth gag is released, and the endotracheal tube is then held in place by the surgeon in one hand as the gag is removed from the mouth with the other in order to prevent accidental extubation.
9 The lips and teeth are inspected for accidental damage and the temporomandibular joint is checked to ensure it has not been dislocated.

Figure 4.2 Bipolar cautery of the right palatine tonsil

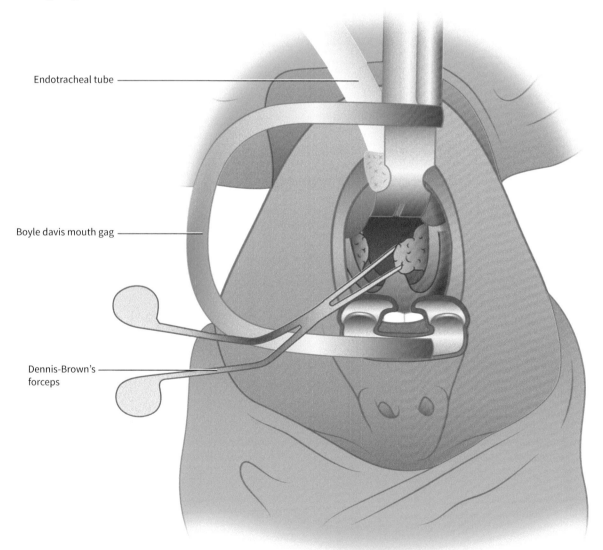

Endotracheal tube

Boyle davis mouth gag

Dennis-Brown's forceps

COMPLICATIONS

Early

- Primary (reactionary) post-tonsillectomy haemorrhage, occurring within 24 hours of surgery due to inadequate haemostasis or slipped tie.
- Temporomandibular joint dislocation.
- Dental injuries—e.g., chipped tooth or loss of tooth (children with loose teeth at higher risk).

Intermediate and late

- Secondary post-tonsillectomy haemorrhage (5–10 days post op), usually due to secondary infection of the tonsillar fossa—can be severe and require return to theatre for haemostasis.
- Pain—can be severe and be referred to the ears.
- Infection.
- Voice change.

POSTOPERATIVE CARE

Inpatient

- Patients can eat and drink normally immediately after surgery.
- Tonsillectomy in children with low weight (<15kg), severe OSA, or complex medical background often requires overnight stay.

Outpatient

- Patients must be advised to return via their nearest A&E if any signs of post-tonsillectomy bleed occur.
- Two weeks off school/work is generally recommended.
- No formal outpatient follow-up is required unless tonsillectomy is performed for OSA or malignancy.

 SURGEON'S FAVOURITE QUESTION

What is the most common histological type of tonsillar malignancy, and what is an important recognised pathogen?

Squamous cell carcinoma and human papilloma virus (HPV) infection.

SURGICAL TRACHEOSTOMY

Andrea McCarthy

DEFINITION

A tracheostomy is a surgical opening that provides an artificial conduit between the trachea and the skin of the neck. It is maintained by the placement of a tracheostomy tube through which ventilation occurs.

✓ INDICATIONS

Elective

- Long-term assisted ventilation (most common).
- To aid in pulmonary toilet (method to clear mucus and secretions from the airway).
- Prophylactically for some head and neck cancers to ensure airway patency (e.g., surgery of the mouth, oropharynx and larynx).
- Congenital abnormalities resulting in obstruction of the upper airways (e.g., Pierre Robin Sequence).

Emergency

- Acute upper airway obstruction (foreign body, anaphylaxis, infection, laryngeal tumour, inhalation injury, maxillofacial trauma, bilateral vocal cord palsy).

✗ CONTRAINDICATIONS

- Anaplastic thyroid cancer.
- Gross anatomical distortion due to neck mass/previous neck surgeries (can make the procedure difficult).

ANATOMY

Gross anatomy

- The trachea is 10 cm long, 2 cm in diameter, and stretches to 15 cm on inspiration. It consists of cervical and thoracic components.
- The trachea begins at the inferior border of the cricoid (C6) and descends to and terminates at the level of the sternal angle (T4/T5).
- The gross structure of the trachea consists of 10–15 'C'-shaped cartilage 'rings' that are completed posteriorly by the trachealis muscle (the cricoid is the only complete ring).
- The trachea is lined with pseudostratified ciliated columnar epithelium.
- Structures that are incised/divided in a tracheostomy, from superficial to deep: skin, subcutaneous tissue/fat, platysma, strap muscles, thyroid, pretracheal fascia, trachea.

- Anatomical relationships:
    › Anteriorly—strap muscles (sternohyoid, and sternothyroid), thyroid isthmus at rings 2–4, and pretracheal fascia, which envelops the thyroid gland.
    › Posterolaterally—recurrent laryngeal nerve, carotid sheath.
    › Laterally—lobes of thyroid.
    › Posteriorly—oesophagus.

Neurovasculature

- Nervous supply—the recurrent laryngeal nerve.
- Arterial supply—inferior thyroid artery and bronchial artery.
- Venous drainage—inferior thyroid vein.
- Lymph drainage—pre- and paratracheal nodes and deep cervical nodes.

Figure 4.3 Anatomical relations of the trachea

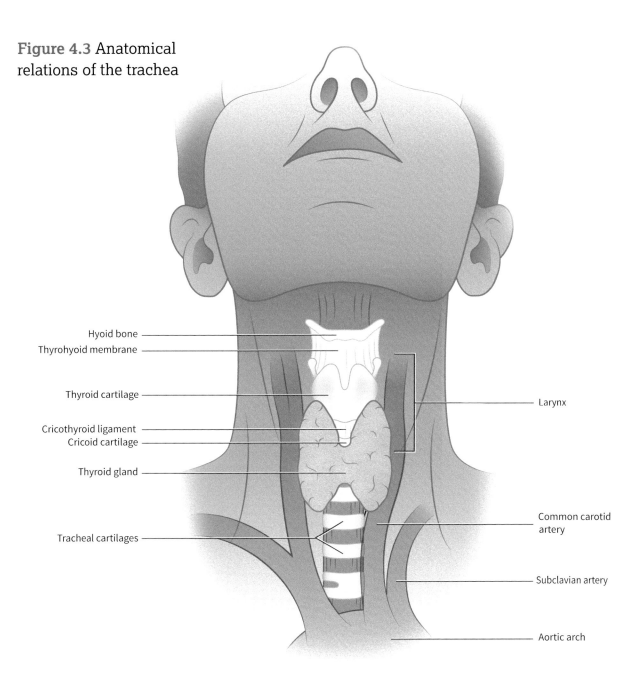

Hyoid bone

Thyrohyoid membrane

Thyroid cartilage

Cricothyroid ligament

Cricoid cartilage

Thyroid gland

Tracheal cartilages

Larynx

Common carotid artery

Subclavian artery

Aortic arch

STEP-BY-STEP OPERATION

Anaesthesia: general or local if unable to intubate.

Position: supine with head and neck extended using shoulder roll and head secured with a ring.

Considerations: Tracheostomies can be either percutaneous, using the Seldinger technique with progressive dilatation, or via traditional open surgery. Percutaneous tracheostomies are frequently performed in Intensive Treatment Unit (ITU) by anaesthetists, whereas open techniques are performed by surgeons either as emergencies or electively. The surgical technique is described below.

1 A 2–3 cm horizontal incision is made midway between the cricoid and the sternal notch. Vertical incisions can be done in emergencies. The horizontal incision confers superior cosmesis, whereas vertical incisions allow for a more bloodless field.

2 Subcutaneous fat is dissected, and the platysma muscle is divided in the same plane as the incision, revealing the midline raphe.

3 The investing fascia is divided in the midline, allowing the strap muscles to be retracted laterally. The thyroid

gland is revealed. Anterior jugular vessels can cross the midline and need to be ligated if encountered.

4 The thyroid gland is retracted superiorly, and the thyroid isthmus is divided in the midline and closed with locking sutures to both stumps to prevent further bleeding. This exposes the trachea situated behind the thyroid gland.

5 Further local anaesthetic can be injected into the tracheal rings and the tracheal lumen itself. Either a vertical incision (always in paediatrics), a window, or a flap can be created through cartilage rings 2–4 (never ring 1).

6 The anaesthetist is always informed prior to cutting into the trachea. They should also retract the endotracheal (ET) tube to prevent bursting the ET

balloon. Diathermy is not used in order to decrease the risk of airway fire.

7 After the incision has been performed, the ET tube cuff is deflated and pulled back until the tip can be seen above the tracheostomy opening. 'Stay sutures', non-absorbable sutures secured to the lateral aspects of the tracheal opening, can be inserted and brought out to be secured with tapes to the neck skin. In an emergency, these can be pulled and the tracheal opening will be brought to the wound surface. In children, the trachea is sutured to the skin with absorbable sutures.

8 The tracheostomy tube is inserted, and the cuff of the tracheostomy tube is inflated. The tube is secured around the neck with collar ties or ribbon gauze.

Figure 4.4 Use of 'Stay sutures' in surgical tracheostomy to secure the position of the trachea

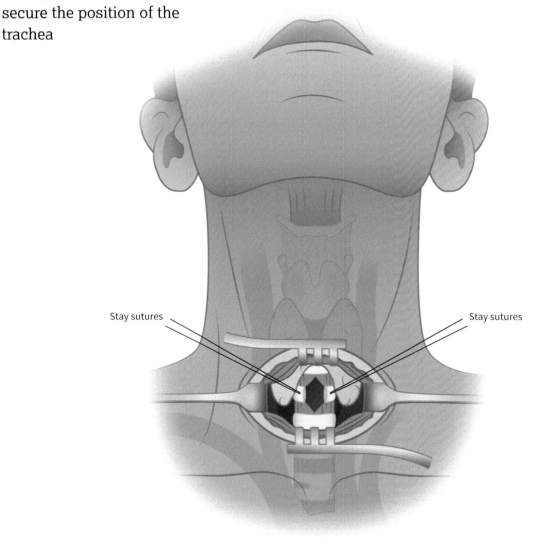

Stay sutures

Stay sutures

COMPLICATIONS

Early

› Bleeding.
› Damage to surrounding structures:
  › Oesophagus—can lead to mediastinitis.
  › Recurrent laryngeal nerve paresis or palsy (hoarse/weak voice) or external branch of superior laryngeal nerve paresis or palsy (loss of high pitch) <1%. If recurrent laryngeal nerve injury is bilateral, a permanent tracheostomy will be required due to airway obstruction from closed vocal cords.
  › Pleura-pneumothorax.
› Air embolus.
› Creation of false passage and resultant surgical emphysema.

Intermediate and late

› Accidental extubation—may result in loss of airway and death.
› Swallowing difficulty.
› Crusting or blockage.
› Local site infection or tracheitis.
› Tracheoesophageal fistula.
› Persistent tracheo-cutaneous fistula after decannulation.
› Tracheal necrosis—may lead to tracheal stenosis.
› Tracheal ulceration.
› Tracheo-innominate artery fistula—can result in massive bleeding.

POSTOPERATIVE CARE

Inpatient

› Usually first night on ITU/High Dependency Unit (HDU), then stepped down to a ward capable of managing tracheostomies.

Outpatient

› Patient education on how to care for their tube and recognise emergency situations (e.g., blockage/displacement).

› The first tube change should be post-op day 7 on the ward.
› Further tube changes are required every 2–3 months.
› Permanently removing a tracheostomy tube in a patient who can safely ventilate orally/nasally must be done by experienced staff. An occlusive dressing is applied, and the tracheal stoma will close completely by secondary intention.

SURGEON'S FAVOURITE QUESTION

What are the additional hazards of tracheostomy in the paediatric population compared to adults?

Mostly, this is due to the differences in anatomy:

› Trachea is less rigid and therefore difficult to palpate and highly mobile.
› Neck is short, limiting the surgical field.
› Closer proximity to the domes of the pleura extending into the neck, which are vulnerable to injury.
› The innominate vein sits higher in children and is susceptible to injury.

SEPTOPLASTY

Alexander Yao

DEFINITION

Surgical straightening of a deviated nasal septum.

✓ INDICATIONS

- Nasal obstruction due to a deviated nasal septum.
- May be performed as a part of other procedures:
  - A septorhinoplasty procedure.
  - To allow access for functional endoscopic sinus surgery or endoscopic skull base procedures.
  - As part of surgical management of epistaxis.
  - Obtaining septal cartilage for use in an autograft.

✗ CONTRAINDICATIONS

- Extensive autoimmune disease affecting the nasal septum—e.g., Granulomatosis with Polyangiitis (GPA).

ANATOMY

Gross anatomy

- The nasal septum consists of:
  - Anterior part: septal cartilage and maxillary crest.
  - Posterior part: perpendicular plate of the ethmoid, vomer, and palatine bone.
- Deviation of the nasal septum from the midline is common and may be asymptomatic. Localised areas of marked deviation are known as spurs. The septum may even deviate in different directions along its length.

Neurovasculature

- Innervation:
  - Superiorly: olfactory nerve.
  - Anteriorly: anterior ethmoidal nerve.
  - Posteriorly: medial posterior superior nasal and nasopalatine nerves.
- Arterial supply:
  - Mainly via the sphenopalatine artery (SPA), as per the rest of the nasal cavity. The SPA supplies, in particular, the posterior septum.

- The SPA anastomoses with:
  - Superior labial artery (septal branch).
  - Greater palatine artery (ascending branch).
  - Anterior and posterior ethmoid arteries.
- This anastomosis forms Kiesselbach's plexus, located on the antero-inferior aspect of the cartilaginous septum in an area known as Little's area.
- Venous drainage:
  - The veins accompany the arteries.
  - Veins drain to the pterygoid plexus, facial vein and ophthalmic veins.
  - Importantly the veins may carry infection to the cavernous sinus which can result in a cavernous sinus thrombosis, carrying a 50% mortality.

Figure 4.5 The nasal septum and re-alignment of septal cartilage

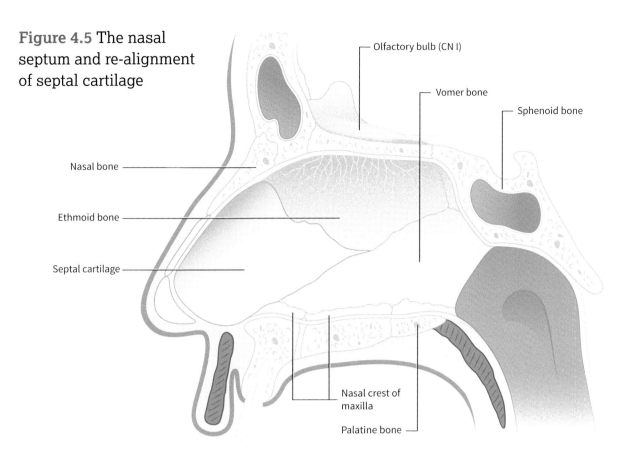

Olfactory bulb (CN I)

Vomer bone

Sphenoid bone

Nasal bone

Ethmoid bone

Septal cartilage

Nasal crest of maxilla

Palatine bone

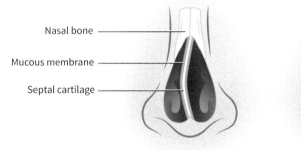
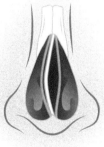
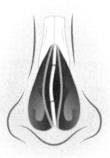

Nasal bone

Mucous membrane

Septal cartilage

STEP-BY-STEP OPERATION

Anaesthesia: general; topical Moffet's solution (cocaine, adrenaline, saline, sodium bicarbonate) may be given locally in the nose preoperatively to vasoconstrict and anaesthetise the nose. Variations of this topical solution can be used depending on surgeon preference.

Position: supine with the head secured with a head ring.

1 Nasal specula (Killian's or Cottle's) are used to inspect the nasal cavity. Both sides of the septum are infiltrated with lidocaine and adrenaline or saline.

2 The mucoperichondrium is incised down to cartilage with a vertical incision at the anterior septal edge. Incision can be placed on left or right depending on the direction and nature of deformity.

3   A Freer's elevator is inserted into the sub-perichondrial plane and used to raise a subperichondrial flap, with care being taken not to tear the flap.

4   A contralateral flap may need to be elevated using the technique described above in severe deviations. The cartilaginous septum can be dislocated off the bony vomer/perpendicular plate of the ethmoid.

5   The areas of cartilaginous and/or bony septal deviation are resected. Care is taken to avoid twisting of the perpendicular plate of the ethmoid (connects to cribriform plate; fractures may cause cerebrospinal fluid [CSF] leaks). Care is also taken not to remove excess cartilage and compromise nasal tip support.

6   Removed septal cartilage can have the deviation corrected through scoring. It can then be replaced, or it can be removed completely.

7   The maxillary crest can be fractured or removed with a gouge to remove any further nasal obstruction.

8   The flaps can be closed with absorbable mattress sutures used to "quilt" the septum, and the incision with an absorbable suture. This reduces the risk of septal haematoma.

9   Silastic nasal splints may be inserted in both nasal cavities and secured to the septum with an anterior stitch to support the septum and prevent scar tissue forming, or nasal packs may be inserted to prevent flap movement and further reduce haematoma risk.

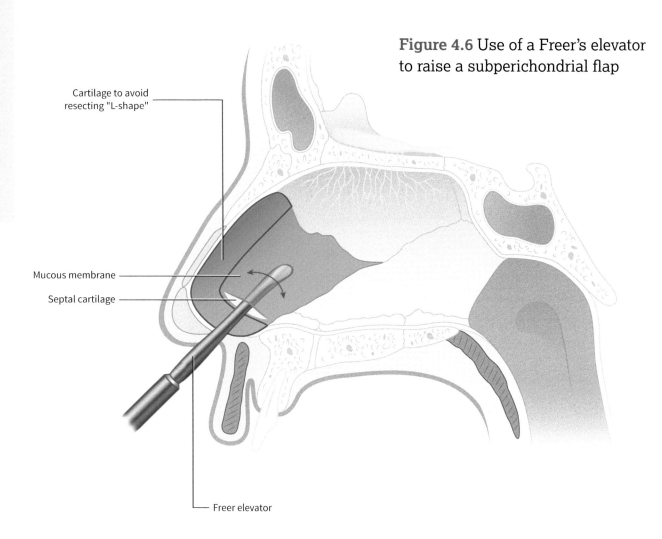

Figure 4.6 Use of a Freer's elevator to raise a subperichondrial flap

Cartilage to avoid resecting "L-shape"

Mucous membrane

Septal cartilage

Freer elevator

COMPLICATIONS

Early
> Bleeding.

Intermediate and late
> Infection.
> Septal haematoma.
> Septal perforation.
> Cosmetic changes—e.g., collapse of the nasal bridge from reduced septal support ("saddle nose" deformity).

> Failure to resolve symptoms.
> Teeth or upper lip numbness.
> Reduction in sense of smell/anosmia resulting from fracture of the cribriform plate.

POSTOPERATIVE CARE

Inpatient
> The operation is typically day-case surgery, or patients are discharged after an overnight stay. Nasal packing, if used, can be removed prior to discharge, or dissolvable packing washed out with saline rinses.

Outpatient
> Nasal splints, if used, can be removed after 1 week in the outpatient setting.
> Outpatient review in 6–8 weeks to assess functional outcome.

💬 SURGEON'S FAVOURITE QUESTION

Why might patients get a "saddle nose" deformity after a septoplasty?

A loss of anterior cartilaginous support of the nose can lead to a sagging of the nose, the classical "saddle nose" deformity. This can be due to either over-resection or necrosis of cartilage.

SUPERFICIAL PAROTIDECTOMY

Nimeshi Jayakody

EAR NOSE AND THROAT

DEFINITION

Surgical removal of the superficial lobe of the parotid gland.

✓ INDICATIONS

- Removal of benign or malignant tumours (most commonly a pleomorphic adenoma—benign tumour).
- Chronic parotitis.
- Sialolithiasis (stones within the salivary ducts).
- Parotid abscess.

✗ CONTRAINDICATIONS

- Multiple parotid cysts in human immunodeficiency virus (HIV) patients—repeated aspirations preferred.

ANATOMY

Gross anatomy

- Anatomical relations:
  - Anterior: overlaps the posterior surface of the masseter.
  - Superior: zygomatic arch.
  - Posterior: external auditory meatus, mastoid, sternocleidomastoid.
  - Inferior: an imaginary line from the mastoid to the greater cornu of hyoid.
- The parotid duct (Stensen's duct) is 5 cm long and opens into the oral cavity opposite the second upper molar. It lies upon the middle third of an imaginary line from the tragus to the commissure of the mouth.

Neurovasculature

- There are two main parts to the parotid: superficial and deep lobes, separated by the facial nerve and its branches.
- Structures running through the parotid gland:
  - Facial nerve—the main branch splits into five branches within the gland, innervating the muscles of facial expression (temporal, zygomatic, buccal, marginal mandibular, cervical).
  - The retromandibular vein.
- Inferior to the gland is the greater auricular nerve.
- Deep to the parotid is the auriculotemporal nerve.
- Arterial supply—branches of external carotid artery.
- Venous drainage—retro-mandibular vein.

130

Figure 4.7 Gross anatomy and relations of the parotid gland

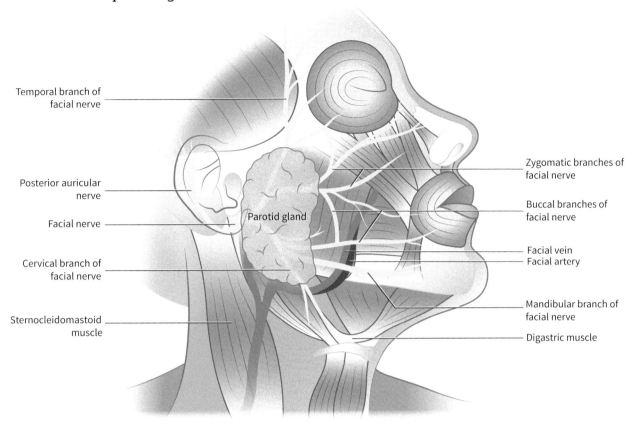

Temporal branch of facial nerve

Posterior auricular nerve

Facial nerve

Cervical branch of facial nerve

Sternocleidomastoid muscle

Parotid gland

Zygomatic branches of facial nerve

Buccal branches of facial nerve

Facial vein
Facial artery

Mandibular branch of facial nerve

Digastric muscle

STEP-BY-STEP OPERATION

Anaesthesia: general.

Position: supine with a shoulder roll and head ring with the head turned to the opposite side.

Considerations: Facial nerve electrodes should be placed onto the myotomes supplied by the branches of the facial nerve for monitoring during the procedure. Increased electrical signals from the electrode indicate close proximity to the facial nerve.

1 The most commonly used incision is the "lazy S" incision. An alternative is the facelift incision.

2 The "lazy S" incision begins anterior to the tragus, following the border of the ear and then along the angle of the mandible into the neck.

3 An anterior skin flap is raised between the parotid capsule and the superficial fat from the posterior-to-anterior border of the parotid gland using careful blunt dissection.

4 The first nerve to be identified is the greater auricular nerve, which is usually divided.

5 The gland is carefully dissected to expose the main branch of the facial nerve using common anatomical landmarks as guides to its exit from the stylomastoid foramen: the posterior belly of digastric, the tragal pointer, and the tympanomastoid suture.

6 Once the main trunk of the facial nerve is identified, the different branches of the nerve are carefully located.

7 The superficial lobe is excised and dissected carefully away from the facial nerve by dividing the tissue above the nerve branches using a harmonic scalpel (the use of ultrasonic vibrations to cut and coagulate the vessels) or using scissors and bipolar diathermy. Careful attention is made to ensure the tumour capsule is not disturbed.

8 The integrity of the facial nerve is checked at the end of the procedure.

9 A closed suction drain is often placed away from the facial nerve.

10 The incision is closed with non-absorbable sutures or staples.

Figure 4.8 Careful excision of the superficial lobe of the parotid gland

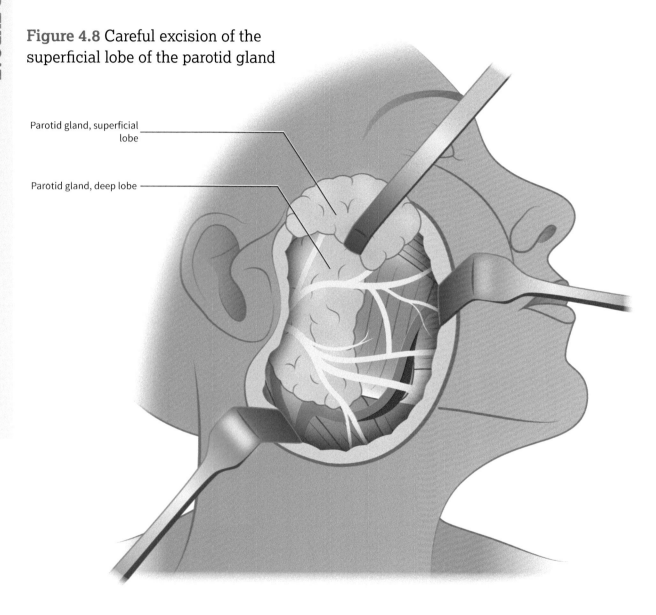

Parotid gland, superficial lobe

Parotid gland, deep lobe

COMPLICATIONS

Early

> Bleeding and haematoma formation.
> Facial nerve palsy causing unilateral facial muscle weakness—can be temporary or permanent (<1%).
> Loss of sensation of the lower pinna due to greater auricular nerve injury—extremely common.

Intermediate and late

> Infection.
> Facial asymmetry.
> Tumour recurrence.
> Sialocele and salivary fistula.
> Gustatory sweating, also known as Frey's syndrome.

POSTOPERATIVE CARE

Inpatient

▸ Drain removed after 24–48 hours or when <30mls in 24 hours.

Outpatient

▸ Sutures can be removed at 5–7 days.
▸ Follow-up appointment to review histology and monitor for side effects. This is within 2 weeks for possible malignant lesions, or 4–6 weeks for benign lesions.

SURGEON'S FAVOURITE QUESTION

In a post-parotidectomy follow-up appointment, a patient mentions that he/she sweats on the side of the surgery when he/she eats or even thinks of food. What is this condition called, and why does it occur?

Frey's syndrome—This is due to aberrant re-innervation of the exposed secreto-motor (parasympathetic) nerves to the skin's sweat glands (instead of to the parotid). This can result in 'gustatory sweating', whereby when you eat, the skin overlying the parotid gland sweats. It can be treated with botulinum toxin injection.

FUNCTIONAL ENDOSCOPIC SINUS SURGERY (FESS)

Alexander Yao

DEFINITION

FESS encompasses a group of diagnostic and therapeutic operations to improve the function of the para-nasal sinuses and nasal cavity and/or provide access to the skull base, orbit, or brain.

✔ INDICATIONS

- Chronic rhinosinusitis (CRS) refractory to medical treatment.
- Recurrent acute sinusitis or acute sinusitis with complications (e.g., intracranial collection, orbital abscess).
- Mucoceles.
- Sinonasal tumours (e.g., squamous cell carcinoma, adenocarcinoma, adenoid cystic carcinoma, olfactory neuroblastoma, antrochoanal polyp, inverted papilloma).
- Nasal polyposis—inflammatory, benign.
- Refractory epistaxis—FESS provides access for cautery +/- sphenopalatine artery ligation.
- Performed in conjunction with other procedures:
  - Eye: orbital decompression, tear duct surgery (dacryocystorhinostomy).
  - Brain: trans-sphenoidal pituitary tumour removal, cerebrospinal fluid (CSF) leak repair in anterior skull base defects or fractures.

✘ CONTRAINDICATIONS

- Where an open approach to the nose, skull base, or eye would be more appropriate.

ANATOMY

- The nasal vestibule is the most anterior part of the nasal cavity and is lined by stratified squamous epithelium.
- The remainder of the nasal cavity is lined by respiratory epithelium, a ciliated pseudostratified columnar epithelium that warms and moistens the air.
- The upper third of the nasal mucosa is innervated by the olfactory bulb (cranial nerve 1) and is responsible for olfaction.
- Turbinates are bony protrusions from the lateral nasal wall covered by respiratory epithelium.
- There are three turbinates in each nasal cavity:
  - Superior.
  - Middle.
  - Inferior.
- The space below each turbinate is called the meatus and is responsible for draining sinuses and air cells.
  - Superior meatus—drains the posterior ethmoid air cells.
  - Middle meatus—drains the maxillary sinus, anterior ethmoid air cells, and the frontal sinus.
  - Inferior meatus—drains the nasolacrimal duct.
  - The sphenoid sinus drains through an ostium on the posterior wall to the superior turbinate.
  - The frontal sinus drains via the frontal recess.
- There are four paired sinuses (air spaces within the skull lined by respiratory epithelium):
  - Maxillary—positioned inferolateral, lies beneath the orbit and above the alveolar process of maxilla.
  - Frontal—positioned superiorly, lies anterior to the frontal lobe and anterior cranial fossa.
  - Ethmoid (anterior and posterior)—sit between the orbits, lying below the cribriform plate and anterior cranial fossa.
  - Sphenoid—the most posteriorly positioned sinus, lies anterior to the hypophyseal fossa (containing the pituitary gland) and the middle cranial fossa. The optic nerve runs within the roof of the sinus.

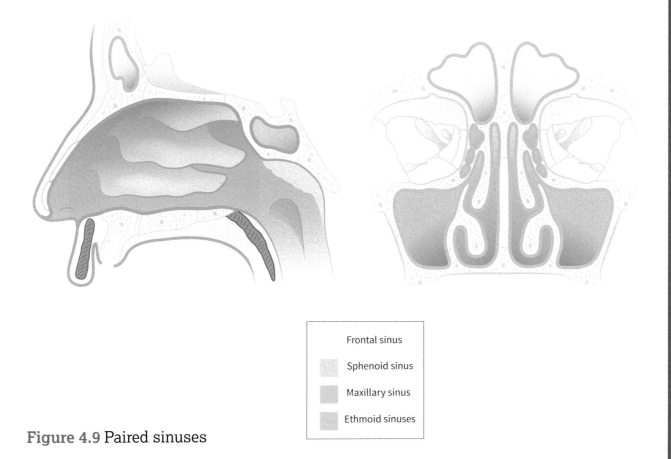

Frontal sinus

Sphenoid sinus

Maxillary sinus

Ethmoid sinuses

Figure 4.9 Paired sinuses

STEP-BY-STEP OPERATION

Anaesthesia: general.

Position: supine, on a head ring; the eyes must not be covered by surgical drapes in order to visualise orbital bleeding, orbital intrusion, or traction on the eye.

Considerations: All patients require a preoperative CT scan of the sinuses for anatomical planning and safety.

1 Local anaesthetic and vasoconstrictor are applied to the nasal mucosa (commonly "Moffett's solution" of sodium bicarbonate, adrenaline, and cocaine) to reduce intraoperative bleeding.

2 A rigid endoscope with a camera attached is passed into the nasal cavity—usually 0°, but 30° or 40° scopes can be used to visualise hidden areas. The surgeon watches on a video screen, illuminating the nasal cavity by holding the endoscope in the non-dominant hand whilst using a variety of FESS instruments in the dominant hand.

3 Nasal polyps can be removed if present.

4 The uncinate process can be removed to expose the maxillary ostium. The ostium can be enlarged with a microdebrider instrument.

5 Depending on the extent of disease, the anterior ethmoid, posterior ethmoid, sphenoid, and frontal sinuses can be opened to improve sinus drainage. The microdebrider or various FESS instruments can be used.

6 Any mucopus can be suctioned out of the sinus with a curved sucker (and sent for microbiology culture) and saline flushing performed if required.

7 The eyes can also be balloted during the operation whilst observing the lateral nasal wall endoscopically for movement (suggesting lamina papyracea dehiscence).

8 Adrenaline-soaked neuropatties (small squares of dressings on long strings) can be inserted to provide vasoconstriction and to stop bleeding.

9 Absorbable nasal packing can be used to reduce bleeding.

Figure 4.10 Passage of a rigid endoscope into the nasal cavity to visually assess air sinuses

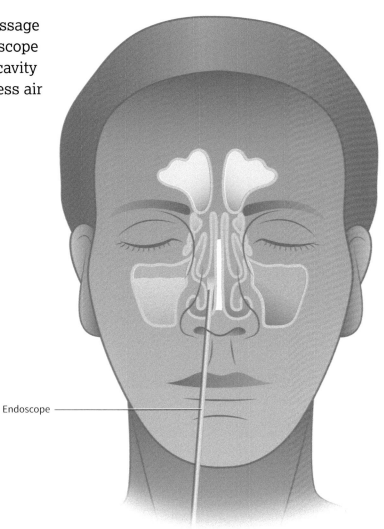

Endoscope

COMPLICATIONS

Early

> Epistaxis.
> Orbital penetration with ocular complications (e.g., diplopia with damage to the extra-ocular muscles, orbital haematoma, and, rarely, blindness if the optic nerve is affected).
> Injury to skull base, causing CSF leak.

Intermediate and late

> Infection within the sinuses or extending to the cranial cavity (e.g., meningitis).
> Synechia or adhesions between mucosal nasal surfaces.
> Epiphora (teary eyes) due to injury to the nasolacrimal duct.
> Failure to improve patient symptoms.

POSTOPERATIVE CARE

Inpatient

▸ Patient is discharged from hospital either on the same day or the day after the operation, ensuring no complications such as CSF leak or orbital damage.

▸ If absorbable nasal packing is used, it will need to be flushed out with saline rinses.

Outpatient

▸ Upon discharge the patient usually commences nasal douching (salty water rinses of the nasal cavity) for a few weeks to prevent crusting and adhesions. Steroid nasal drops for CRS can then be recommenced.

▸ 1–2 weeks off work is recommended. The patient should be advised to avoid excessive activity, blowing their nose, swimming, and contact sports for at least a month.

▸ Routine outpatient appointment in 4–6 weeks postoperatively.

SURGEON'S FAVOURITE QUESTION

How do you define chronic rhinosinusitis?

This is a group of disorders characterised by inflammation of the nose and sinuses. It is defined by:

▸ Two or more of the following four symptoms, of which one must be either obstruction or rhinorrhoea:

  › Nasal obstruction

  › Rhinorrhoea

  › Facial pain/pressure

  › Smell loss/reduction

▸ **And** symptoms lasting for more than 12 weeks

▸ **And** objective evidence of inflammation from:

  › CT scan

  › Nasendoscopy.

SUCTION DIATHERMY ADENOIDECTOMY (ALSO KNOWN AS SUCTION ELECTROCAUTERY OR SUCTION COAGULATION)

Katrina Mason

DEFINITION
Surgical removal of the adenoids using suction and diathermy under direct vision.

✓ INDICATIONS

- Nasal obstruction due to adenoidal hypertrophy causing Obstructive Sleep Apnoea (OSA), often performed in conjunction with tonsillectomy ("adenotonsillectomy").
- Chronic otitis media with effusion (OME), 'glue ear'.
- Recurrent acute otitis media (the adenoids may harbour chronic infection or physically obstruct the eustachian tube from draining the middle ear cavity).
- Recurrent or chronic adenitis and/or rhinosinusitis refractory to medical treatment.

✗ CONTRAINDICATIONS

- Children at increased risk of velopharyngeal insufficiency (VPI)—improper closing of the soft palate against the posterior pharyngeal wall during speech and swallowing, leading to regurgitation of food/air and hypo-nasal speech. At-risk groups include:
    › Cleft palate.
    › Muscle weakness or neurological disorders with hypotonic conditions.
    › Short palate.
- Severe uncorrected bleeding disorders.
- Patients at risk of atlanto-axial subluxation (e.g., Down's Syndrome, Achondroplasia)—often, modified positioning and spine stabilisation techniques can be employed.

ANATOMY

Gross anatomy

- The adenoids are glands of dense lymphoid tissue. They are large in young children and atrophy by adulthood.
- The adenoids sit on the medioposterior wall of the nasopharynx slightly above the level of the soft palate.
- They form part of Waldeyer's ring of lymphoid tissue in the pharynx.
- Anatomical boundaries of the adenoids are:
    › Anterior—nasal cavity and nasal choanae (the posterior nasal apertures).
    › Posterior—superior pharyngeal constrictor muscle.
    › Lateral—eustachian tube openings.
    › Superior—skull base.
    › Inferior—oropharynx.

Neurovasculature

- Nerve supply is by the glossopharyngeal nerve (CN IX).
- Arterial supply:
    › Ascending palatine artery, a branch of the facial artery responsible for supplying the soft palate and palatine glands.
    › Ascending pharyngeal, a branch of the maxillary artery that also supplies the pharynx.
    › Tonsillar branch of the facial artery supplying the palatine tonsil.
- Venous drainage is via the pharyngeal and pterygoid plexus, which ultimately drain to the internal jugular vein.
- Lymphatic drainage is to the retropharyngeal and parapharyngeal lymph nodes, which drain to the upper jugular nodes.

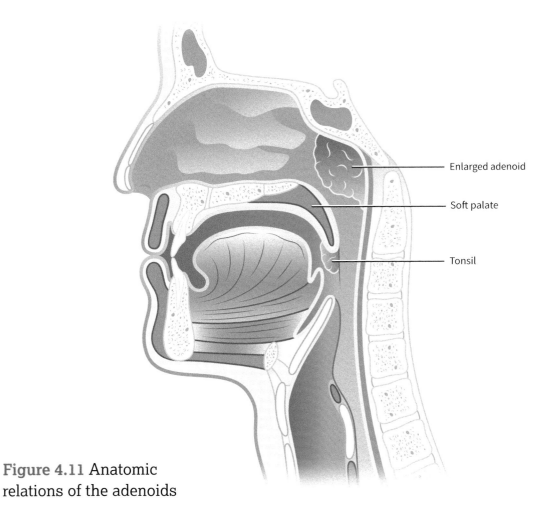

Figure 4.11 Anatomic
relations of the adenoids

- Enlarged adenoid
- Soft palate
- Tonsil

STEP-BY-STEP OPERATION

Anaesthesia: general; patients are often intubated to secure the 'shared airway'/protect from aspiration
of blood.
Position: supine with a shoulder roll/sandbag under the shoulder blades to extend the neck and head.
Considerations: Indirect visualisation using a mirror is the traditional technique, but endoscopic visualisation can be
used. If using indirect visualisation, the surgeon wears a head-mounted light.

1 A Boyle-Davis mouth gag with a mounted mouth
guard is used to open the mouth, protect the teeth, and
expose the oropharynx.

2 One or two flexible suction catheters are passed
through the nose into the oral cavity and pulled out of
the mouth, then secured with a clamp. This 'loop' of
catheter pulls the palate and uvula out of the field of
vision.

3 A small circular dental mirror is inserted into the
mouth and is used to visualise the adenoidal tissue
behind the palate throughout the surgery.

4 The suction diathermy probe (a long, thin instrument
that combines diathermy and integrated suction)
is bent at a slight (20°) angle to allow for the
cauterisation of adenoidal tissue in the posterior
nasopharynx.

5 Working along the midline, the adenoidal tissue is
simultaneously burnt/coagulated with the diathermy
and suctioned out into a vacuum system.

6 Gentle, controlled movements are repeated along the
length of the adenoids, removing the bulk of the tissue
whilst being careful not to cauterise the eustachian

tube cushions laterally. Often, a small inferior rim of adenoid tissue is left to prevent VPI.

7 When the choanae are clearly visible and the nasopharynx has a smooth contour, haemostasis is ensured, and the procedure is complete.

8 The mouth gag is released. The endotracheal tube is then held in place by the surgeon in one hand as the gag is removed from the mouth with the other in order to prevent accidental extubation. The teeth and lips are checked for iatrogenic trauma.

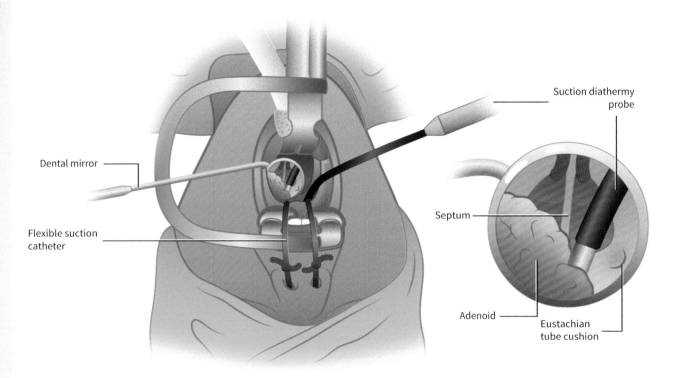

Figure 4.12 Use of suction diathermy to gently excise adenoid tissue under direct vision with a dental mirror

COMPLICATIONS

Early

> Primary (within 24 hours) or secondary (delayed) haemorrhage.
> Burns to nasopharynx or surrounding structures leading to scarring.
> Temporomandibular joint dislocation.
> Dental injuries (e.g., chipped tooth or loss of tooth— children with loose teeth are at higher risk).
> Velopharyngeal insufficiency.

Intermediate and late

> Infection.
> Halitosis.
> Neck injury ranging from stiffness to torticollis to, extremely rarely, Grisel's syndrome (see below).
> Adenoid tissue regrowth and recurrence of symptoms.

POSTOPERATIVE CARE

Inpatient

> Adenoidectomy is usually a day procedure, but patients who have OSA may require overnight stay.

> Postoperative antibiotics and nasal drops may be prescribed.

Outpatient

> One week off school is generally recommended.

> Outpatient follow-up depends upon indication, usually 6 weeks post-procedure.

 SURGEON'S FAVOURITE QUESTION

What is Grisel's syndrome?

Subluxation of the atlanto-axial joint not associated with trauma; it may be caused by pathological relaxation of the transverse ligament of the atlanto-axial joint by, for example, pharyngitis, adenotonsillitis, post adenotonsillectomy, or cervical abscess.

MANIPULATION OF FRACTURED NASAL BONES

Angelina Jayakumar

EAR NOSE AND THROAT

DEFINITION

The manipulation of fractured nasal bones to restore cosmetic form and mechanical function of the nose following trauma.

✓ INDICATIONS

> Simple, non-comminuted fractures of the nasal bones or nasal-septal complex causing external nasal deformity and/or nasal obstruction. Patients should be seen within one week of injury, with surgery within two weeks prior to bone healing in unfavourable shape.

✗ CONTRAINDICATIONS

> Severe comminuted or open fractures of the nasal bones and septum—more formal surgical closure may be required.
> Beyond three to four weeks, simple manipulation is not possible due to fibrous bony union. Instead, a rhinoplasty may be required, which must be delayed for six months.

ANATOMY

Gross anatomy

> The nose consists of the external nose and the nasal cavity, separated into two sides by the septum in the midline.
> The external nose can be artificially divided into thirds.
> › Upper third—two paired nasal bones that attach superiorly to the frontal bone and laterally to the maxilla. The procerus muscle, running supero-inferiorly, overlies the upper third.
> › Middle third—the upper lateral cartilages, attached to the infero-lateral border of the nasal bones. The cartilaginous portion of the nasal septum joins in the midline. The nasalis muscle runs laterally and overlies the middle third.
> › Lower third—laterally runs the minor and major alar cartilages and fibro-fatty tissue, which together form the nostrils.

Neurovasculature

> Sensory innervation to the nose and nasal cavity is provided by the ophthalmic and maxillary branches of the trigeminal nerve.
> The external nose is supplied by terminal branches of both the internal and external carotid:
> › The superior portion is supplied by the dorsal nasal artery, a branch of the ophthalmic artery, and the external nasal branch of the anterior ethmoid artery.
> › The inferior portion is supplied by the lateral nasal artery, a branch of the angular artery, and columellar branches of the superior labial artery, both of which arise from the facial artery.

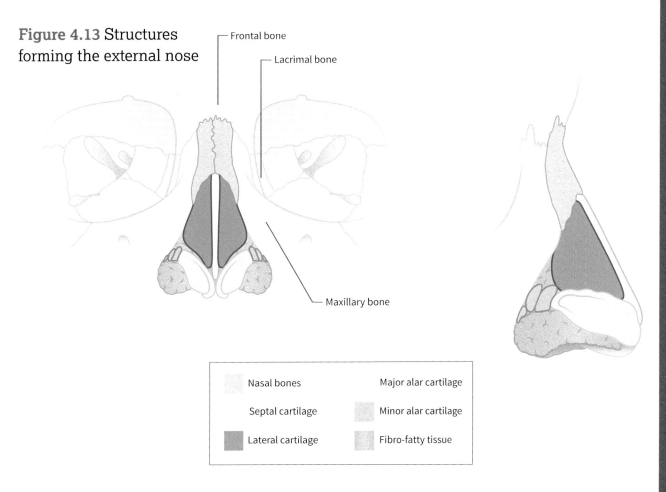

Figure 4.13 Structures forming the external nose

— Frontal bone

— Lacrimal bone

— Maxillary bone

Nasal bones   Major alar cartilage

Septal cartilage   Minor alar cartilage

Lateral cartilage   Fibro-fatty tissue

STEP-BY-STEP OPERATION

Anaesthesia: general or local.

Position: supine.

1 A Boies elevator is inserted into the nostril ipsilateral to the depressed nasal bone. It is then used to apply controlled force to elevate the fragment in the opposite direction to the fracturing force (usually antero-laterally).

2 The opposite nasal bone, usually laterally displaced, should initially be displaced further in the direction of fracture, then reduced back towards the midline/medial position with digital pressure.

3 If digital pressure or elevators do not work, Walsham forceps can be used. They are inserted into one nasal cavity at a time, one blade of the forceps beneath the bone and the other blade opposed on the outer skin surface. The fractured bone is grasped between the blades and manipulated into position.

4 For septal deviations, the forceps can be placed between the nostrils and used to elevate the dorsum and disimpact and realign the septum.

5 The nasal bones are then splinted into position by applying a layer of surgical tape followed by a rigid nasal splint, either Plaster of Paris or a thermoplastic splint.

6 If the septum was reduced, then an internal silastic splint on either side of the septum may be placed and sutured into the septum.

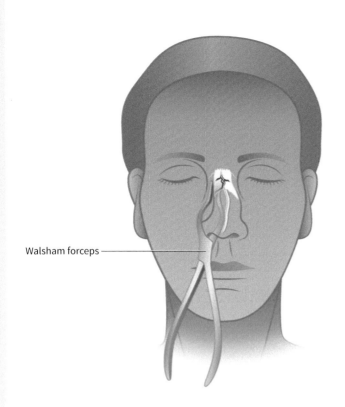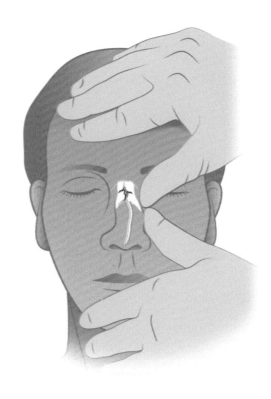

Walsham forceps

Figure 4.14 Manipulation of a fractured nasal septum with Walsham forceps and digital manipulation

COMPLICATIONS

Early
▸ Bleeding, which can cause peri-orbital bruising.

Intermediate and late
▸ Infection.
▸ Failure of manipulation, which can result in a persistent deformity—these patients can then be offered rhinoplasty surgery.
▸ Septal manipulation can cause:
  › A septal haematoma—this needs to be evacuated, as it can lead to tissue necrosis, septal abscess, and/or perforation.

› Nasal-septal deviation and subsequent nasal obstruction.
› Cerebrospinal fluid leak caused by fractures through the cribriform plate—rare, as small fractures seal spontaneously with conservative management (95% within two weeks).
› Anosmia through damage to olfactory receptors in the roof of the nose (very rare).

POSTOPERATIVE CARE

Inpatient

▸ This is a day-case procedure, with patients typically not requiring an overnight admission.

Outpatient

▸ The patient can be seen in clinic in 1 week for removal of nasal splints or, if an external splint only, the patient can remove this themselves.

▸ Routine outpatient follow up at 4-6 weeks is optional.

▸ Whilst bones are healing and malleable, exercise is not recommended for 2 weeks and contact sports for 6 weeks postoperatively.

💬 SURGEON'S FAVOURITE QUESTION

What nerve should you block when applying local anaesthetic?

The external nasal nerve, which is a branch of the anterior ethmoid nerve, which is a branch of the nasociliary nerve, which in turn is a branch of the ophthalmic (V1) branch of the trigeminal nerve.

MYRINGOTOMY AND TYMPANOSTOMY TUBE GROMMET INSERTION

Ivana Capin and Katrina Mason

DEFINITION
Insertion of a ventilation tube across the tympanic membrane (TM).

✓ INDICATIONS

- Otitis media with effusion (OME), aka 'glue ear', causing hearing loss that does not resolve over three months of observation (can lead to speech and language delay and behaviour problems).
- Atelectatic or retracted TMs, which are at risk of cholesteatoma formation due to chronic negative middle ear pressures (e.g., eustachian tube dysfunction).
- Facilitate use of intra-tympanic steroids e.g. for Meniere's disease
- Acute otitis media (AOM) with complications: sepsis, mastoiditis, meningitis, intracranial abscess, facial nerve palsy.
- Recurrent AOM with middle ear effusion.

✗ CONTRAINDICATIONS

- Suspected intratympanic glomus tumour.

ANATOMY

Gross anatomy
- Sections of the ear:
  - External—pinna, external auditory canal.
    - Function—amplifies and transmits sound to middle ear.
  - Middle—ossicles (malleus, incus, stapes).
    - Function: amplifies and transmits sound to inner ear.
  - Inner—semicircular canals, vestibule, cochlea.
    - Function: conducts sound to the brain via conversion of mechanical wave to electrical signals and assists in balance.
- The tympanic membrane is an oval, transparent membrane separating the middle and external ear and is composed of three layers:
  - Outer epithelial layer (ectoderm)—lined by stratified squamous epithelium continuous with the skin of the ear canal.
  - Middle fibrous layer (mesoderm)—contains outer radiating and inner circular fibres.
  - Inner mucous layer (endoderm)—a single layer of squamous epithelium continuous with the lining of the middle ear cavity.

- The TM is divided into two parts:
  - Pars flaccida—above the malleolar folds.
  - Pars tensa—the rest of the drum.
- The manubrium (handle) of the malleus attaches to the TM, which is held in place by a ring of cartilage (annulus).
- The eustachian tube connects the middle ear to the nasopharynx, allowing for equalisation of atmospheric pressure across the TM.

Neurovasculature
- The sensory nerve supply to the TM includes:
  - Auriculotemporal nerve (mandibular branch of trigeminal nerve).
  - Auricular branch of vagus nerve (Arnold nerve).
  - Tympanic branch of glossopharyngeal nerve (Jacobson nerve).
- The blood supply is derived from the stylomastoid branch of the posterior auricular, deep auricular, and anterior tympanic branches from the maxillary artery.
- Venous drainage comprises veins on the superficial aspect of the TM draining to the external jugular vein, and veins from the deep surface of the TM draining to the transverse sinus and dural veins.

Figure 4.15 Anatomy of the middle and inner ear and components of the tympanic membrane

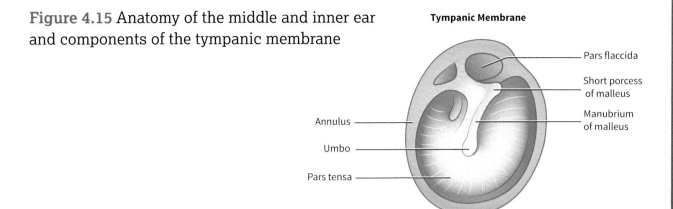

Tympanic Membrane

Pars flaccida

Short porcess of malleus

Manubrium of malleus

Annulus

Umbo

Pars tensa

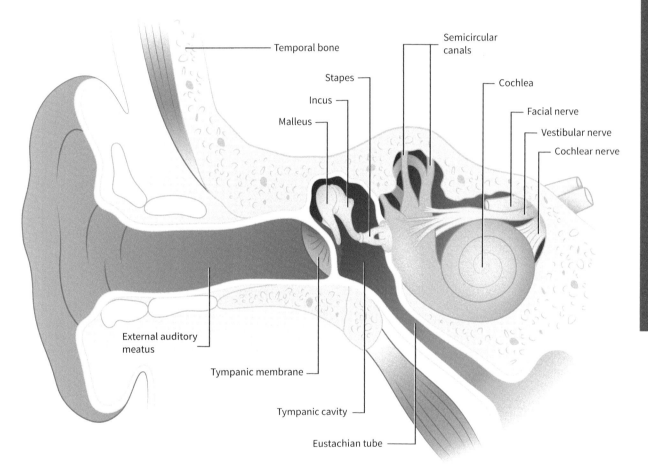

Temporal bone

Semicircular canals

Stapes

Cochlea

Incus

Facial nerve

Malleus

Vestibular nerve

Cochlear nerve

External auditory meatus

Tympanic membrane

Tympanic cavity

Eustachian tube

STEP-BY-STEP OPERATION

Anaesthesia: general; can be undertaken using local anaesthesia in compliant adults.

Position: supine with a head ring to support the head, and the head tilted slightly away from the surgeon.

Considerations: Prior to surgery, patients should have an up-to-date audiological assessment of hearing—pure tone audiometry and tympanometry.

1 Microscope assistance is used to magnify the small operating field. An aural speculum is inserted into the canal and wax removed using suction or fine ear instruments (e.g., a wax hook or crocodile forceps).

2 The entire TM should be visualised for unexpected disease and to identify the location of grommet placement. Most grommets are placed in the antero-inferior portion of the pars tensa but can be placed in any location except the postero-superior quadrant, which overlies the incus and stapes.

3 A Myringotome (fine knife) is used to make a small 2 mm incision ('myringotomy') in a radial direction in the TM.

4 Fluid from the middle ear can be suctioned through the incision with a fine suction tip. If infection is present, this can be flushed with saline and suctioned.

5 The grommet is held by the crocodile forceps and placed through the incision under direct vision.

6 Often, a fine needle is needed to push the grommet so that is sits across the TM.

7 Topical antimicrobial eardrops can be dropped into the canal and middle ear through the grommet.

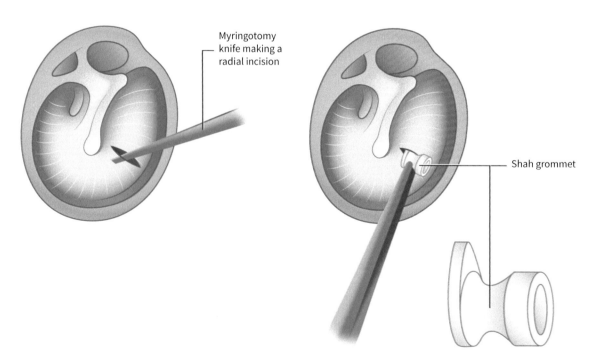

Myringotomy knife making a radial incision

Shah grommet

Figure 4.16 Use of a myringotomy knife to make a small incision in the pars tensa for the insertion of a shah grommet

COMPLICATIONS

Early

> Pain.

> Bleeding.

> Injury to incudo-stapedial joint (if misplaced in the postero-superior quadrant).

> Grommet accidentally placed within or migrating to the middle ear space.

Intermediate and late

> Infection.

> Early extrusion or failure to extrude (grommets usually extrude within 6–18 months).

> Persistent TM perforation.

> Tympanosclerosis (scarring of the TM).

> Focal atrophy at the site of insertion—increases risk of retraction pocket and cholesteatoma formation.

> Deterioration in hearing.

> Blocked grommets.

POSTOPERATIVE CARE

Inpatient

> A day-case surgery.

Outpatient

> Antibiotic ear drops for 3–5 days, water precautions for 2 weeks.

> The first outpatient follow up is usually 6 weeks after surgery with audiological hearing assessment.

> Regular outpatient review every 6 months with audiological hearing assessment until the grommets have fallen out, the TM has healed, and/or the preoperative condition has resolved.

🗨❓ SURGEON'S FAVOURITE QUESTION

Which groups of children are at increased risk of OME?

Children who are more prone to eustachian tube dysfunction, such as children with Down's Syndrome, those with craniofacial disorders or cleft palate. Bone-conducting hearing aids are an alternative to surgery for these patients.

5 ENDOCRINE

JAMES GLASBEY, KATRINA MASON

TOTAL THYROIDECTOMY

James Glasbey

DEFINITION
Complete removal of the thyroid gland.

✓ INDICATIONS

- Compressive symptoms—airway obstruction and dysphagia, most commonly from a multinodular goitre.
- Total thyroidectomy for thyroid malignancy is indicated in:
  - Papillary or follicular cancer with a primary tumour >4 cm, extrathyroidal extension, or metastases to lymph nodes or distant sites.
  - Papillary or follicular cancer with a tumour <4 cm with abnormalities in the contralateral lobe or when postoperative radioiodine is indicated.
  - Multifocal papillary microcarcinoma (more than five foci).
  - Medullary carcinoma.
  - Metastasis in the thyroid—usually from renal cell carcinoma or melanoma (very rare).
- Hyperthyroidism refractory to medical therapy, or patients with contraindications to radioiodine treatment e.g. pregnant women.
- Moderate-to-severe Graves' ophthalmopathy. Surgery is preferred over radioiodine since radioiodine may exacerbate Graves' ophthalmopathy.

✗ CONTRAINDICATIONS

- Uncontrolled preoperative hyperthyroidism (risk of 'thyroid storm').
- Locally advanced anaplastic carcinoma.
- Hemithyroidectomy/unilateral lobectomy is preferred in small tumours <4 cm or indeterminate or suspicious nodules.

ANATOMY

Gross anatomy

- The thyroid is a butterfly-shaped endocrine gland that sits in the midline of the neck.
- Components of the adult thyroid gland:
  - Central 'isthmus'—overlying the second and third cartilaginous tracheal rings.
  - Two lateral lobes—projecting laterally from the isthmus down to the sixth tracheal ring (the superior and inferior parts of which are called the 'poles').
- A superior pyramidal lobe, an embryological remnant, may also be present.
- The adult thyroid is invested in the pretracheal fascia, blending superiorly with the larynx. The gland therefore moves cranially with tongue protrusion and on swallowing.

Neurovasculature

- On either side of the thyroid, within the trachea-oesophageal grooves, lies the recurrent laryngeal nerve (RLN). This nerve supplies the intrinsic muscles of the larynx. Deep to the upper pole of the thyroid sits the external branch of the superior laryngeal nerve, which supplies the cricothyroid muscle and contributes to vocal strength and pitch.
- The superior thyroid arteries (a branch of the external carotid artery) supply the superior thyroid poles.
- The inferior thyroid arteries (a branch of the thyrocervical trunk of the subclavian artery) supply the inferior thyroid poles.
- The superior, middle, and inferior thyroid veins drain the thyroid gland.
- The thyroid lymph fluid drains to the lateral deep cervical nodes and pre- and paratracheal lymph nodes.

Figure 5.1 Neurovasculature innervations and relations of the thyroid gland

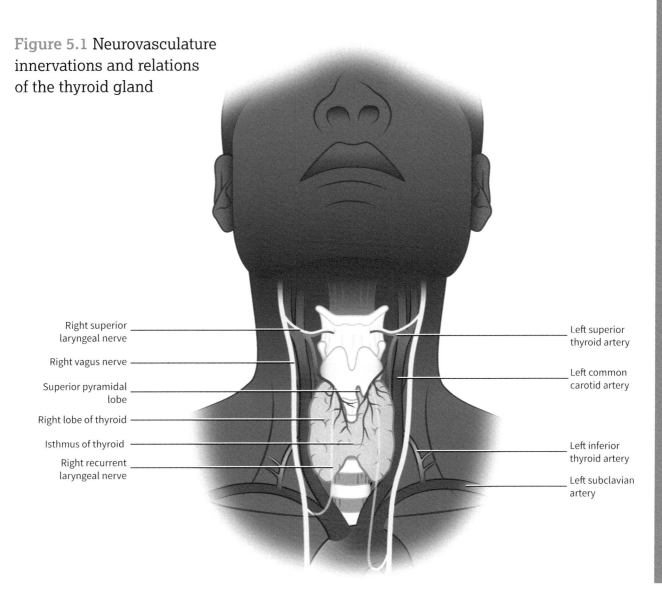

Right superior laryngeal nerve

Right vagus nerve

Superior pyramidal lobe

Right lobe of thyroid

Isthmus of thyroid

Right recurrent laryngeal nerve

Left superior thyroid artery

Left common carotid artery

Left inferior thyroid artery

Left subclavian artery

STEP-BY STEP OPERATION

Anaesthesia: general.

Position: reverse trendelenburg with a shoulder roll and head ring to extend and expose the neck.

Considerations: A neural integrity monitor electromyogram endotracheal tube is used to detect vocal fold movement from laryngeal nerve stimulation during the procedure.

1 A transverse 'collar' incision is made two finger-breadths above the sternal notch and extending to the medial border of the sternocleidomastoid on either side.

2 The skin and platysma are divided. Superior and inferior subplatysmal flaps are raised.

3 The strap muscles are exposed and separated with dissection down through the pale midline raphe onto the thyroid. Lateral sub-strap dissection is then performed until the common carotid is encountered-the lateral extent of dissection.

4 The middle thyroid vein, if present, is ligated and divided. The upper pole is mobilised, and the superior vessels isolated, ligated, and divided.

5 RLN is located in the tracheoesophageal groove and identified and protected. This step is assisted by neurostimulation to confirm the nerve. The neighbouring inferior thyroid artery is secured and double-ligated.

6 The RLN is then traced cranially and dissected off the thyroid until it enters the larynx posterior to the cricothyroid joint.

7 The parathyroid glands (and their vasculature) are identified and preserved if possible.

8 The same steps of lateral sub-strap dissection, mobilisation and ligation of superior pole, dissection and preservation of RLN and parathyroids are

153

repeated on the contralateral lobe. The thyroid gland can then be dissected off the trachea.

9   Haemostasis is checked with head down tilt and a Valsalva manoeuvre. One or two drains are placed.

10 The strap muscles and platysma are closed with absorbable sutures and the skin with non-absorbable sutures or clips.

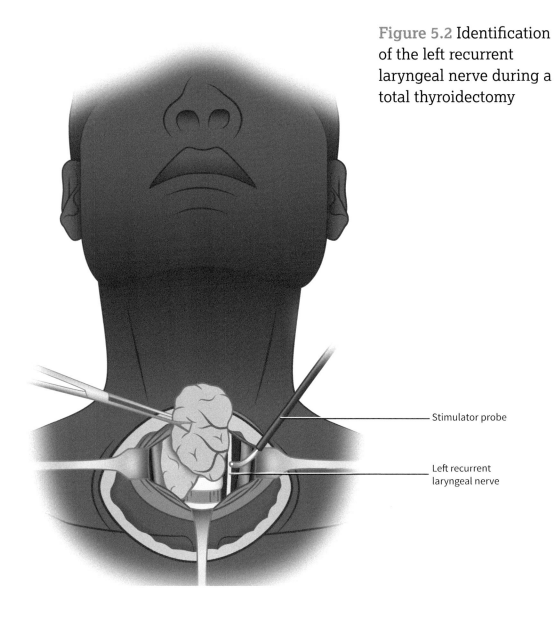

Figure 5.2 Identification of the left recurrent laryngeal nerve during a total thyroidectomy

Stimulator probe

Left recurrent laryngeal nerve

COMPLICATIONS

Early

›   Haematoma—can cause acute life-threatening airway obstruction from tracheal compression and oedema.

›   RLN paresis or palsy (hoarse/weak voice) or external branch of superior laryngeal nerve paresis or palsy (loss of high pitch) <1%. If RLN injury is bilateral, a tracheostomy may be required due to airway obstruction from closed vocal cords.

›   Thyroid 'storm'—intraoperative hyperpyrexia, sweating, tachycardia, heart failure.

›   Pneumothorax.

›   Horner's syndrome.

›   Oesophageal perforation or tracheal injury.

›   Hypothyroidism.

Intermediate and late

›   Hypocalcaemia due to hypoparathyroidism caused by accidental removal of or damage to the parathyroid glands.

›   Seroma.

›   Chyle leak.

POSTOPERATIVE CARE

npatient

›   Calcium and parathyroid hormone (PTH) levels checked the same day, with calcium and vitamin D replacement as appropriate.

›   Patients undergoing surgery for benign disease should be commenced on a weight-appropriate dose of levothyroxine.

›   Patients requiring post-op radioiodine ablation >3 weeks post-op are commenced on liothyronine (T3).

›   Drains removed when <30ml in 24 hours.

Outpatient

›   Follow-up appointment 4 weeks postoperatively for benign disease or 2 weeks for malignant disease to plan further oncological treatment.

›   Levothyroxine dose is titrated to thyroid-stimulating hormone (TSH) level at 6 weeks.

ⓘ SURGEON'S FAVOURITE QUESTION

Describe the embryology of the thyroid gland. Why is it important?

The thyroid bud is a diverticulum (pouch) that projects through the floor of the pharynx. The thyroid tissue descends to its adult locality, leaving the foramen caecum of the tongue and pyramidal lobe of the thyroid in its wake. Thyroid remnants can be found along this tract, such as lingual thyroid, thyroglossal cysts, and ectopic thyroid tissue.

PARATHYROIDECTOMY

James Glasbey

DEFINITION
Removal of a single or multiple parathyroid glands. Can be performed using open or minimally invasive techniques.

✓ INDICATIONS

> Symptomatic primary hyperparathyroidism (HPT) or parathyroid crisis caused by a parathyroid adenoma.
> Asymptomatic primary HPT with (a) raised serum calcium levels (variable cut-offs) and (b) objective evidence of end organ damage; reduced glomerular filtration rate or bone density T-score <-2.5.
> Parathyroid cancer.

✗ CONTRAINDICATIONS

Absolute
> Familial hypocalciuric hypercalcaemia: urine calcium <200mg/day[1].

Relative
> Known contralateral recurrent laryngeal nerve injury—bilateral recurrent laryngeal nerve palsy results in acute airway obstruction from closed vocal cords and will require a tracheostomy.
> Symptomatic cervical disc spondylopathy.

ANATOMY

Gross anatomy

> The parathyroids are very small (5 mm) glands that typically lie in upper and lower pairs. They can vary in number from two to six in total and have a characteristic tan-brown colour.
> The superior parathyroid glands originate from the fourth branchial pouch. They only migrate a short distance, located close to the inferior thyroid artery in the adult, and tend to have a posterior lie.
> The inferior parathyroid glands arise from the third branchial pouch, along with the thymus. Typically, the thymus is said to 'point' to the glands. Whilst the thymus descends into the thorax, the inferior parathyroids lie either (a) underneath the lower pole of the thyroid (90%) or (b) along the tract of the inferior

thyroid veins (10%). This can be as far inferior as the anterior mediastinum.
> Parathyroid adenomas can be identified preoperatively using ultrasound scan, 99-c sestamibi scintigraphy, and CT.

Neurovasculature

> The inferior thyroid artery (from the thyrocervical trunk of the subclavian artery) supplies the superior parathyroid glands. The inferior parathyroids receive their blood supply from either the inferior thyroid artery or the variable thyroid ima artery.
> Small veins from the parathyroid glands drain into neighbouring superior, middle, and inferior thyroid veins.
> Lymph from the parathyroid drains to the lateral deep cervical nodes and paratracheal lymph nodes.

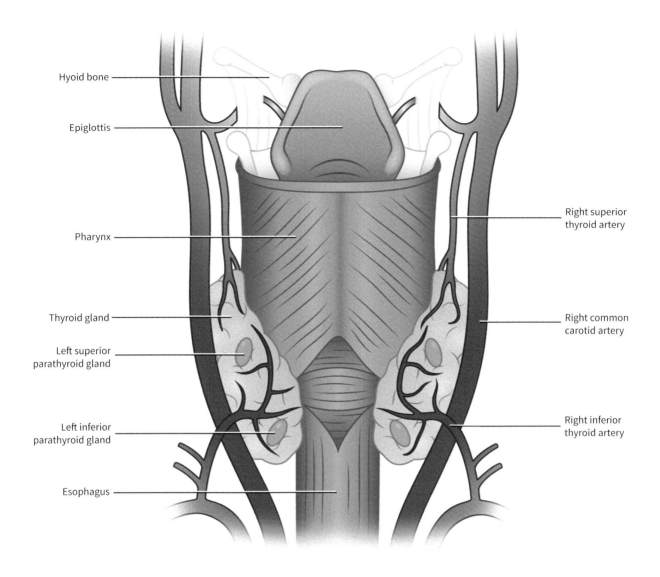

Hyoid bone

Epiglottis

Pharynx

Thyroid gland

Left superior
parathyroid gland

Left inferior
parathyroid gland

Esophagus

Right superior
thyroid artery

Right common
carotid artery

Right inferior
thyroid artery

Figure 5.3 Vasculature and anatomical location of the parathyroid glands

STEP-BY-STEP OPERATION

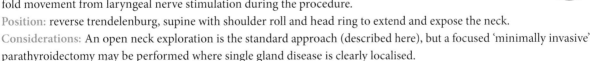

Anaesthesia: general; a neural integrity monitor electromyogram endotracheal tube is used to detect vocal fold movement from laryngeal nerve stimulation during the procedure.

Position: reverse trendelenburg, supine with shoulder roll and head ring to extend and expose the neck.

Considerations: An open neck exploration is the standard approach (described here), but a focused 'minimally invasive' parathyroidectomy may be performed where single gland disease is clearly localised.

1 A transverse 'collar' incision is made two finger-breadths above the sternal notch and extending to the medial border of the sternocleidomastoid on either side.

2 The skin and platysma are divided. Superior and inferior subplatysmal flaps are raised.

3 The strap muscles are exposed and separated with dissection down through the pale midline raphe onto the thyroid. Lateral sub-strap dissection is then performed until the common carotid is encountered.

4 A thyroid lobe is anteromedially displaced to locate the parathyroid gland.

5 The recurrent laryngeal nerve is located in the tracheoesophageal groove and identified and protected. This step is assisted by neurostimulation to confirm the nerve.

6 Once located, single or multiple enlarged glands are removed. If all four are enlarged, at least three are resected, typically leaving half a gland in situ.

7 Intra-operative frozen sections or rapid parathyroid hormone (PTH) assays (intra-operative PTH reduction of >50% from baseline) may be utilised to confirm correct identification of an adenoma.

8 Haemostasis is achieved meticulously, using diathermy cautiously around the recurrent laryngeal nerve. A drain can be placed.

9 The strap muscles and platysma are closed with absorbable sutures and skin with non-absorbable sutures or clips.

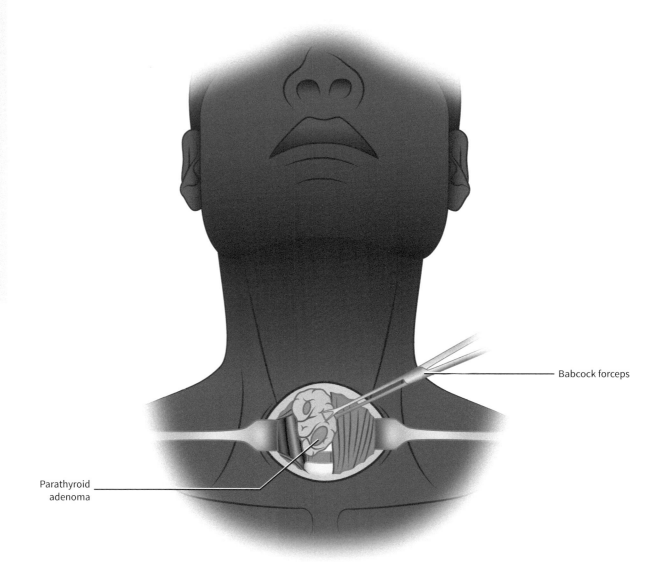

Babcock forceps

Parathyroid adenoma

Figure 5.4 Identification of abnormal parathyroid glands

COMPLICATIONS

Early

- Recurrent laryngeal nerve palsy (hoarse/weak voice) or external branch of superior laryngeal nerve palsy (loss of high pitch) <1%.
- Haematoma—can cause acute life-threatening airway obstruction from tracheal compression and oedema.

Intermediate and late

- Transient hyperthyroidism.
- Temporary hypocalcaemia (usually resolves within 6 weeks to 1 year).

- Permanent hypocalcaemia (higher risk with multiglandular resection).
- Prolonged, severe hypocalcaemia or 'hungry bone syndrome'; can develop in the presence of normal or even elevated parathyroid hormone postoperatively.
- Persistent hyperparathyroidism (1–5%); commonly due to incomplete excision, supernumerary, or ectopic parathyroid tissue.

POSTOPERATIVE CARE

Inpatient

- Minimal 6-hour postoperative observation to exclude cervical haematoma prior to discharge if no drain used.
- PTH and serum calcium levels are checked prior to discharge and abnormal calcium levels corrected. Additional vitamin D supplementation may be required.
- Drain (if used) removed when <30ml output in 24 hours.
- Next-day discharge is common for a routine uncomplicated surgery; however, renal HPT patients

often require several days to allow for careful biochemical monitoring and correction.

Outpatient

- Follow-up appointment for wound review and biochemical profiling 4 weeks post-op.
- A single 6-month follow-up appointment for serum calcium testing and confirmation of cure may be acceptable in those with a single adenoma. More regular, long-term follow-up is recommended in multiglandular disease.

❓ SURGEON'S FAVOURITE QUESTION

With which multiple endocrine neoplasia (MEN) syndrome(s) is primary hyperparathyroidism associated?

Parathyroid hyperplasia is present in 90% of patients with MEN1A (pancreatic tumours, pituitary adenoma, parathyroid hyperplasia). It is also found in 50% of patients with MEN2A (medullary thyroid carcinoma, phaeochromocytoma, parathyroid hyperplasia).

ADRENALECTOMY

James Glasbey

DEFINITION
Removal of the adrenal gland(s), either laparoscopically or openly.

✓ INDICATIONS

Unilateral adrenalectomy

> Any non-functioning tumour >4 cm in size, or <4 cm and growing by >1 cm per year.
> Phaeochromocytoma.
> Conn's syndrome failing medical management.
> Cushing's syndrome due to a secretory adenoma.
> Adrenocortical or adrenomedullary carcinoma (primary tumours).
> Solitary metastasis to adrenal glands from another primary site.

Bilateral adrenalectomy

> Bilateral adrenal tumours.

> Hypersecretion due to a primary pituitary adenoma (e.g., Cushing's disease).

✗ CONTRAINDICATIONS

Absolute
> Medically untreated phaeochromocytoma.

Relative contraindications for a laparoscopic approach
> Primary carcinoma of the adrenal cortex.
> Radiographic evidence of tumour invasion.
> Tumour size >15cm.
> Severe cardiac disease.
> Extensive prior upper abdominal surgery.

ANATOMY

Gross anatomy
> The adrenal glands (or 'suprarenal' glands) sit above and medial to the upper poles of each kidney, directly below the diaphragm.
> The left adrenal gland sits posterior to the stomach. The right sits behind the right lobe of the liver, just medial to the inferior vena cava (IVC).

Neurovasculature
> Each adrenal gland receives blood supply from three arteries:
>> Superior suprarenal artery—a branch of the inferior phrenic artery.
>> Middle suprarenal artery—a direct branch of the abdominal aorta.
>> Inferior suprarenal artery—a branch of the renal artery.
> The adrenal glands drain into a single main suprarenal vein on either side.
>> The longer, left suprarenal vein joins the left renal vein before emptying into the IVC.

> The short, right suprarenal vein drains directly to the IVC.
> Lymphatic drainage is to the para-aortic nodes.

Histology
> Microscopically, the adrenal glands consist of two developmentally distinct territories: an outer *cortex* (developing from the mesoderm of the urogenital ridge) and an inner *medulla* (developing from the neural crest ectoderm).
> The outer cortex secretes steroid hormones and can be divided into three functional regions:
>> The zona glomerulosa, which produces mineralocorticoids (e.g., aldosterone).
>> The zona fasciculata, which produces glucocorticoids (e.g., cortisol).
>> The zona reticularis, which produces androgens (e.g., dehydroepiandrosterone).
> The inner medulla consists of chromaffin cells innervated by sympathetic preganglionic fibres. These produce adrenaline and noradrenaline.

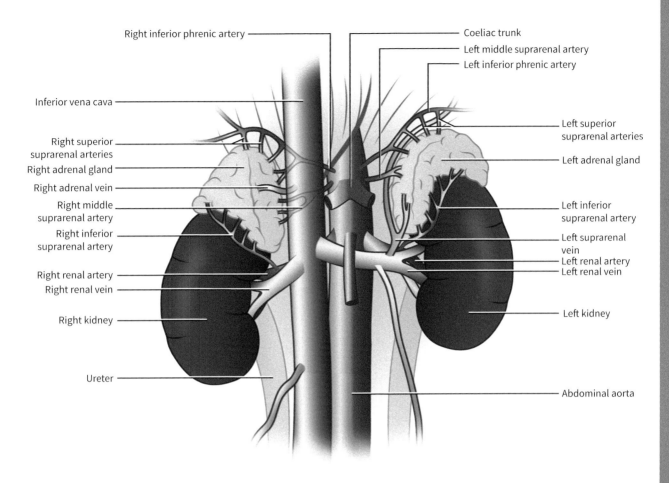

Figure 5.5 Vasculature and relations of the adrenal glands

STEP-BY-STEP OPERATION

Anaesthesia: general.

Position: lateral decubitus position with the table tilted 15° downwards to laterally flex the spine; secured with beanbags, pads, and clamps.

Considerations:

▸ Cushing's syndrome (immunosuppression)—prophylactic antibiotics.

▸ Conn's syndrome—spironolactone.

▸ Phaeochromocytoma—alpha-blockers (e.g., phenoxybenzamine (always started first) and beta-blockers (e.g., labetalol).

1 Four trocars are placed in the right subcostal area and the midline, spaced 9–12 cm apart. Pneumoperitoneum is achieved to an insufflation pressure of 13–15 mmHg.

2 The peritoneal reflection of the right hepatic triangular ligament is incised, allowing the liver to be retracted medially. The duodenum may also need to be mobilised.

3 The anterior renal fascia (Gerota's fascia) is opened from the right kidney up to the diaphragm, reaching 4–6 cm above the superior pole of the kidney.

4 With the right kidney exposed, the adipose tissue medial to the kidney can be dissected up to the IVC.

5 The lateral wall of the IVC is dissected and exposed.

6 The right adrenal vein and any accessory veins are identified along the lateral wall of the IVC.

7 The multiple small adrenal arteries arising from the aorta, phrenic, and renal arteries are identified and ligated.

8 The lateral periadrenal adipose tissue containing the adrenal gland is dissected from the diaphragm and right kidney *en bloc*, taking care not to disrupt the tumour capsule if present. This is then separated circumferentially from the IVC.

9 The tissue is placed in an endoscopic bag and removed from a single, large port site, without rupture of the tumour.

10 Large port sites are closed with a single anchoring suture. Fascia and skin closure are achieved with non-absorbable sutures.

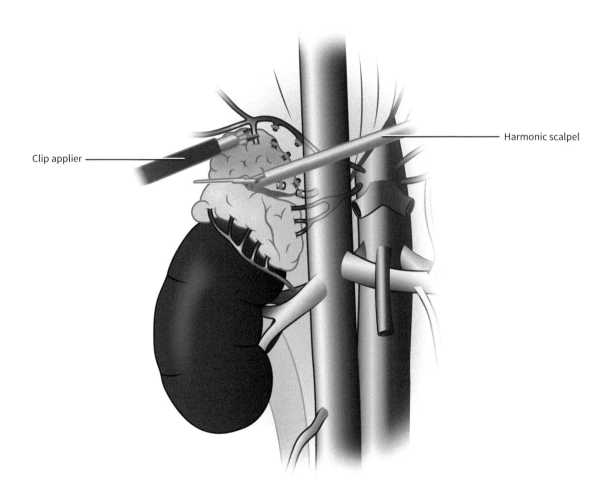

Clip applier

Harmonic scalpel

Figure 5.6 Dissection and *en bloc* removal of an adrenal tumour (within its capsule)

COMPLICATIONS

Early

- Haemodynamic instability—particularly phaeochromocytoma, where vasoconstriction renders patient relatively volume deplete, and massive catecholamine release due to manipulation of tumour can lead to refractory hypertension +/- catecholamine-induced cardiomyopathy.
- Bleeding.
- Visceral injury.
- Tumour capsule rupture resulting in dissemination of malignancy.

Intermediate and late

- Phaeochromocytoma—heart failure and hypertension.
- Cushing's syndrome—increased risk of generic postoperative complications, including wound infection, Deep Vein Thrombosis (DVT) and Pulmonary Embolism (PE), pneumonia, pain, and ileus.
- Renovascular hypertension and reduced renal function.
- Nelson's syndrome—rapid enlargement of a pituitary adenoma following removal of both adrenal glands (rare).
- Adrenal insufficiency (rare).

POSTOPERATIVE CARE

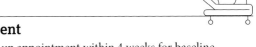
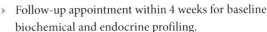
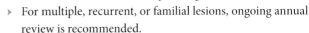

Inpatient

- Routine high-dependency care is advised in phaeochromocytoma excision.
- Careful fluid and glucose infusion titration is used to prevent hypotensive episodes.
- Lifelong glucocorticoid and mineralocorticoid replacement therapy is necessary following bilateral adrenalectomy to avoid adrenal insufficiency.

Outpatient

- Follow-up appointment within 4 weeks for baseline biochemical and endocrine profiling.
- For multiple, recurrent, or familial lesions, ongoing annual review is recommended.

 ## SURGEON'S FAVOURITE QUESTION

What is the 'rule of 10s' for phaeochromocytoma? How does it present?

10% of phaeochromocytomas are of extra-adrenal origin, 10% occur in childhood, 10% are bilateral, and 10% are malignant. They classically present with a triad of episodic headaches (sudden-onset, pounding), tachycardia (and/or palpitations), and sweating. Patients may also have neurofibromas, a concurrent medullary carcinoma of the thyroid, or parathyroid hyperplasia as part of an MEN2A/2B syndrome.

6 VASCULAR

MADELAINE GIMZEWSKA AND ESTHER PLATT

CAROTID ENDARTERECTOMY

Madelaine Gimzewska

DEFINITION

The removal of plaque from the carotid artery in carotid artery atherosclerosis.

✔ INDICATIONS

- Endarterectomy is preferred over medical management alone or stenting (no longer commonly performed in the UK):
  - Patients presenting with transient ischaemic attack or non-disabling stroke and carotid stenosis of 70–99% who meet the following criteria.
  - Life expectancy 5+ years.
  - Surgically accessible lesion.
  - No prior ipsilateral endarterectomy.
  - Combined perioperative risk of stroke and death is <6% for surgeon and centre.
- Endarterectomy is considered in asymptomatic patients who meet the following criteria:
  - Life expectancy 5+ years.
  - ≥ 80% stenosis despite intensive medical therapy.

- Combined perioperative risk of stroke and death is <3% for surgeon and centre.

✘ CONTRAINDICATIONS

Relative

- Major disabling stroke.
- 'Hostile neck' (head and neck cancer, previous neck dissection, previously irradiated neck, cervical spine disease with fixed neck flexion).
- Severe recurrent carotid stenosis.
- Atypical lesion location that is surgically inaccessible.
- Contralateral vocal cord paralysis.

Absolute

- Asymptomatic complete carotid occlusion.

ANATOMY

Gross anatomy

- The right common carotid artery is a branch of the brachiocephalic artery. The left common carotid artery is a direct branch of the aorta aortic arch.
- The carotid sheath is derived from the deep cervical fascia. It contains the common carotid artery (CCA), the internal jugular vein (IJV), and the vagus nerve. The carotid sheath runs deep to the platysma and sternocleidomastoid (SCM).
- At the level of C3/C4 (the level of the superior thyroid cartilage), the CCA divides into:
  - The external carotid artery (ECA)—the arterial supply of the face and scalp. The ECA has multiple branches: superior thyroid, ascending pharyngeal, lingual, facial, occipital, posterior auricular, maxillary, and superficial temporal.
  - The internal carotid artery (ICA)—responsible for supplying the anterior circulatory system of the brain. It normally has no branches in the neck.
  - Carotid baroreceptors that respond to alterations in blood pressure are located at the origin of the ICA

and lie within the adventitia. They are innervated by a branch of the glossopharyngeal—the sinus nerve of Hering.

Anatomical relations

- In close proximity to the ICA are:
  - The marginal and mandibular branch of CN VII (Facial).
  - CN IX (Glossopharyngeal).
  - CN X (Vagus).
  - CN XII (Hypoglossal).
- The glossopharyngeal nerve crosses the ICA superficially and runs deep to the ECA as it travels lateral to medial.
- The hypoglossal nerve descends between the ICA and IJV before looping across the ICA and ECA deep to the posterior belly of the digastric muscle.
- The vagus nerve descends the neck within the carotid sheath lateral to the ICA.
- The recurrent laryngeal nerve (a branch of the vagus nerve) descends within the carotid sheath medial to the ICA.

Figure 6.1 Branches of the external carotid artery

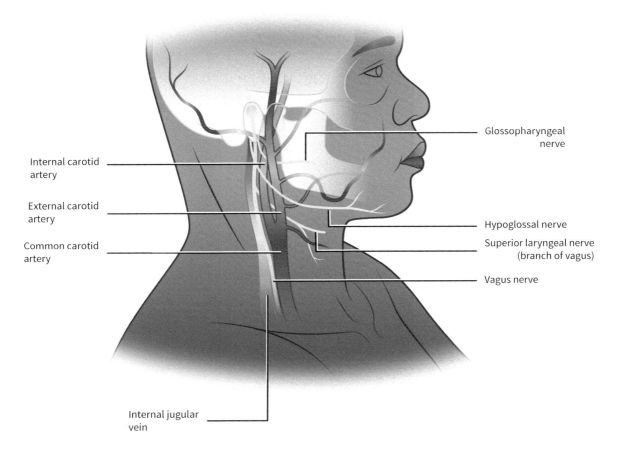

- Internal carotid artery
- External carotid artery
- Common carotid artery
- Internal jugular vein
- Glossopharyngeal nerve
- Hypoglossal nerve
- Superior laryngeal nerve (branch of vagus)
- Vagus nerve

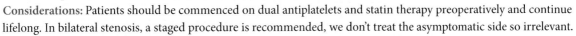
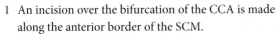

STEP-BY-STEP OPERATION

Anaesthesia: general or local/regional with a superficial cervical plexus block.

Position: supine with the neck extended and face turned to the contralateral side.

Considerations: Patients should be commenced on dual antiplatelets and statin therapy preoperatively and continue lifelong. In bilateral stenosis, a staged procedure is recommended, we don't treat the asymptomatic side so irrelevant.

1 An incision over the bifurcation of the CCA is made along the anterior border of the SCM.

2 The subcutaneous tissues and platysma are divided, and the SCM is reflected postero-laterally. The carotid sheath is exposed.

3 The IJV is identified; the facial vein is identified, ligated, and divided to provide access; the IJV is then retracted laterally or medially.

4 The CCA, ICA, and ECA are dissected free from surrounding tissues and encircled with slings ready for clamping.

5 Immediately prior to the clamping, a bolus of IV heparin is administered. Clamps are then placed on the ICA first (above the plaque preventing embolisation), and then on the CCA (below the plaque) and the ECA.

6 A longitudinal arteriotomy (incision) is made along the full length of the diseased CCA and ICA.

7 If using a general anaesthetic, a shunt may be placed from the common carotid below the level of the clamp to the ICA above the clamp. With local anaesthetic, the patient is monitored for evidence of neurological compromise whilst the ICA is clamped. A shunt can be used to restore blood flow if required.

8 The plaque is removed from the lumen of the artery by dissection in the layers of the deep media. Care is taken to create a smooth and tapered transition between normal artery and the endarterectomised section in order to prevent subsequent arterial dissection.

9 The artery is then closed either primarily, or with a patch (commonly either bovine pericardium or synthetic material such as Dacron) to increase vessel diameter.

10 The wound is closed in layers; skin can be closed with either a subcuticular suture or metal clips; a drain can be inserted.

Figure 6.2 Excision of atherosclerotic plaque at the site of an arteriotomy in the ICA

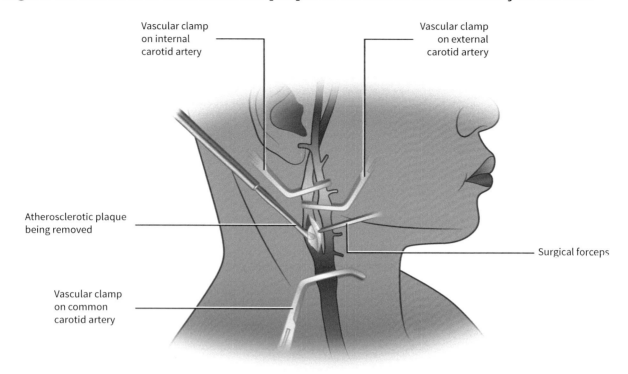

Vascular clamp on internal carotid artery

Vascular clamp on external carotid artery

Atherosclerotic plaque being removed

Surgical forceps

Vascular clamp on common carotid artery

COMPLICATIONS

Early

- Intra/postoperative stroke.
- Myocardial infarction.
- Mortality (0.5–3%).
- Bleeding or haematoma—can result in a compressive airway obstruction requiring an emergency haematoma evacuation.
- Infection.
- Nerve damage:
  - Hypoglossal nerve—tongue weakness, deviates towards side of damage—difficulty in speaking and swallowing.
  - Glossopharyngeal nerve—difficulty swallowing.
  - Mandibular branch of the facial nerve—asymmetrical smile.
  - Recurrent laryngeal nerve—vocal cord palsy.

Intermediate and late

- Hyperperfusion syndrome (rare) as a result of rapid reperfusion of previously hypoxic areas of the brain. Presents with headache, focal motor seizures and intra-cerebral haemorrhage.
- Ongoing neurological deficit from peri-operative stroke or nerve damage.
- Re-stenosis of the artery.
- Patch infection.

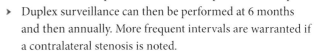

POSTOPERATIVE CARE

Inpatient

▸ Hourly neurological observations in a High Dependancy Unit (HDU) setting are required for 24 hours postoperatively.

▸ Patients should be monitored with an arterial line in place to allow for accurate control of blood pressure, as this is commonly labile for the first 12–24 hours.

▸ Drain (if inserted) removed once <20 ml in 24 hours.

Outpatient

▸ Routine follow up in 4–8 weeks with repeat carotid duplex.

▸ Duplex surveillance can then be performed at 6 months and then annually. More frequent intervals are warranted if a contralateral stenosis is noted.

 SURGEON'S FAVOURITE QUESTIONS

What are the branches of the ECA?

Superior thyroid, ascending pharyngeal, lingual, facial, occipital, posterior auricular, maxillary, superficial temporal. "**Some Anatomists Like Freaking Out Poor Medical Students.**"

OPEN ABDOMINAL AORTIC ANEURYSM REPAIR

Madelaine Gimzewska

DEFINITION

Open surgical repair of an infrarenal abdominal aortic aneurysm (AAA).

✓ INDICATIONS

- Elective repair of AAA if one of the following conditions apply:
  - A diameter of over 5.5 cm indicates the risk of rupture is higher than repair (Diameter expanding greater than 10 mm per year).
- Urgent repair is indicated in symptomatic aneurysms.
- Emergency repair is indicated in an AAA rupture.
- Some cases of aneurysms caused by microbiological infection (mycotic aneurysms).

✗ CONTRAINDICATIONS

- Elective repair—those unlikely to survive or recover from the operation. The decision is based on comorbidities, life expectancy, quality of life, cardiopulmonary reserve, and exercise tolerance.
- Emergency repair—when considered futile or against the patient's expressed wishes.

ANATOMY

- The thoracic aorta transitions into the abdominal aorta as it passes through the diaphragm's aortic hiatus at the level of T12. The abdominal aorta descends along the posterior wall of the abdomen, anterior to the vertebral column.
- The abdominal aorta has nine branches that supply the abdominal viscera:
  1. Right and left phrenic artery—supplies the diaphragm.
  2. Coeliac trunk—supplies the liver, stomach, oesophagus, duodenum, and pancreas (foregut).
  3. Right and left suprarenal arteries—supply the adrenal glands.
  4. Superior mesenteric artery (SMA)—supplies the small bowel from the lower half of the duodenum to the first two-thirds of the transverse colon.
  5. Right and left renal arteries—supply the kidneys (the right renal artery is longer than the left).
  6. Right and left gonadal arteries—supply the testicles in males and the ovaries in females.
  7. Inferior mesenteric artery (IMA)—supplies the large intestine from the splenic flexure to the level of the upper rectum.
  8. Median sacral artery—supplies the sacrum and coccyx.
  9. Lumbar arteries (L1–L4)—supply the lumbar vertebrae.
- At the level of L4, the abdominal aorta bifurcates into the left and right common iliac arteries.
- The common iliac arteries bifurcate into the internal iliac artery (supplying the pelvis) and the external iliac artery (supplying the leg).
- The external iliac artery becomes the common femoral artery as it emerges from under the inguinal ligament. The common femoral artery gives rise to the profunda femoris and the superficial femoral artery (SFA) in the thigh.

Figure 6.3 Branches and bifurcations of the abdominal aorta

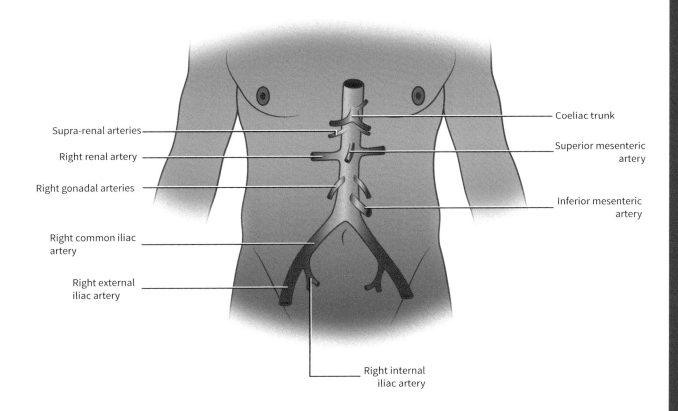

STEP-BY-STEP OPERATION

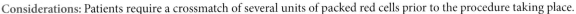

Anaesthesia: general anaesthesia, often with an epidural for postoperative pain relief.

Position: supine.

Considerations: Patients require a crossmatch of several units of packed red cells prior to the procedure taking place.

1. A transverse or midline laparotomy incision is made.
2. The small bowel and omentum are covered in damp swabs and are then retracted to one side.
3. The retroperitoneal cavity is exposed, and the retroperitoneal duodenum is mobilised towards the patient's right side.
4. The aorta is visualised, and the neck of the aneurysm and the iliac vessels are dissected to gain full proximal and distal exposure. A bolus of IV heparin is administered.
5. Proximal control is obtained by clamping the aorta above the level of the aneurysm. Distal control is obtained by the clamping of both iliac arteries.
6. A longitudinal incision along the anterior surface of the aneurysm is made, and the aneurysm sac is opened. Special care is taken to avoid the origin of the IMA. Once incised, thrombus and debris from within

the sac are removed. Back-bleeding is controlled from the lumbar arteries by over-sewing.

7. The prosthetic (Dacron) graft is sutured in from the proximal normal aorta to either the normal post-aneurysmal aorta (using a straight tube graft) or into the normal iliac arteries (using a bifurcated graft).
8. The proximal clamp is briefly removed, and the graft is flushed with heparin (this removes any thrombus and prevents more thrombus developing). This is repeated just before finishing the distal anastomosis to remove any further thrombus from the graft.
9. The distal limb pulses are assessed using Doppler, and the feet are checked for perfusion.
10. The aneurysm sac and retroperitoneum are closed over the graft, and the bowel is checked for evidence of ischaemia. The abdominal cavity is then closed in layers.

VASCULAR

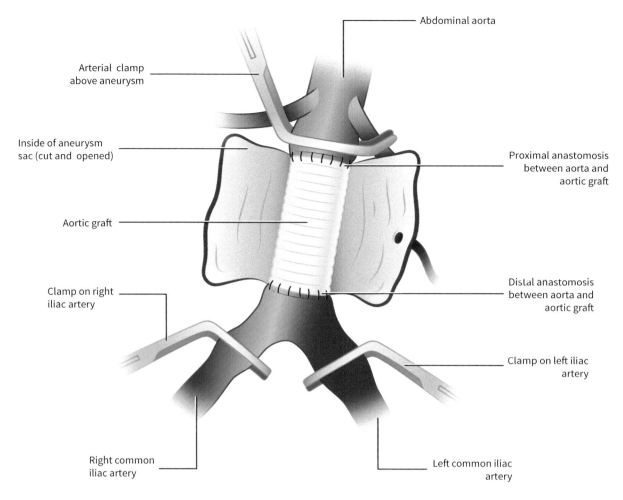

Arterial clamp above aneurysm

Abdominal aorta

Inside of aneurysm sac (cut and opened)

Proximal anastomosis between aorta and aortic graft

Aortic graft

Distal anastomosis between aorta and aortic graft

Clamp on right iliac artery

Clamp on left iliac artery

Right common iliac artery

Left common iliac artery

Figure 6.4 The anastomosis of a straight tubed Dacron graft at the site of an abdominal aortic aneurysm

COMPLICATIONS

Early

> Myocardial infarction—a major complication of the aortic surgery, particularly related to sudden periods of hypotension when clamps are removed and distal perfusion is restored.
> Bleeding.
> Lower limb ischaemia due to distal embolisation or thrombosis (trash foot).
> Renal, bowel and spinal ischaemia.
> Damage to ureters or bowel.
> Paralytic ileus.

Intermediate and late

> Graft infection.
> Incisional hernia.
> Aorto-enteric fistula.
> 30-day mortality for elective repair (5%).
> 30-day mortality for emergency repair (50%).
> Sexual dysfunction due to pelvic nerve damage.

POSTOPERATIVE CARE

Inpatient

▸ Initially, patients should be cared for on either Intensive Care Unit (ICU)/High Dependency Unit (HDU).

▸ A clear diet is started Day 1 postoperatively and built up as tolerated.

Outpatient

▸ Patients attend vascular clinic 6 weeks postoperatively.

▸ Unlike endovascular aneurysmal repair (EVAR), patients who have undergone an open abdominal AAA repair do not require routine long-term follow-up or repeat imaging; however, some guidelines do suggest CT imaging after 4–5 years to assess for pseudoaneurysm formation at the site of anastomosis.

❓ SURGEON'S FAVOURITE QUESTION

At what level does the aorta pass behind the diaphragm?

The level of the 12th thoracic vertebra.

ENDOVASCULAR ANEURYSM REPAIR (EVAR)

Madelaine Gimzewska

DEFINITION

Repair of an abdominal aortic aneurysm (AAA) using a minimally invasive endovascular technique.

✓ INDICATIONS

> Elective repair of AAA if one of the following conditions apply:
>> A diameter of over 5.5 cm indicates the risk of rupture is higher than repair (Diameter expanding greater than 10 mm per year).
> Urgent repair is indicated in symptomatic aneurysms.
> Immediate repair is indicated in an AAA rupture.
> Emergency cases of aneurysms caused by microbiological infection (mycotic aneurysms).

✗ CONTRAINDICATIONS

> Unsuitable aortic anatomy (as identified on CT angiogram—e.g., tortuous aorta, iliac arteries too small).
> eGFR <30 ml/min—however, CO_2 angiography or small doses of iodinated contrast and the use of fusion imaging techniques can negate this contraindication.

ANATOMY

> The thoracic aorta transitions into the abdominal aorta as it passes through the diaphragm's aortic hiatus at the level of T12. The abdominal aorta descends along the posterior wall of the abdomen, anterior to the vertebral column.
> The abdominal aorta has nine branches that supply the abdominal viscera:
> 1. Right and left phrenic artery—supplies the diaphragm.
> 2. Coeliac trunk—supplies the liver, stomach, oesophagus, duodenum, and pancreas (foregut).
> 3. Right and left suprarenal arteries—supply the adrenal glands.
> 4. Superior mesenteric artery (SMA)—supplies the small bowel from the lower half of the duodenum to the first two-thirds of the transverse colon.
> 5. Right and left renal arteries—supply the kidneys (the right renal artery is longer than the left).
> 6. Right and left gonadal arteries—supply the testicles in males and the ovaries in females.
> 7. Inferior mesenteric artery (IMA)—supplies the large intestine from the splenic flexure to the level of the upper rectum.
> 8. Median sacral artery—supplies the sacrum and coccyx.
> 9. Lumbar arteries (L1–L4)—supply the lumbar vertebrae.
> At the level of L4, the abdominal aorta bifurcates into the left and right common iliac arteries.
> The common iliac arteries bifurcate into the internal iliac artery (supplying the pelvis) and the external iliac artery (supplying the leg).
> The external iliac artery becomes the common femoral artery as it emerges from under the inguinal ligament. The common femoral artery gives rise to the profunda femoris and the superficial femoral artery (SFA) in the thigh.
> The common femoral arteries are routinely used for endovascular access. Each femoral artery is located at the mid-inguinal point (medially halfway between the anterior superior iliac spine (ASIS) and the pubic symphysis).
> The deep inguinal ring lies on the midpoint of the inguinal ligament (halfway between the ASIS and the pubic tubercle). The femoral artery lies at the mid-inguinal point.
> The femoral artery runs medial to the femoral nerve and lateral to the femoral vein (NAVY—nerve, artery, vein, Y fronts from lateral to medial).

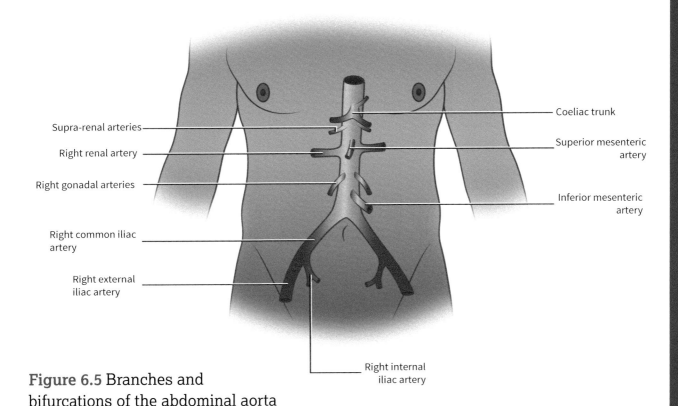

Figure 6.5 Branches and bifurcations of the abdominal aorta

Labels (clockwise from top right): Coeliac trunk, Superior mesenteric artery, Inferior mesenteric artery, Right internal iliac artery, Right external iliac artery, Right common iliac artery, Right gonadal arteries, Right renal artery, Supra-renal arteries

STEP-BY-STEP OPERATION

Anaesthesia: general, regional or local.

Position: supine.

Considerations: EVAR is conducted in an interventional suite or hybrid theatre (a surgical theatre equipped with image intensifier).

1 Femoral arteries are accessed through specific percutaneous devices or through cutdowns (incisions in both groins with dissection of the surrounding tissues to expose and control both femoral arteries).

2 Once exposed, the arteries are cannulated and a catheter and wire combination is advanced through the femoral arteries. Typically via the right femoral artery, a stiff wire is positioned with its tip in the descending thoracic aorta above the AAA. Via the left femoral artery, a diagnostic catheter is inserted to a level just above the AAA. Through this runs (contrast dye is injected in the aorta and radiographs taken) are performed to demonstrate the anatomy of the aorta and the aneurysm.

3 The main body of the graft is then inserted over the stiff guide wire with the proximal end of the graft being deployed into the infrarenal landing zone (hooks anchor the graft to the aortic wall). Once the proximal portion of the graft is anchored, the remaining graft is deployed.

4 A contrast run is performed in the right iliac artery, and measurements of the vessel are taken.

5 An appropriately sized right iliac limb is deployed so that the proximal portion anchors into the aortic graft whilst the distal end lies within the right common iliac artery. The left iliac limb is then deployed via the left femoral artery.

6 The proximal and distal ends of the graft system and all junctions are gently ballooned (a catheter-deployed balloon is briefly expanded across the junction to fully seal the graft to the artery wall).

7 Further contrast runs are performed to assess the seal of the graft.

8 The femoral artery sheaths and all wires are removed, and the arteries are repaired. The incisions are then closed in layers.

Figure 6.6 Positioning of the main body and the right and left limbs of an EVAR graft within a AAA.

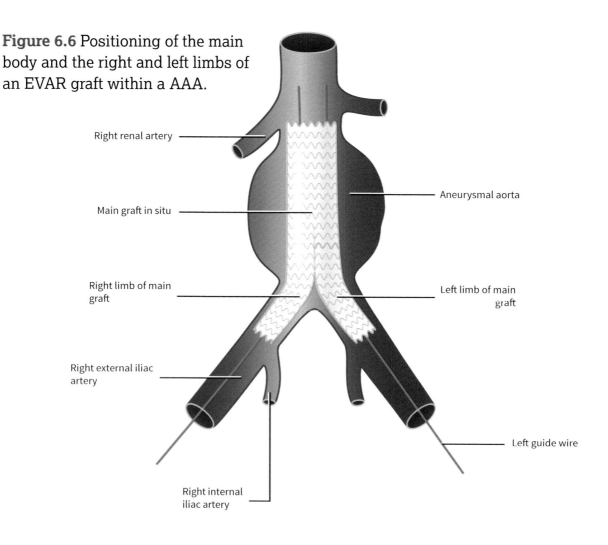

Right renal artery

Main graft in situ

Right limb of main graft

Right external iliac artery

Right internal iliac artery

Aneurysmal aorta

Left limb of main graft

Left guide wire

COMPLICATIONS

Early

> Renal, bowel, and spinal ischaemia.
> Leg ischaemia due to distal embolisation or thrombosis (may require embolectomy, thrombectomy, bypass, or, rarely, amputation).
> Contrast-induced nephropathy.
> Complications of femoral access—pseudoaneurysm, haematoma, distal embolisation.

Intermediate and late

> Infection of either the wound or graft.
> Graft migration.
> Renal damage due to multiple contrast CT scans required for follow-up.

> Aorto-enteric fistula.
> Endoleaks:
> > Ia—failure of seal between graft and aneurysm neck.
> > Ib—failure of seal between graft and iliac vessels at distal end of the graft.
> > II—flow of blood into the aneurysm sac from back-bleeding vessels (typically lumbar vessels).
> > III—failure of a seal between components of the graft device.
> > IV—leaking through the graft material.
> > V—growth of the aneurysm sac with no identifiable (types I–IV) leak.

POSTOPERATIVE CARE

Inpatient

▸ Ruptured AAA patients should initially be cared for in Intensive Care Unit (ICU)/High Dependency Unit (HDU).

▸ Elective patients are suitable for ward-level care.

▸ It is important to ensure that adequate maintenance fluids are prescribed to limit renal damage following CT contrast.

Outpatient

▸ Stent surveillance—to monitor for signs of the AAA increasing in size or signs of metal fatigue. Most commonly, CT angiogram is used for 1 year, and then a combination of ultrasound and plain radiographs are used to assess for leaks and stent fractures and to measure sac size.

SURGEON'S FAVOURITE QUESTION

What is the difference between a 'true' aneurysm and a pseudoaneurysm?

A true aneurysm is a focal dilatation of all three layers of the arterial wall. A pseudoaneurysm is formed by blood collecting between the tunica media and tunica adventitia of the artery wall, frequently caused by injury to the vessel.

ENDOVASCULAR ANEURYSM REPAIR (EVAR)

RADIOCEPHALIC FISTULA FORMATION

Madelaine Gimzewska

DEFINITION

Surgical formation of an abnormal connection between an artery and a vein—an arteriovenous (AV) fistula, used for vascular access in haemodialysis treatment.

✓ INDICATIONS

> Patients requiring long-term vascular access for haemodialysis.

✗ CONTRAINDICATIONS

> Vascular anatomy unsuitable for fistula formation—e.g., small vascular diameter or atherosclerotic disease of the artery. A vein luminal diameter of ≤2.5 mm and an arterial luminal diameter of ≤2 mm.

> Damaged veins from cannulation and blood sampling. Patients approaching the need for dialysis should have their veins protected, and blood samples should be taken from the back of the hands.

ANATOMY

> Cephalic vein:
>> The cephalic vein is a superficial vein of the anterolateral arm that drains the dorsal network of the hand.
>> Within the anterior cubital fossa, the cephalic vein communicates with the basilic vein via the median cubital vein.
>> The cephalic vein drains into the axillary vein at the deltopectoral groove.
> Radial artery:
>> The radial artery is a branch of the brachial artery. The brachial artery bifurcates into the radial and ulnar arteries just distal to the antecubital fossa.

>> The radial artery runs along the anterolateral aspect of the forearm, supplying the posterior forearm and lateral hand.
>> Within the hand, the radial artery anastomoses with the ulnar artery to form the superficial and deep palmar arches.
> The superficial branch of the radial nerve lies lateral to the radial artery, and care must be taken to avoid injury during the formation of a radiocephalic fistula.

Figure 6.7 Arterial supply and venous drainage of the upper limb

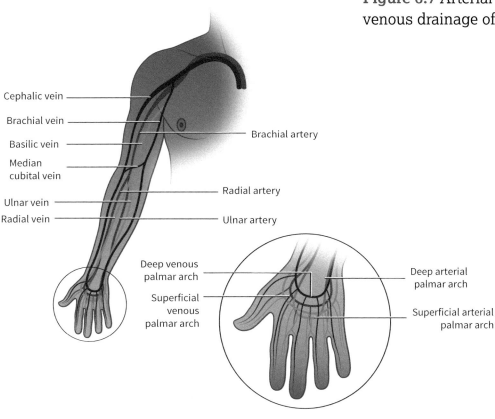

Cephalic vein

Brachial vein

Basilic vein

Median cubital vein

Ulnar vein

Radial vein

Brachial artery

Radial artery

Ulnar artery

Deep venous palmar arch

Superficial venous palmar arch

Deep arterial palmar arch

Superficial arterial palmar arch

STEP-BY-STEP OPERATION

Anaesthesia: general, local, or a regional nerve (brachial plexus) block.

Position: supine, with the arm supinated on an arm board angled at 90° to the patient's torso.

Considerations: Prior to surgery, patients undergo duplex imaging to assess the suitability of their vasculature for a fistula. Within theatre, ultrasound-guided preoperative markings may be performed.

1 A 5–7 cm incision is made running over and longitudinal to the cephalic vein, 2–3 cm proximal to the wrist.

2 Through this incision, both the cephalic vein and the radial artery are visualized and accessed.

3 The cephalic vein is mobilised, and branches are ligated.

4 The cephalic vein is then divided distally at the wrist. The distal end is left tied off, and a clamp is left on the proximal end. The vein is then flushed with heparinised saline (causing dilation).

5 The radial artery is exposed and dissected from surrounding tissue; care is taken to preserve the superficial branch of the radial nerve.

6 Clamps are applied to the radial artery, one proximal and one distal to the site where the cephalic vein will be anastomosed.

7 A longitudinal arteriotomy is performed on the radial artery.

8 An end (end of vein) to side (side of artery) anastomosis is performed using non-absorbable monofilament sutures.

9 The arterial clamps are removed, and blood flow is restored.

10 Adequate flow through the fistula is confirmed (a palpable thrill), and the wound is closed in layers.

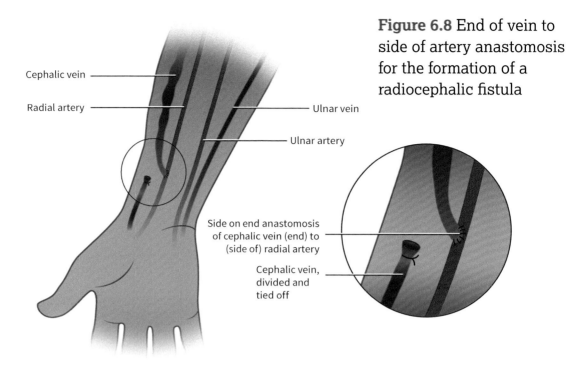

Figure 6.8 End of vein to side of artery anastomosis for the formation of a radiocephalic fistula

Cephalic vein

Radial artery

Ulnar vein

Ulnar artery

Side on end anastomosis of cephalic vein (end) to (side of) radial artery

Cephalic vein, divided and tied off

COMPLICATIONS

Early

> Bleeding and haematoma formation.

> Damage to surrounding structures, specifically the superficial branch of the radial nerve.

> Thrombosis of fistula resulting in failure.

> Early and severe steal syndrome (rarely).

Intermediate and late

> Wound infection.

> Failure of fistula to mature (early fistula failure).

> Excessive vein dilation.

> Stenosis within the vein reducing blood flow and ultimately causing thrombosis.

> Failure of an established fistula due to thrombosis (late fistula failure).

> Steal syndrome—whereby blood is shunted away from the distal circulation and up the AV fistula, causing ischaemic symptoms within the hand.

> Congestive cardiac failure if blood flow through the fistula is very high.

POSTOPERATIVE CARE

Inpatient

> Patients are discharged on the day of surgery.

Outpatient

> Arterialisation of the vein will take approximately 6 weeks. Patients are seen in clinic prior to the AV fistula being used for haemodialysis.

> Patients are warned that tourniquets and blood pressure cuffs, as well as cannulation and venepuncture, should be avoided on the arm with the fistula.

> If there is any concern about the fistula, such as thrombosis, aneurysm, or stenosis, it can be investigated with duplex ultrasound.

SURGEON'S FAVOURITE QUESTION

Why do we make a first attempt at forming a fistula as distally as possible down the arm?

Fistulas have a high failure rate with time, and thus if the first fistula is formed as distally as possible, subsequent attempts can be made, each time moving more proximally.

BELOW KNEE AMPUTATION (BKA)

Madelaine Gimzewska

DEFINITION

Amputation of the lower limb below the level of the knee.

✓ INDICATIONS

Summarised as

- Dead:
  - Potentially life-threatening lower limb ischaemia or necrosis with no safe options for revascularisation.
  - Non-salvageable limb following trauma.
- Dying:
  - Potentially life-threatening infection of the lower limb despite optimal antimicrobial therapy.
  - Malignant tumour of the lower limb (e.g., osteosarcoma).
- Damn nuisance:
  - A lower limb that hampers the functionality of the patient.

✗ CONTRAINDICATIONS

- Patients who are not expected to be independently mobile postoperatively. In these patients, an above knee amputation is more suitable, as the likelihood of successful stump healing is significantly higher for above knee amputation compared to below knee amputation.
- Amputations requested by patients with body dysmorphic syndrome.

ANATOMY

- The lower leg has four compartments: anterior (extensor), lateral (peroneal), superficial posterior (flexor), and deep posterior (flexor).
- The compartments are separated by three fascial layers: the interosseous membrane, the transverse intermuscular septum, and the anterior intermuscular septum.
- Superficial posterior compartment:
  - The superficial posterior compartment is separated from the lateral compartment by the posterior intermuscular septum and from the deep posterior compartment by a fascial layer.
  - Contains the soleus, gastrocnemius, and plantaris muscles.
  - The deep soleal veins are contained in this compartment.
- Deep posterior compartment:
  - The deep posterior compartment is separated from superficial compartment by the posterior intermuscular septum, and from the anterior compartment by the interosseous membrane.
  - Contains the tibialis posterior, flexor hallucis longus, and flexor digitorum longus.

- Importantly, the tibial nerve and the posterior tibial artery descend in the posterior compartment.
- The lateral compartment:
  - The lateral (peroneal) compartment is bounded by the anterior intermuscular septum (anteriorly), the posterior intermuscular septum (posteriorly), and the fibula (medially).
  - It contains the peroneal artery and is supplied by the superficial peroneal nerve together with the deep peroneal nerve, which arises from the bifurcation of the common peroneal nerve as it winds around the head of the fibula.
- The anterior compartment:
  - The anterior compartment is bounded medially by the lateral surface of the tibia and laterally by the extensor surface of the fibular and anterior intermuscular septum.
  - Contains tibialis anterior and extensor digitorum longus.
  - It contains the deep peroneal nerve and anterior tibial artery as it descends the lower leg before transitioning into the dorsalis pedis artery on the dorsal surface of the foot.

Figure 6.9 Compartments of the lower limb (below the knee)

Tibialis posterior

Tibialis anterior

Extensor digitorum longus

Anterior tibial artery

Fibularis brevis and longus

Deep fibular nerve

Superficial fibular nerve

Fibula

Flexor hallucis longus

Gastrocnemius, lateral head

Cutaneous vein

Sural communicating nerve

Short saphenous vein

Tibia

Popliteus

Flexor digitorum longus

Posterior tibial artery and nerve

Long saphenous vein

Fibular artery

Gastrocnemius, medial head

Soleus

Plantaris

Sural nerve

| Anterior compartment | Lateral compartment | Deep posterior compartment | Superficial posterior compartment |

STEP-BY-STEP OPERATION

Anaesthesia: general or regional.

Position: supine with the affected limb exposed and marked.

Considerations: use of a tourniquet—e.g., in patients with bleeding diatheses, patients who are unable to receive blood transfusion (Jehovah's Witness), and young trauma patients (well- vascularised muscle tissue). Stumps can be fashioned in a variety of ways: Burgess flap (long posterior flap), skew flap, or equal anterior-posterior fish-mouth flap. The Burgess flap, the most commonly used flap, is described below.

1 The Burgess flap is marked 10–12 cm distal to the tibial tuberosity. The anterior incision extends across the anterior two-thirds of the leg, and the posterior incision is made more distally and comprises the remaining one-third of the circumference of the leg. It is made long enough so that this posterior flap can wrap over the stump. The transition between the anterior and posterior flaps is gently curved to reduce redundant skin.

2 Muscle and soft tissues of the anterior and lateral compartments are divided.

3 The vascular bundles (anterior tibial and peroneal) are suture-ligated as they are encountered. The long saphenous vein is identified and ligated.

4 The tibial and peroneal nerve are sharply divided and allowed to retract into the soft tissues. The sural nerve is sharply divided 5 cm proximal to the skin edge.

5 The tibia is skeletalised using a periosteal elevator and divided using an oscillating bone saw two fingers' breadth proximal to the skin incision. The cut end is rasped and smoothed over.

6 The fibula is then cut 2 cm proximal to the tibia.

7 Muscles of the deep posterior compartment are then divided at the same level as the tibia. The posterior flap is created using gastrocnemius, superficial tissues, and skin. If it is too bulky, soleus can be excised to allow tension-free closure.

8 The tourniquet is released, and haemostasis is obtained with sutures and/or cautery. A drain can be inserted between the stump and the flaps.

9 The posterior flap is then brought up over the end of the stump to meet the anterior flap, and the muscle fascia is sutured to the tibial periosteum. The fascia and skin are closed in layers.

10 The stump is then dressed simply for protection during healing. Constrictive circumferential dressings should be avoided. The knee is immobilised in a splint or dressing to prevent postoperative knee contracture.

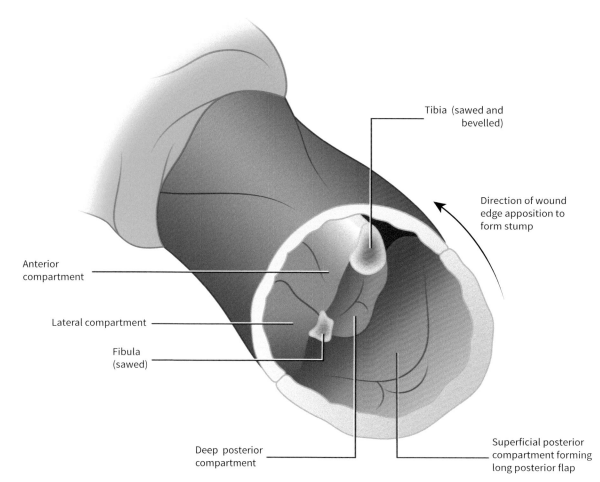

Figure 6.10 Cut surfaces of the tibia, fibula and anterior and posterior compartments in a BKA

COMPLICATIONS

Early
> Bleeding and haematoma formation.

Intermediate and late
> Flap necrosis.
> Mortality—most commonly due to cardiovascular events.
> Infection of the wound or surrounding soft tissues.

> Stump pain.
> Deep Vein Thrombosis (DVT)/Pulmonary Embolism (PE).
> Wound dehiscence and non-healing stump wound.
> Phantom limb pain.
> Flexion contracture of the knee.
> Neuromas.
> Pressure sores from immobility or prosthesis.

POSTOPERATIVE CARE

Inpatient
> The drain is removed when output has fallen to <30mls/24hrs.
> Adequate pain control is critical to aid stump healing—patients often require patient-controlled analgesia following amputation and are started early on neuropathic analgesia.
> Postoperative physiotherapy and occupational therapy services provide vital support and rehabilitation for patients undergoing lower limb amputations.

Outpatient
> Specialist rehabilitation services should be engaged to optimise the opportunity of mobilisation with a prosthetic. A special moulding elastic sock ('Juzo' sock) can be applied from 1 week to help shape the stump ahead of fitting for prostheses; prostheses can be fitted once the stump has fully healed (usually a minimum of 6 weeks).

❓ SURGEON'S FAVOURITE QUESTION

What factors must be considered when deciding upon an amputation level?

1) Likelihood of postoperative ambulation with a BK stump (patient physiology, pre-existing contractures).

2) Likelihood of stump healing (depends on extent of disease/trauma).

ABOVE KNEE AMPUTATION (AKA)

Madelaine Gimzewska

DEFINITION

Amputation of the lower limb between the hip and the knee (transfemoral amputation).

✓ INDICATIONS

Summarised as

- Dead:
  - Potentially life-threatening lower limb ischaemia or necrosis with no safe options for revascularisation.
  - Non-salvageable limb following trauma.
- Dying:
  - Potentially life-threatening infection of the lower limb despite optimal antimicrobial therapy.
- Malignant tumour of the lower limb (e.g., osteosarcoma).
- Damn nuisance:
  - A lower limb that hampers the functionality of the patient.

✗ CONTRAINDICATIONS

- Amputations requested by patients with body dysmorphic syndrome.

ANATOMY

Gross anatomy

- The upper portion of the lower limb is divided into three compartments.
- Anterior compartment—contains the sartorius and quadriceps femoris muscles (comprising the three vastus muscles and rectus femoris), pectineus, iliopsoas, and iliacus. These muscles act to extend the knee.
- Medial compartment—contains the hip flexors (gracilis, obturator externus, adductor brevis, adductor longus, and adductor magnus).
- Posterior compartment—contains the hamstrings (biceps femoris, semitendinosus, and semimembranosus).
- The femur supports the thigh, articulating with the pelvis superiorly and the tibia and patella complex inferiorly.

Neurovasculature

- The sciatic nerve innervates the posterior compartment and is found posterior to the femur.
- The obturator nerve innervates the medial compartment of the thigh.
- The femoral nerve innervates the anterior compartment of the thigh.
- The superficial femoral artery (SFA) and vein (SFV) run in the adductor canal between the anterior and medial compartments.
- The profunda femoris artery and vein run close to the femur in the medial compartment, with branches supplying the muscles of the thigh.
- The great saphenous vein (GSV) runs along the medial aspect of the thigh.

Figure 6.11 Compartments of the lower limb (above the knee)

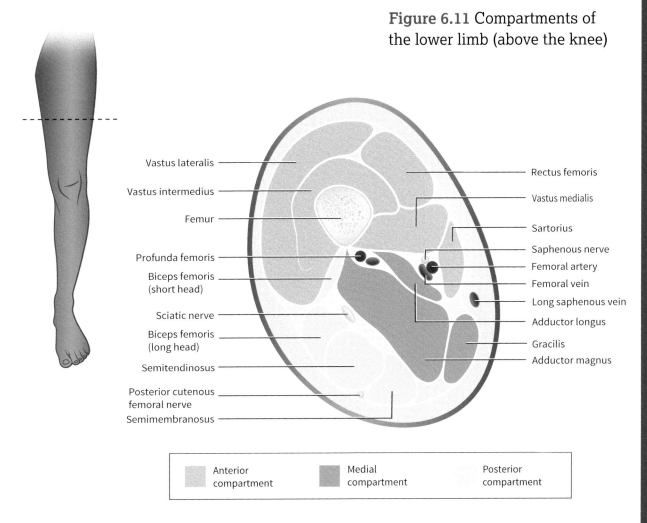

Vastus lateralis

Vastus intermedius

Femur

Profunda femoris

Biceps femoris (short head)

Sciatic nerve

Biceps femoris (long head)

Semitendinosus

Posterior cutenous femoral nerve

Semimembranosus

Rectus femoris

Vastus medialis

Sartorius

Saphenous nerve

Femoral artery

Femoral vein

Long saphenous vein

Adductor longus

Gracilis

Adductor magnus

| Anterior compartment | Medial compartment | Posterior compartment |

STEP-BY-STEP OPERATION

Anaesthesia: general or regional.

Position: supine with the affected limb exposed and marked; bolster placed under ipsilateral buttock.

Considerations: use of a tourniquet—e.g., in patients with bleeding diatheses, patients who are unable to receive blood transfusion (Jehovah's Witness), and young trauma patients (well-vascularised muscle tissue).

1 The skin is prepped and a transversely oriented 'fish-mouth' incision is made proximal to the knee. The anterior and posterior flaps are generally of equal length with the level of bone division 12–15 cm above the superior margin of the knee joint to ensure adequate soft tissue.

2 The fascia and muscles of the anterior and medial compartment are divided with a 'raking' incision; special attention is paid to identifying the GSV (encountered early) and the SFA/SFV bundle (encountered late) so that they can be ligated securely.

3 The femur is skeletalised using a periosteal elevator and divided using an oscillating bone saw two fingers' breadth proximal to the skin incision, ensuring

adequate soft tissue cover. Rasping is generally not required, as the overlying muscle mass is large, but can be considered in a particularly thin patient.

4 The remaining muscles of the posterior compartment are then divided.

5 Special attention is paid to identifying the sciatic nerve, which is then sharply cut and allowed to retract naturally. A sciatic nerve catheter may be inserted to deliver local anaesthetic to the divided sciatic nerve.

6 If used, the tourniquet is then released, and any additional bleeding points are identified and dealt with by either ligation or cautery; a drain can be inserted between the anterior and posterior muscle flaps.

7 The hip is flexed prior to closing the wound; if tension on the wound is seen, the femur should be shortened.

8 The fascia and skin are then closed in layers, with special attention paid to not create 'dog ears'

(out-pouchings of tissue) where the anterior and posterior flaps meet.

9 The stump is then dressed simply for protection during healing. Constrictive circumferential dressings should be avoided.

Figure 6.12 Above knee amputation using 'fish-mouth' incision

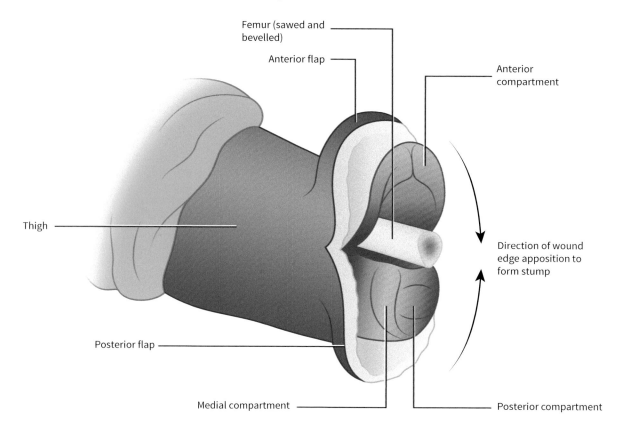

Femur (sawed and bevelled)

Anterior flap

Anterior compartment

Thigh

Direction of wound edge apposition to form stump

Posterior flap

Medial compartment

Posterior compartment

COMPLICATIONS

Early
> Bleeding and haematoma formation.

Intermediate and late
> Deep Vein Thrombosis (DVT)/Pulmonary Embolism (PE).
> Infection of the wound or surrounding soft tissues.
> Flap necrosis.

> Mortality—most commonly due to cardiovascular events.
> Stump pain.
> Phantom limb pain.
> Wound dehiscence and a non-healing stump wound.
> Neuroma formation.
> Pressure sores from immobility.

POSTOPERATIVE CARE

Inpatient

› If inserted, the drain is removed when output has fallen to <30mls/24hrs.

› Adequate pain control is critical to aid stump healing— patients often require patient-controlled analgesia following amputation and are started early on neuropathic analgesia.

› Postoperative physiotherapy and occupational therapy services provide vital support and rehabilitation for patients undergoing lower limb amputations.

Outpatient

› Specialist rehabilitation services should be engaged to optimise the opportunity of mobilisation with a prosthetic (if the patient is likely to mobilise).

› Some centres encourage air-cushioned prosthetic mobilisation for selected individuals within two weeks of the AKA.

❓ SURGEON'S FAVOURITE QUESTION

What percentage of patients are able to mobilise with a prosthetic following an AKA compared to a below knee amputation (BKA)?

Approximately one-third for AKA and two-thirds for BKA.

FEMORAL-POPLITEAL BYPASS GRAFT

Madelaine Gimzewska

DEFINITION

The use of a graft to bypass a section of symptomatic occlusive femoral-popliteal artery disease

---

✓ INDICATIONS

> Patients with critical limb ischaemia or lower limb claudication following failure of medical management who have a diseased superficial femoral artery (SFA) or proximal popliteal artery.

✗ CONTRAINDICATIONS

> Inadequate inflow (insufficient blood flow into the area of stenosis).

> Inadequate outflow (a poor quality distal popliteal artery supplying distal vessels).

> Advanced ischaemic disease requiring amputation.

ANATOMY

> The abdominal aorta bifurcates into the common iliac arteries at the level of L4.

> The common iliac arteries bifurcate into the internal and external iliac arteries, which are responsible for supplying the pelvis and legs, respectively.

> As the external iliac artery passes deep to the inguinal ligament, it transitions to become the common femoral artery (CFA), which immediately emits two branches to the head of the femur (the medial and lateral circumflex arteries).

> The CFA then bifurcates into the profunda femoral artery (PFA) and the SFA.

> The SFA supplies the leg; as it descends through the adductor hiatus, it becomes the popliteal artery, which then passes into the popliteal fossa.

> Within the popliteal fossa, the popliteal artery bifurcates into the anterior tibial artery and the tibioperoneal trunk.

> The tibioperoneal trunk then divides into the posterior tibial and peroneal arteries, which descend the remainder of the leg through the posterior compartment.

> The anterior tibial artery passes through a hiatus in the interosseous membrane between the tibia and fibula and then descends in the anterior compartment of the leg before becoming the dorsalis pedis artery.

> The dorsalis pedis artery, together with the lateral and medial plantar arteries (branches of the posterior tibial artery), supplies blood to the foot.

Figure 6.13 Divisions and branches of the common iliac artery

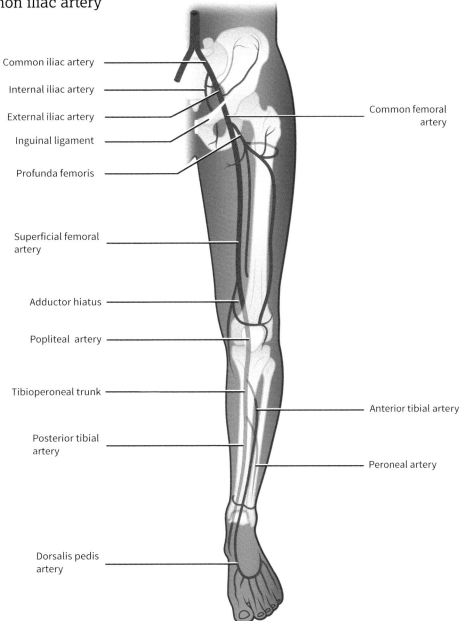

Common iliac artery

Internal iliac artery

External iliac artery

Inguinal ligament

Profunda femoris

Superficial femoral artery

Adductor hiatus

Popliteal artery

Tibioperoneal trunk

Posterior tibial artery

Dorsalis pedis artery

Common femoral artery

Anterior tibial artery

Peroneal artery

STEP-BY-STEP OPERATION

Anaesthesia: general

Position: supine

1 The CFA is identified by palpation, and a groin incision is made longitudinally to expose the CFA, SFA, and PFA, which are then dissected from the surrounding tissues.

2 Sloops are placed around the proximal segment of the CFA and around the SFA and PFA to ready them for clamping later.

3 An incision is made at the site of distal anastomosis:

a For an above knee popliteal artery bypass—the incision is made over the medial aspect of the distal thigh, anterior to the sartorius, exposing the popliteal artery just below the adductor magnus.

b For a below knee popliteal artery bypass—the incision is made along the posterior border of the medial aspect of the tibia.

4 The popliteal artery is then dissected and, using sloops, proximal and distal control are obtained.

5   An incision is made along the length of the great saphenous vein, which is then dissected out from the underlying subcutaneous tissue. The proximal and distal ends of the vein are then clamped, and the branches are ligated.

6   The vein graft can either be left in its natural position (in situ) or be tunnelled more deeply beneath the sartorius muscle in the thigh, then between the two heads of gastrocnemius behind the knee to reach the popliteal artery below the knee. If it is tunnelled, the vein is usually reversed so that the valves do not impede the flow of blood. If the graft is to be left in situ or, if tunnelled, not reversed, then a valvulotome instrument is used to obliterate the valves (if using a prosthetic graft, then steps 5 and 6 are omitted). During a fem-pop bypass, most surgeons will reverse the vein and tunnel deeply. Using an in-situ vein

bypass is more advantageous when the bypass is being extended down to the calf arteries (e.g., the posterior tibial artery), as the vein needs less preparation and this avoids any discrepancy in vessel size that can occur when a reversed vein is used.

7   A bolus of IV heparin is administered.

8   Clamps are applied proximally and distally to the site of anastomosis of the CFA/SFA, and the graft is anastomosed. The graft is run to ensure good flow and to check for any leaks.

9   The vein (or prosthetic graft) is then tunnelled deeply or left in situ, and the distal anastomosis onto the popliteal artery is performed.

10 The clamps are removed, allowing blood to flow through the graft. Distal pulses and foot temperature are checked. The wounds are then closed in layers.

Figure 6.14 Use of a valvulotome to prepare the GSV for anastomosis as a bypass graft

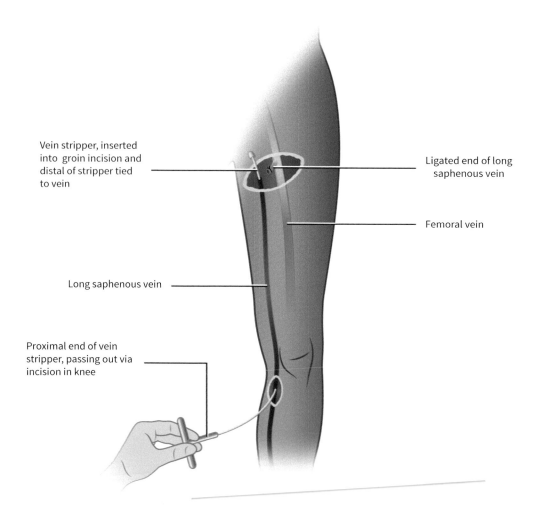

Vein stripper, inserted into groin incision and distal of stripper tied to vein

Ligated end of long saphenous vein

Femoral vein

Long saphenous vein

Proximal end of vein stripper, passing out via incision in knee

Figure 6.15 Femoral-Popliteal bypass graft using the GSV

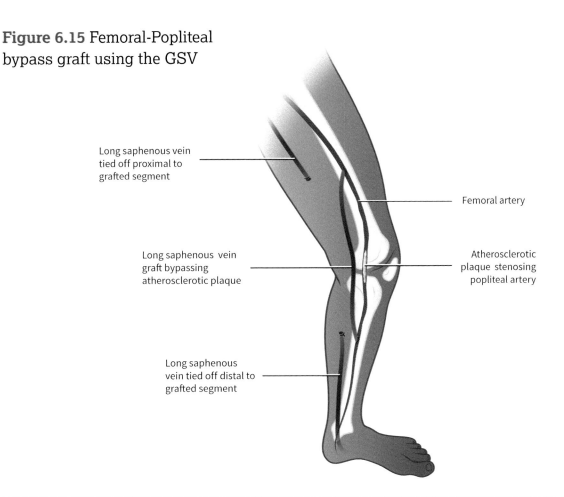

Long saphenous vein tied off proximal to grafted segment

Femoral artery

Long saphenous vein graft bypassing atherosclerotic plaque

Atherosclerotic plaque stenosing popliteal artery

Long saphenous vein tied off distal to grafted segment

COMPLICATIONS

Early
> Bleeding
> Haematoma
> Graft failure
> Nerve damage

Intermediate and late
> Graft infection
> Graft stenosis and/or occlusion
> Wound infection
> Seroma formation
> False aneurysm formation
> Graft occlusion

POSTOPERATIVE CARE

Inpatient
> Patients are encouraged to mobilise day 1 postoperatively.
> Patients are discharged 2–4 days postoperatively with antiplatelet agents (typically clopidogrel).

Outpatient
> Outpatient review at 6 weeks to assess clinical response and to perform duplex ultrasound surveillance of the graft.
> All efforts must be made to modify lifestyle and vascular risk factors in order to maximise long-term benefit and graft longevity.

 SURGEON'S FAVOURITE QUESTION

Where does the SFA become the popliteal artery?

When it passes through the adductor magnus hiatus.

EMBOLECTOMY

Madelaine Gimzewska

DEFINITION
Removal of embolus from a blood conduit, most commonly an artery.

✓ INDICATIONS

- Emergency:
  - Acute upper limb ischaemia caused by brachial artery occlusion (less likely limb threatening but often causes limb claudication).
  - Acute lower limb ischemia caused by the blockage of an artery (aorta, iliac, femoral, or popliteal) by an embolism.

✗ CONTRAINDICATIONS

- Acute arterial thrombosis in a patient with chronic peripheral arterial disease—these cases should be considered for alternative techniques (e.g., bypass, endarterectomy, or balloon angioplasty with or without stenting).
- Non-viable limb—in these cases, an amputation should be performed or end-of-life care provided.

ANATOMY

Gross anatomy

- The abdominal aorta bifurcates into the common iliac arteries at the level of L4.
- The common iliac arteries bifurcate into the internal and external iliac arteries, which are responsible for supplying the pelvis and legs, respectively.
- As the external iliac artery passes deep to the inguinal ligament, it transitions to become the common femoral artery (CFA), which immediately emits two branches to the head of the femur (the medial and lateral circumflex arteries).
- The CFA then bifurcates into the profunda femoral artery (PFA) and superficial femoral artery (SFA).
- The SFA supplies the leg; as it descends through the adductor hiatus, it becomes the popliteal artery, which then passes into the popliteal fossa.
- Within the popliteal fossa, the popliteal artery bifurcates into the anterior tibial artery and the tibioperoneal trunk.

- The tibioperoneal trunk then divides into the posterior tibial and peroneal arteries, which descend the remainder of the leg through the posterior compartment.
- The anterior tibial artery passes through a hiatus in the interosseous membrane between the tibia and fibular and then descends in the anterior compartment of the leg before becoming the dorsalis pedis artery.
- The dorsalis pedis artery, together with the lateral and medial plantar arteries (branches of the posterior tibial artery), supply blood to the foot.

Pathology

- Limb arterial emboli may originate from any proximal arterial flow location—from the left atrium to the segment of artery immediately proximal to the embolism.

Figure 6.16 Divisions and branches
of the common iliac artery

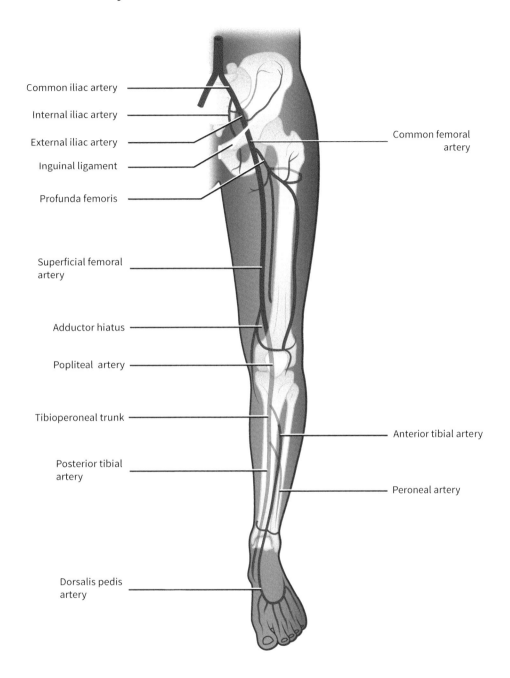

Common iliac artery

Internal iliac artery

External iliac artery

Inguinal ligament

Profunda femoris

Common femoral
artery

Superficial femoral
artery

Adductor hiatus

Popliteal artery

Tibioperoneal trunk

Anterior tibial artery

Posterior tibial
artery

Peroneal artery

Dorsalis pedis
artery

STEP-BY-STEP OPERATION

Anaesthesia: general or local.

Position: supine.

1 The artery through which the embolectomy will be performed is exposed (most commonly the CFA and, more rarely, the below-knee popliteal artery in cases of lower limb emboli or the brachial artery in upper limb emboli).

2 Proximal and distal arterial control is established by applying vascular slings to the artery on either side of the intended arteriotomy site. The slings are held under tension.

VASCULAR

3 IV heparin is given if the patient has not been heparinised preoperatively.

4 An arteriotomy is performed proximal to the site of the embolism (longitudinal arteriotomies are used in severely diseased arteries, but in arteries with little disease, a transverse incision is preferred, as a longitudinal incision requires a patch for closure to prevent stenosis).

5 A Fogarty catheter (2–4 French) is passed into the distal arterial segment and guided past the site of anticipated occlusion.

6 The balloon is inflated beyond the embolism, then the catheter is gently withdrawn in a continuous fashion, adjusting the balloon pressure en route as required (the clot will be captured by the balloon and is pulled out of the arteriotomy).

7 This process is then repeated, both distally and proximally, until no further clots remains.

8 A heparin saline flush is then administered into the artery.

9 Proximal inflow is checked by releasing tension on the proximal vascular sling or clamp, and steps 6–8 are repeated as required. An on-table angiogram may be performed to confirm the degree of arterial patency. If the risk of compartment syndrome is high, prophylactic fasciotomies are performed.

10 The artery is once again flushed with heparin and the arteriotomy closed (primary closure or using patch). Heparin is then continued postoperatively.

Figure 6.17 Passing of a Fogarty catheter to clear a distal embolus

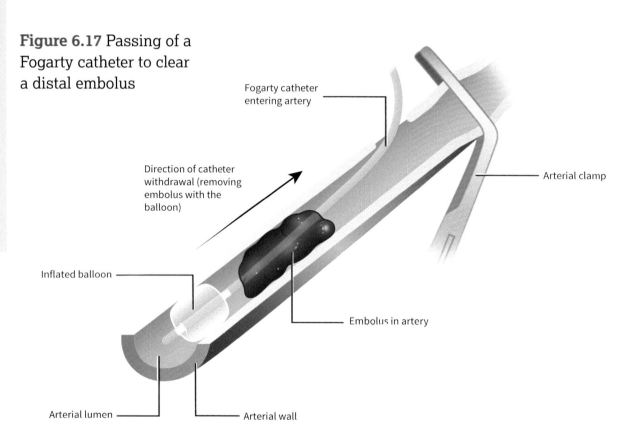

Fogarty catheter entering artery

Direction of catheter withdrawal (removing embolus with the balloon)

Arterial clamp

Inflated balloon

Embolus in artery

Arterial lumen

Arterial wall

COMPLICATIONS

Early

▸ Reperfusion injury causing compartment syndrome.
▸ Bleeding—can range from a small haematoma to active bleeding from the wound requiring a return to theatre.
▸ Haematoma.
▸ Nerve injury.
▸ Recurrent embolisation.

Intermediate and late

▸ Wound infection.
▸ Lymph leak.
▸ Re-occlusion.

POSTOPERATIVE CARE

Inpatient

▸ Patients should be continued on an anticoagulant postoperatively (usually heparin) and then be commenced on anticoagulation therapy prior to discharge.

▸ In order to appropriately inform the patient of the duration of anticoagulation, the source/cause for the thromboembolism should be investigated prior to discharge (echocardiogram, 24hr ECG tape, CT/MR angiogram of the proximal arterial tree, and thrombophilia screening).

Outpatient

▸ Follow-up in vascular clinic is not routinely required unless further disease amenable to intervention has been identified.

🗨 SURGEON'S FAVOURITE QUESTION

What is the purpose of commencing anticoagulation preoperatively?

The aim of anticoagulation is to reduce the chance of further emboli and to prevent thrombus forming around the occluding embolus, making the ischaemia worse and making it more difficult to treat.

FEMORAL ENDARTERECTOMY

James Cragg

DEFINITION
Removal of an atherosclerotic plaque from a stenosed or occluded femoral artery. It may be undertaken in isolation or be undertaken to facilitate a bypass procedure.

✓ INDICATIONS

▸ Intermittent claudication causing intolerable symptoms despite a trial of medical management.
▸ Patients with critical limb ischaemia (rest pain, ulceration, gangrene, and tissue loss) and proven femoral arterial stenosis or occlusion.

✗ CONTRAINDICATIONS

▸ Patients with multi-level disease not amenable to revascularisation. In this situation, the improvement in perfusion would be inadequate for the underlying problem or the patient is not considered fit enough to tolerate the procedure with an acceptable risk of complications.

ANATOMY

▸ The external iliac artery becomes the common femoral artery (CFA) at the mid-inguinal point (halfway between the pubic symphysis and the anterior superior iliac spine (ASIS) within the femoral triangle).
▸ The femoral triangle contains, from lateral to medial: the femoral nerve, artery, and vein (NAV-Y fronts). The iliopsoas, pectineus, and adductor longus muscles form the floor of the femoral triangle; the roof is formed by the fascia lata. Its lateral border is the medial border of sartorius, medial border of adductor longus, and superior border of the inguinal ligament.
▸ Within the femoral triangle, the CFA immediately emits two branches to the head of femur—the medial and lateral circumflex arteries. The CFA then bifurcates into the profunda femoral artery (PFA) and the superficial femoral artery (SFA).

▸ The SFA supplies the leg; as it descends through the adductor hiatus, it becomes the popliteal artery, which then passes into the popliteal fossa.
▸ Within the popliteal fossa, the popliteal artery bifurcates into the anterior tibial artery and the tibioperoneal trunk.
▸ The tibioperoneal trunk then divides into the posterior tibial and peroneal arteries, which descend the remainder of the leg through the posterior compartment.
▸ The anterior tibial artery passes through a hiatus in the interosseous membrane between the tibia and fibula and then descends in the anterior compartment of the leg before becoming the dorsalis pedis artery.
▸ The dorsalis pedis artery, together with the lateral and medial plantar arteries (branches of the posterior tibial artery), supplies blood to the foot.

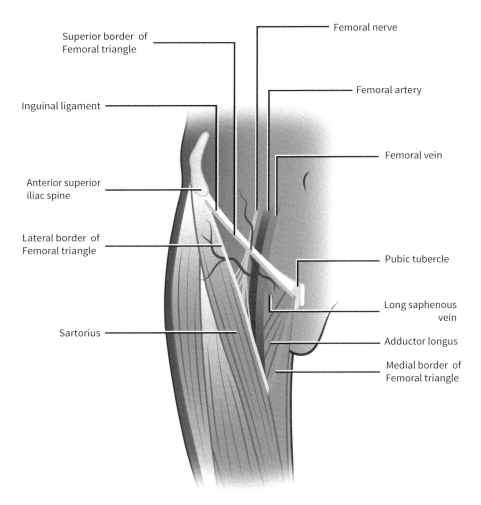

Superior border of Femoral triangle

Femoral nerve

Inguinal ligament

Femoral artery

Anterior superior iliac spine

Femoral vein

Lateral border of Femoral triangle

Pubic tubercle

Long saphenous vein

Sartorius

Adductor longus

Medial border of Femoral triangle

Figure 6.18 Borders and contents of the femoral triangle

STEP-BY-STEP OPERATION

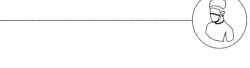

Anaesthesia: general or neuraxial (epidural or spinal).
Position: supine.

1 The femoral artery is located by palpating the femoral pulse. The pulse may not be palpable in a heavily calcified artery; in this instance, the incision is guided by anatomical landmarks and/or ultrasound.

2 A longitudinal incision is made over the CFA, which is then dissected from the surrounding tissues.

3 The dissection is continued inferiorly to expose the PFA and SFA. Once exposed, they are slooped for later clamping.

4 Side branches of the CFA are dissected and controlled with slings to prevent back-bleeding during the endarterectomy.

5 The patient is administered a bolus of IV heparin and the slooped CFA, PFA, and SFA are clamped.

6 An incision is made along the length of the diseased artery (a longitudinal arteriotomy) to reveal any atherosclerotic plaque surrounding the lumen.

7 The plaque is then removed from the inside of the arterial wall using blunt dissection.

8 The artery is closed by either primary intention (rarely) or by using a patch (autologous vein patch, bovine pericardium, Dacron, or Gore-Tex) to prevent a stenosis (by closing directly) and to slightly increase the vessel diameter.

9 Just before the completion of the arterial closure, the clamps are removed and reapplied sequentially to ensure any clot is flushed out of the arteriotomy.

10 The arterial clamps are removed, the distal pulses are checked, and the foot is assessed for perfusion. The wound is then closed in layers.

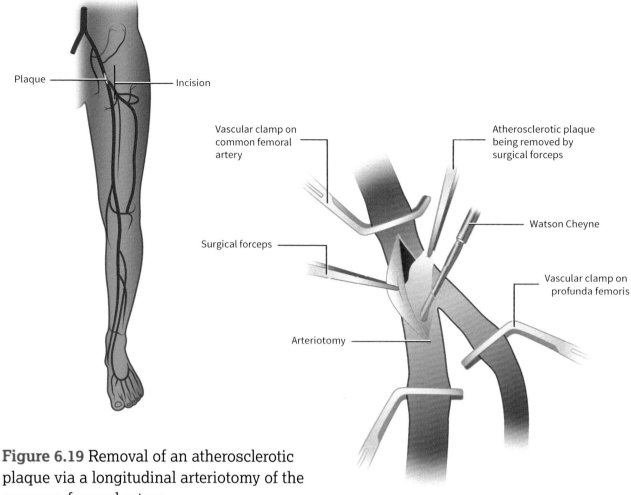

Figure 6.19 Removal of an atherosclerotic plaque via a longitudinal arteriotomy of the common femoral artery

COMPLICATIONS

Early

> Bleeding.
> Haematoma.
> Arterial thrombosis.
> Distal embolisation/trash foot.

Intermediate and late

> Leak of lymphatic fluid.
> Wound infection.
> Patch infection.
> Re-occlusion.
> Pseudoaneurysm.

POSTOPERATIVE CARE

Inpatient

> Patients typically discharged after 1–2 days.
> Anticoagulant medication (clopidogrel) and high-dose statins are commenced prior to discharge.

Outpatient

> Patients are followed up in vascular clinic at 6 weeks.

SURGEON'S FAVOURITE QUESTIONS

What is the difference between the mid-inguinal point and the midpoint of the inguinal ligament?

The mid-inguinal point is halfway between the pubic symphysis and the ASIS and is the location of the femoral artery. The midpoint of the inguinal ligament, between the ASIS and the pubic tubercle, marks the deep ring.

ENDOVENOUS LASER TREATMENT FOR VARICOSE VEINS (EVLT)

James Cragg

DEFINITION

Laser ablation of varicose veins.

✓ INDICATIONS

Symptomatic varicose veins (pain, leg heaviness, swelling, itching):

> Persistent veins unresponsive to 3 months of medical management.

> Documented reflux within the truncal superficial veins—i.e., great saphenous vein (GSV) or short saphenous vein (SSV).

✗ CONTRAINDICATIONS

Relative contraindications

> Pre-existing cellulitis over the puncture site(s).

> Previously failed EVLT.

> Previous deep vein thrombosis.

Absolute contraindications

> Previous phlebitis (indicating the vein for treatment is occluded).

> Acute deep vein thrombosis.

> Pregnancy.

ANATOMY

> The superficial venous system of the leg comprises the GSV and the SSV.

> The GSV arises from the dorsal venous arch of the foot and the dorsal vein of the great toe.

> The GSV ascends along the medial aspect of the lower leg, anterior to the medial malleolus and across the posterior border of the medial condyle of the femur, before then running along the medial border of sartorius to anastomose with the common femoral (deep) vein at the saphenofemoral junction (SFJ) in the femoral triangle.

> The long saphenous nerve runs adjacent to the GSV and transmits sensation from the antero-medial leg and knee.

> The SSV arises from the dorsal venous arch of the foot and the dorsal vein of the little toe and passes posterior to the lateral malleolus and ascends the posterior aspect of the calf. It then passes between the two heads of gastrocnemius and drains into the popliteal (deep) vein in the popliteal fossa.

> The sural nerve runs adjacent to the SSV in the distal calf and transmits sensation from the lateral foot and fifth toe.

> Named perforating veins run between the deep and superficial systems. They are: Hunter's, Dodd's, Boyd's, and Cockett's.

Figure 6.20 Venous drainage
of the lower limb

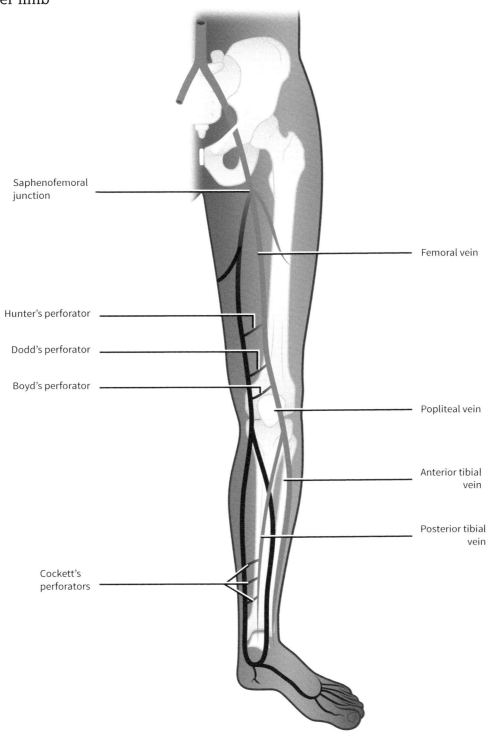

Saphenofemoral
junction

Femoral vein

Hunter's perforator

Dodd's perforator

Boyd's perforator

Popliteal vein

Anterior tibial
vein

Posterior tibial
vein

Cockett's
perforators

VASCULAR

STEP-BY-STEP OPERATION

Anaesthesia: local anaesthetic around the puncture site.
Position: prone for SSV and supine for GSV treatment.

1 Ultrasound is used to map the course of the vein and identify an appropriate segment for treatment.

2 Dilute local anaesthetic is injected into and around the puncture site (most commonly the most distal straight section of vein available).

3 A needle is passed into either the GSV or SSV, through which a guide wire is passed up into the vein. The needle is then removed.

4 A sheath is then passed over the guide wire, and the wire is removed, leaving the sheath in situ. The laser fibre is passed through the sheath (a red light can be seen through the skin above where the tip of the probe lies).

5 The position of the tip of the probe is checked with ultrasound (at least 2 cm distal to the SFJ within the GSV).

6 To compress the wall of the vein against the laser probe and to protect tissues, dilute local anaesthetic (typically 250 mls) is injected under ultrasound guidance around the entire length of the vein.

7 The laser fibre is switched on and is then progressively withdrawn down the length of the vein at a rate of 10 seconds per 1 cm.

8 Foam sclerotherapy injections or direct avulsion of tortuous tributaries not treated by the laser can be performed subsequently.

9 Direct pressure is applied to the puncture sites to control bleeding.

10 Compression bandaging should be applied and left in place for 48 hours, to then be replaced by thigh-length compression stockings.

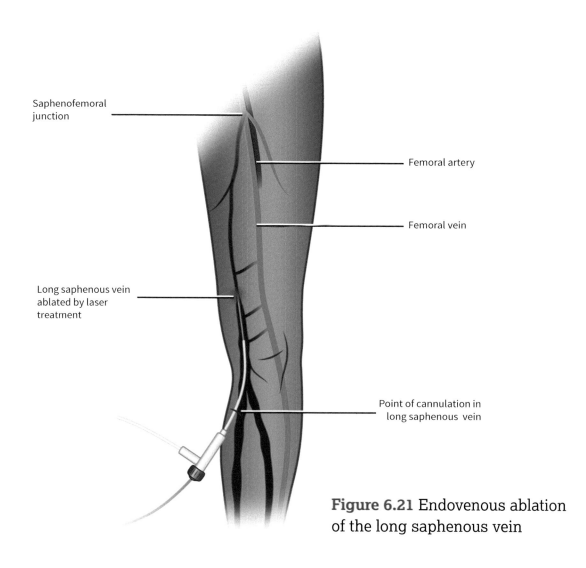

Saphenofemoral junction

Femoral artery

Femoral vein

Long saphenous vein ablated by laser treatment

Point of cannulation in long saphenous vein

Figure 6.21 Endovenous ablation of the long saphenous vein

COMPLICATIONS

Early

- Superficial thrombophlebitis.
- Bleeding.
- Haematoma.
- Thermal injury to the skin and surrounding tissues.

Intermediate and late

- Infection of the wound or deeper soft tissues.
- Permanent skin discolouration secondary to thermal injury.
- Damage to the saphenous nerve resulting in numbness, chronic pain, or neuropathy.
- Deep Vein Thrombosis (DVT).
- Recurrence of varicosities.

POSTOPERATIVE CARE

Inpatient

- EVLT is usually performed as a day case, and patients are discharged once the local anaesthesia has worn off and pain is adequately controlled with simple analgesia whilst mobilising.

Outpatient

- Compression stockings are worn for at least 7 days postoperatively.
- No routine follow-up is required unless the need for further intervention is considered likely.

❓ SURGEON'S FAVOURITE QUESTION

What does the term 'laser' stand for?

The term 'laser' is an acronym for 'light amplification by stimulated emission of radiation'.

7 UROLOGY

EVGENIA THEODORAKOPOULOU

TRANS-URETHRAL RESECTION OF THE PROSTATE (TURP)

Kirsty Dawson

DEFINITION
Endoscopic removal of the inner portion of the prostate gland via the urethra.

✓ INDICATIONS

- Benign Prostatic Hypertrophy (BPH) causing refractory or chronic bladder outlet obstruction unresponsive to medical management.
- Recurrent urinary tract infections and urinary retention due to bladder outlet obstruction.
- Recurrent frank haematuria caused by prostatic pathology.
- Symptomatic relief in prostate cancer where radical prostatectomy is not possible.

✗ CONTRAINDICATIONS

- Active urinary infection.
- Coagulopathy.
- Where a TURP procedure would last longer than 60–90 minutes (e.g., grossly enlarged prostate).
- Presence of complex urethral disease (e.g., strictures or hypospadias) that may prevent instrumentation.

ANATOMY

Gross anatomy
- The prostate is a walnut-sized exocrine gland surrounding the prostatic urethra in males.
- The prostate lies posterior to the pubic symphysis, inferior to the bladder, and anterior to the rectum.
- The ejaculatory ducts enter the postero-superior prostate, opening into the verumontanum (colliculus seminalis) of the urethra. Resection distal to the verumontanum during TURP increases the risk of damaging the urethral sphincter.

Neurovasculature
- The prostate's autonomic nerve supply arises from the the inferior hypogastric plexus.
- The prostate receives its arterial supply from the inferior vesical artery (a branch of the internal iliac artery), which bifurcates into the:
  - Urethral artery—supplies the transitional zone of the prostate.
  - Capsular artery— supplies the glandular tissue of the prostate.

- The prostate drains via the prostatic plexus, which receives blood via the dorsal vein of the penis and then communicates with the pudendal and vesical plexuses. It drains into the internal iliac vein.

Histology
- The prostate is composed of glandular and non-glandular (muscle or fibrous) tissue.
- It comprises four histological zones:
  1. Central—surrounds the ejaculatory ducts.
  2. Peripheral—most prostatic cancers arise here.
  3. Anterior fibromuscular stroma.
  4. Transitional—surrounds the urethra and is the site of BPH; comprises two lateral and one median lobe.
- Hypertrophy of the transition zone causes obstruction of the prostatic urethra, compressing the peripheral fibromuscular tissue to create a surrounding 'surgical capsule'.

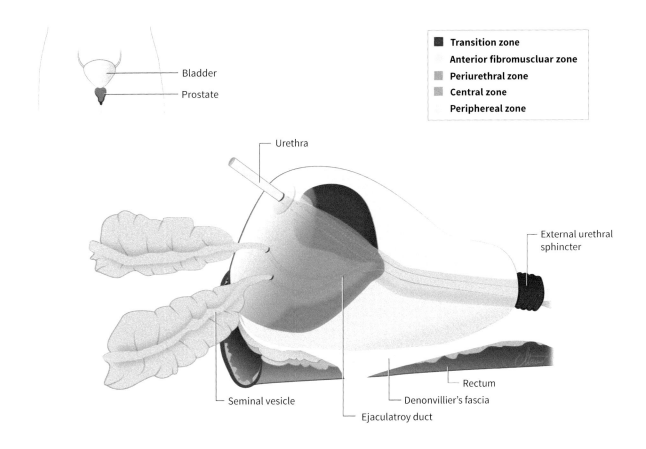

Transition zone
Anterior fibromuscluar zone
Periurethral zone
Central zone
Periphereal zone

Bladder

Prostate

Urethra

External urethral sphincter

Rectum

Denonvillier's fascia

Seminal vesicle

Ejaculatroy duct

Figure 7.1 Gross anatomy and histology of the prostate gland

STEP-BY-STEP OPERATION

Anaesthesia: general or spinal.

Position: lithotomy.

Considerations: Preoperatively, patients should have a sterile urine sample confirmed by urinalysis. At induction, a dose of IV antibiotics is administered.

1 The urethral meatus of the penis is lubricated with local anaesthetic gel. A narrow meatus may first require dilatation.

2 The resectoscope is passed into the lower urinary tract through the meatus, and continuous irrigation of the lower urinary tract is commenced.

3 As the resectoscope is passed throughout the lower urinary tract and into the bladder, all components of the tract are examined to exclude other pathology (e.g., tumours/urethral stricture/bladder calculi).

4 The verumontanum is identified and used as the distal landmark to avoid damage to the external sphincter.

5 Using a diathermy loop, the prostate is resected. If using monopolar diathermy, salt-free irrigation solution should be used to prevent the conduction of current through the fluid.

6 The bladder is irrigated with an Ellik evacuator to retrieve the prostatic fragments for histological analysis.

7 Prior to the removal of instruments, the tract is carefully observed for bleeding, as haemostatic control must first be achieved.

8 A large-bore three-way catheter is then inserted for postoperative bladder irrigation.

UROLOGY

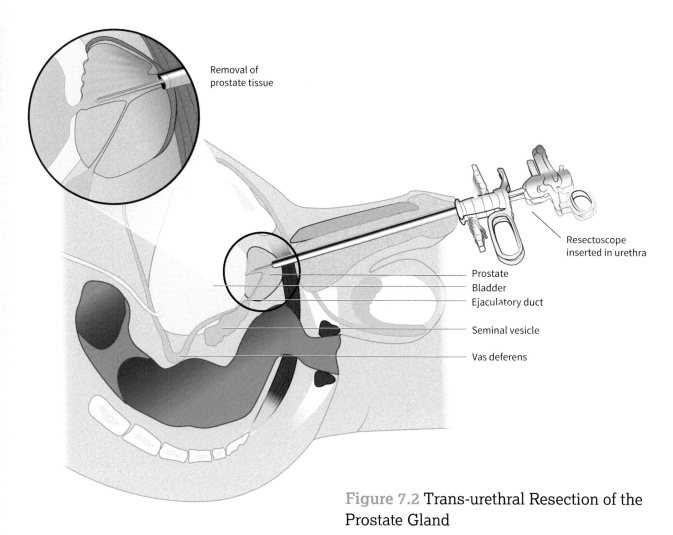

Removal of
prostate tissue

Resectoscope
inserted in urethra

Prostate
Bladder
Ejaculatory duct

Seminal vesicle

Vas deferens

Figure 7.2 Trans-urethral Resection of the
Prostate Gland

COMPLICATIONS

Early

‣ Urinary tract infection.
‣ Haemorrhage and clot retention, commonly presenting as haematuria or loss of urine output.
‣ Transurethral resection (TUR) syndrome—excessive absorption of irrigation fluid causing volume overload, electrolyte disturbance (hyponatraemia and hyperkalaemia), disseminated intravascular coagulopathy, and acute renal failure.

Intermediate and late

‣ Urinary incontinence—injury to the external sphincter, which can be temporary or permanent.
‣ Impotence—injury to the prostatic plexus.
‣ Retrograde ejaculation—injury of the internal sphincter system.
‣ Urethral injury with resultant strictures.
‣ Bladder perforation.
‣ Rectal injury—most common in cases of previous prostate resection or radiotherapy.

POSTOPERATIVE CARE

Inpatient

> The large-bore three-way catheter should remain in situ 6–24 hours after surgery with continuous irrigation to remove blood clots and debris from the prostate and urethra. If bleeding persists, the catheter may remain in until the urine becomes clear.

> Patients are commonly discharged after 1–2 days.

> A trial without catheter (TWOC) is attempted prior to discharge, if this fails, patients are re-catheterised, discharged with the catheter in situ, and return to clinical for a repeat TWOC in 1 week.

Outpatient

> Patients are seen in outpatient clinic at 4–6 weeks.

> Patients should be advised they may still experience symptoms of increased urinary frequency and clots for up to 6 weeks.

SURGEON'S FAVOURITE QUESTION

What are the symptoms of BPH?

These are known as lower urinary tract symptoms (LUTS) and include: sensation of incomplete voiding, hesitancy, straining, poor flow, terminal dribbling, urgency, frequency, nocturia and dysuria.

TRANS-URETHRAL RESECTION OF BLADDER TUMOUR (TURBT)

Louis Hainsworth

DEFINITION

Endoscopic access of the bladder via the urethra for diagnostic, staging, and therapeutic purposes.

✓ INDICATIONS

- Biopsy to investigate suspected bladder malignancy, or to guide treatment.
- Removal of macroscopic non-invasive bladder tumours.
- Debulking of large tumours prior to further treatment (e.g., chemotherapy/radiotherapy).
- Palliation of symptoms in advanced disease.

✗ CONTRAINDICATIONS

- Active urinary tract infection.
- Carcinoma in situ (tumours are often diffuse and therefore difficult to identify and remove).
- Untreated coagulopathy.

ANATOMY

Gross anatomy

- The bladder is a highly distensible muscular structure lying posterior to the pubic symphysis.
- The bladder wall consists of four distinct layers:
  1. Mucosa—composed of transitional epithelium (urothelium).
  2. Lamina propria.
  3. Muscular layer—detrusor muscle/muscularis propria, the fibres of which are organised in three layers: inner longitudinal layer, middle circumferential layer, outer longitudinal layer.
  4. Perivesical soft tissue.
- The trigone is a triangular region of the bladder bordered by the internal urethral opening and the right and left ureteric openings. The superior border of the trigone (interureteric ridge) is folded and raised, lying between the ureteral orifices.
- The urethra runs from the neck of the bladder to the external urethral orifice. In females, it is approximately 4–5 cm long, running along the pelvic floor, and firmly attached to the anterior vaginal wall. In males, it is approximately 20 cm long, passing through the prostate, pelvic floor, perineal membrane, and penis. It is therefore divided into three sections: prostatic, membranous, and spongy.

Neurovasculature

- The parasympathetic fibres are motor to the detrusor muscle and inhibitory to the internal urethral sphincter.
- The sympathetic fibres innervate the neck and trigone of the bladder.
- The obturator nerve (L2–4) is responsible for sensation of the medial thigh and motor innervation of the hip adductors. Intraoperative stimulation of the obturator nerve during a TURBT can result in violent adductor muscle spasming, causing an increased risk of bladder wall perforation. As such, an obturator nerve block may be used to minimise this risk.
- The bladder receives its arterial supply via the superior and inferior vesical arteries (branches of the internal iliac arteries).
- Additional supply is from the obturator and inferior gluteal artery and the uterine and vaginal arteries in females.
- The venous drainage of the bladder is via a plexus terminating in the internal iliac veins.

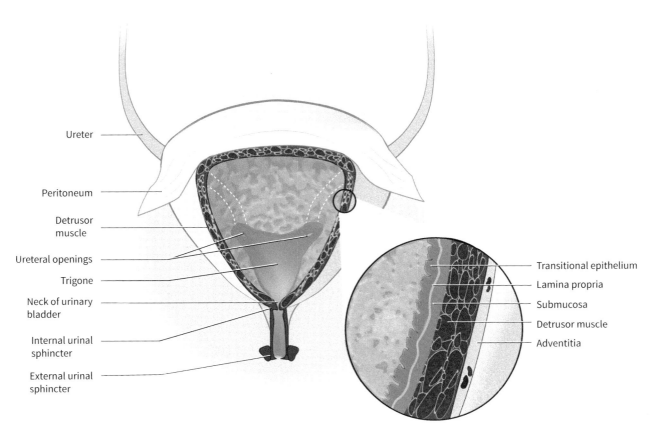

Figure 7.3 Gross anatomy and histology of the bladder

STEP-BY-STEP OPERATION

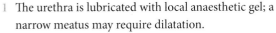

Anaesthesia: general or spinal.

Position: lithotomy.

Considerations: Preoperatively, patients should have a sterile urine sample confirmed by urinalysis. At induction, a dose of IV antibiotics is administered.

1 The urethra is lubricated with local anaesthetic gel; a narrow meatus may require dilatation.

2 A resectoscope is passed via the urethral meatus into the bladder, and continuous irrigation of the lower urinary tract is initiated (to allow for adequate distention for visualisation and access). To avoid over-distension of the bladder, fluid and electrolyte status should be monitored carefully.

3 Once the resectoscope is within the bladder, the whole bladder is surveyed to identify the location, number, and size of tumours.

4 Using diathermy, vessels supplying the tumour(s) are coagulated to reduce bleeding during the resection.

5 The resectoscope is then used to separate the tumour base from the bladder wall and to obtain diagnostic samples (importantly, samples of the tumour margin must also be taken to determine complete resection and enable staging).

6 Diathermy is used to coagulate any remaining bleeding points.

7 Following resection, the specimen is collected with a bladder syringe or Ellik evacuator.

8 A final survey of the lower urinary tract is performed to ensure haemostasis, and the resectoscope is removed.

9 A large-bore three-way catheter is then inserted for postoperative bladder irrigation.

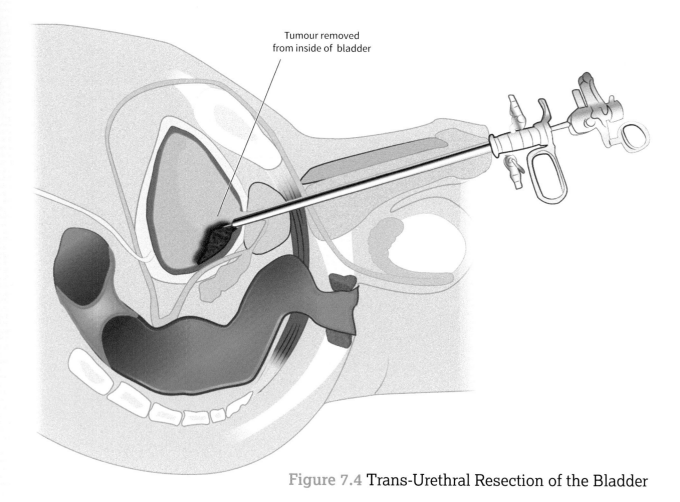

Tumour removed
from inside of bladder

Figure 7.4 Trans-Urethral Resection of the Bladder

COMPLICATIONS

Early

> Urinary tract infection.
> Haemorrhage and clot retention, commonly presenting as haematuria or loss of urine output.
> Transurethral Resection (TUR) Syndrome— excessive absorption of irrigation fluid causing volume overload, electrolyte disturbance (hyponatraemia and hyperkalaemia), disseminated intravascular coagulopathy, and acute renal failure.

Intermediate and late

> Urinary incontinence (temporary or permanent) due to injury to the external urethral sphincter.
> Impotence due to injury to the prostatic plexus.
> Retrograde ejaculation due to injury of the internal sphincter system.
> Urethral injury with resultant strictures.
> Bladder perforation.
> Vesicoureteral reflux.
> Obstructive uropathy with hydronephrosis.

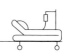

POSTOPERATIVE CARE

Inpatient

> The large-bore three-way catheter should remain in situ 6–24 hours after surgery with continuous irrigation to remove blood clots and debris from the prostate and urethra. If bleeding persists, the catheter may remain in until the urine becomes clear.

> Uncomplication procedures can be performed as a day case.

Outpatient

> Further follow-up depends on histological findings and indications of surgery.

![icon] **SURGEON'S FAVOURITE QUESTION**

Where do squamous cell bladder cancers most commonly develop?

The urothelium of the trigone and lateral walls.

NEPHRECTOMY

Darren Chan and Evgenia Theodorakopoulou

DEFINITION

Surgical removal of all or part of the kidney, through an open or laparoscopic approach. Nephrectomy may be:

› Simple—only the kidney is excised.
› Radical—structures surrounding the kidney (peri-renal fascia, adrenal glands, peri-renal fat, and lymphatics) are also excised.
› Partial/nephron-sparing surgery (NSS)—the kidney is partially resected, preserving as much of the renal parenchyma as possible.

✓ INDICATIONS

› Radical nephrectomy:
  › Renal cell carcinoma (RCC).
  › Palliation for advanced/metastatic malignancy to relieve pain/haematuria/paraneoplastic syndrome.
› Simple nephrectomy:
  › Recurrent, severe renal calculi failing medical and first-line surgical management.
  › Chronic and severe pyelonephritis that fails to respond adequately to medical management.
  › Hypertension secondary to renal artery disease (nephrosclerosis).
  › Obstructive uropathy with non-functioning kidney.
  › Congenital anomalies—polycystic kidney disease causing significant symptoms.

› Living-donor transplantation (donor nephrectomy).
› Trauma.
› Partial nephrectomy/NSS:
  › Small, solitary, localised tumours.
  › Same indications as for simple or radical nephrectomy where a simple or radical approach would result in renal failure—bilateral disease, single functioning kidney, existing/imminent renal impairment.
  › Segmental parenchymal damage due to calculus and trauma.

✗ CONTRAINDICATIONS

› Advanced/metastatic disease where nephrectomy would not have therapeutic/palliative benefit.

ANATOMY

Gross anatomy

› The kidneys are paired retroperitoneal structures extending from the T12–L3 vertebral levels.
› The right kidney is positioned slightly lower than the left kidney due to the liver positioned superiorly on the right side.
› The kidneys, adrenals, and their surrounding peri-renal fat are enveloped by peri-renal (Gerota's) fascia, a dense connective tissue sheath.
› The renal parenchyma is divided into the outer cortex and the inner medulla, which feeds into the renal hilum, a recessed area containing the renal artery and vein, renal pelvis, hilar fat, and lymphatic tissue.

Neurovasculature

› The kidneys receive their innervation via the renal plexus with sympathetic fibres causing vasoconstriction.
› The kidneys receive their blood supply via the left and right renal arteries (branches of the abdominal aorta). Each renal artery branches into segmental vessels, which undergo multiple divisions, supplying the renal parenchyma and becoming the afferent glomerular arterioles.
› The right renal artery is lower than the left and has a longer course, passing posterior to the inferior vena cava (the renal arteries run posterior to the veins).
› The kidneys drain into the left and right renal veins, which drain into the inferior vena cava (IVC).
› The left renal vein is longer and receives tributaries from the phrenic, adrenal, and gonadal veins.

> Lymphatic drainage is into the lateral aortic (lumbar) nodes.

Histology

> The nephron is the functional unit of the kidney.

> Filtration commences at the renal corpuscle of the nephron (Bowman's capsule and glomerulus).

> The subsequent draining sequence is as follows: renal corpuscles → renal tubules → collecting ducts → papillae of renal pyramids → 10–12 minor calyxes → 3–4 major calyxes → renal pelvis.

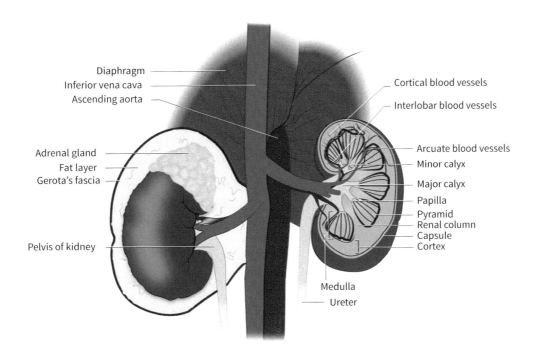

Figure 7.5 Gross anatomy and histology of the kidney

STEP-BY-STEP OPERATION

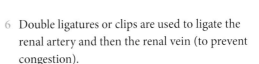

Anaesthesia: general.

Position: lateral decubitus.

1 A 10–12 cm incision is made into the flank, accessing the peritoneum.

2 The colon is freed by incising laterally along the white line of Toldt (an avascular plane in the lateral reflection of the posterior parietal peritoneum over the mesentery of the ascending and descending colon) and is then reflected medially to expose Gerota's fascia (in left-sided nephrectomies, the splenocolic and lienophrenic ligaments are divided, enabling mobilisation of the spleen to minimise risk of injury).

3 The intra-abdominal viscera, vessels, and lymph nodes are examined for metastatic disease.

4 Gerota's fascia is dissected to access the kidney and adrenal gland. The peri-nephric fat is excised to visualise the hilar structures.

5 The renal vein is palpated to identify a tumour thrombus (if present, this necessitates ligation close to or at the IVC).

6 Double ligatures or clips are used to ligate the renal artery and then the renal vein (to prevent congestion).

7 The ureter is identified and ligated. This is then followed by the gonadal and adrenal vessels, lymphatics. and nerves. This process allows for mobilisation of the kidney, adrenals. and surrounding peri-renal fat/fascia.

8 The kidney and surrounding tissue are removed from the peritoneum and sent for histological analysis.

9 Surgical drains may be inserted, and chest drains may be required if a pleural injury during a flank approach has resulted in a significant pneumothorax.

10 Prior to closure, it is important to ensure haemostasis. The mesentery is first closed, followed by a two-layer closure for the abdominal wounds (to minimise risk of herniation).

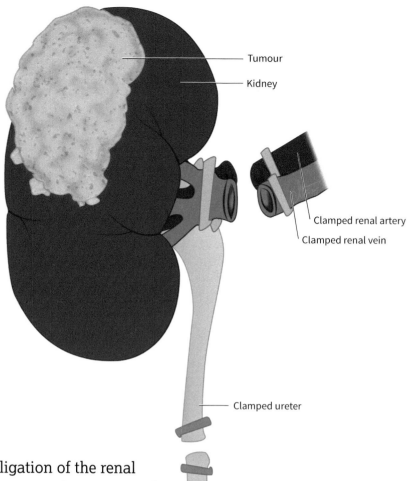

Tumour

Kidney

Clamped renal artery

Clamped renal vein

Clamped ureter

Figure 7.6 Clip ligation of the renal artery, vein and ureter prior to removal of the kidney

COMPLICATIONS

Early

- Pneumothorax.
- Haemorrhage.
- Damage to adjacent organs/blood vessels.
- Renal impairment—usually transient due to intra-operative ischaemia/parenchymal loss.

Intermediate and late

- Urinary fistula/leak.
- Ureteral obstruction.
- Incisional hernia.
- Infection.

POSTOPERATIVE CARE

Inpatient

- Judicious fluid status and electrolyte monitoring.
- Patients are commonly discharged after 2–7 days.

Outpatient

- Outpatient follow-up at 4–6 weeks to monitor recovery and check urinalysis, renal function, and blood pressure. These parameters are then checked 6–12 monthly.

- Strenuous activities should be avoided for 6 weeks postoperatively.
- Yearly monitoring for tumour recurrence if performed for renal cell carcinoma.

SURGEON'S FAVOURITE QUESTION

What are the features of paraneoplastic syndrome in renal cell carcinoma?

Paraneoplastic syndrome comprises a cluster of widespread symptoms secondary to malignancy. RCC-induced paraneoplastic symptoms include hypercalcaemia, poly-cythaemia, Stauffer syndrome/hepatic dysfunction pyrexia, cachexia, and hypertension.

SCROTAL EXPLORATION AND ORCHIDOPEXY

Louis Hainsworth

DEFINITION
Surgical exploration of the contents of the scrotum to assess and treat underlying pathology.

✓ INDICATIONS

> Clinical or radiological suspicion of testicular torsion.
> Scrotal abscesses requiring drainage.
> Large symptomatic epididymal cysts.

✗ CONTRAINDICATIONS

> Untreated coagulopathy.

ANATOMY

Gross anatomy
> The scrotum:
  › A dual-chambered pouch lying between the penis and anus responsible for housing the testes.
  › The scrotum consists of a thin layer of skin overlying the dartos muscle, which contracts and relaxes to bring the testes closer to and further away from the abdomen, controlling scrotal temperature for optimal sperm viability.
  › Deep to the dartos lie the external, middle, and internal spermatic fascia.
> The spermatic cord:
  › The spermatic cord starts at the deep inguinal ring, travels through the inguinal canal, and exits via the superficial inguinal ring to enter the testis.
  › It contains multiple key structures:
    ▫ three arteries—testicular, deferential, and cremasteric.
    ▫ three nerves—genital branch of the genitofemoral nerve, autonomic fibres, and the ilioinguinal nerve (note that the ilioinguinal nerve does not actually run within the cord, but alongside it).
    ▫ three supportive structures—vas deferens, pampiniform plexus, and lymphatic vessels.
    ▫ three coverings—external spermatic fascia, cremaster muscle/fascia, and internal spermatic fascia.
> The testes:
  › The testes are paired organs lying within the scrotum, separated by the scrotal septum.

> The tunica vaginalis surrounds the testes in two layers (viscera and parietal). Deep to the tunica vaginalis lies the tunica albuginea, the tough, fibrous covering of the testes.
> The testicular parenchyma is composed of 250–350 lobules, separated by septa of connective tissue that arise from the mediastinum testis (a vertical septum derived from the tunica albuginea).
> The lobules contain seminiferous tubules, which join to form the rete testis, which in turn forms the efferent ducts that allow sperm to enter the epididymal head.
> Epididymis:
  › The epididymis is a highly convoluted tubule extending from the upper to the lower pole of the testis where it becomes the vas (ductus) deferens.
  › The vas deferens joins the duct of the seminal vesicle to form the ejaculatory duct, which empties into the verumontanum of the urethra.

Neurovasculature
> The testes received their autonomic innervation via the testicular plexus.
> Arterial supply is from the testicular arteries, arising from the abdominal aorta.
> The testes drain through a network of 8–12 veins that form the pampiniform plexus. The plexus then converges to form the right (drains into the inferior vena cava) and left (drains into the renal vein) testicular veins.

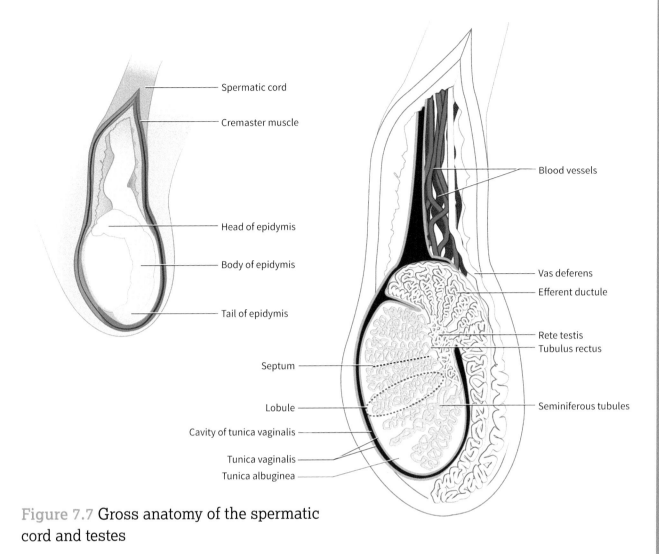

Figure 7.7 Gross anatomy of the spermatic cord and testes

Labels (left figure): Spermatic cord · Cremaster muscle · Head of epidymis · Body of epidymis · Tail of epidymis · Septum · Lobule · Cavity of tunica vaginalis · Tunica vaginalis · Tunica albuginea

Labels (right figure): Blood vessels · Vas deferens · Efferent ductule · Rete testis · Tubulus rectus · Seminiferous tubules

STEP-BY-STEP OPERATION

Anaesthesia: general.

Position: supine.

1. The scrotal skin is stretched over the testis, and a midline raphe or bilateral transverse incision is made through the scrotal skin, the dartos muscle, and the spermatic fasciae.
2. After entering the ipsilateral scrotal compartment, the tunica vaginalis is incised.
3. The testis is then delivered out of the incision.
4. The spermatic cord and testis are examined for a twisted cord and a blue/black testicle.
5. If torsion is apparent, then the cord is untwisted and the affected testicle is wrapped in a warm swab.
6. Following a few minutes, perfusion to the testicle is reassessed by observing its colour, using Doppler to assess for adequate flow, and making a small incision in the tunica albuginea and observing for fresh bleeding.
7. If the testis is unsalvageable/non-viable, an orchidectomy is performed.
8. Orchidopexy is prophylactically undertaken for both salvaged and contralateral testes to prevent future torsion (the testis is secured to the inner wall of the scrotum with fine non-absorbable sutures).
9. Haemostatic control is achieved, and the testis is repositioned into the hemiscrotum in the correct anatomical position (epididymis placed posteriorly, and sinus of testes placed laterally).
10. The dartos muscle and skin are closed in layers.

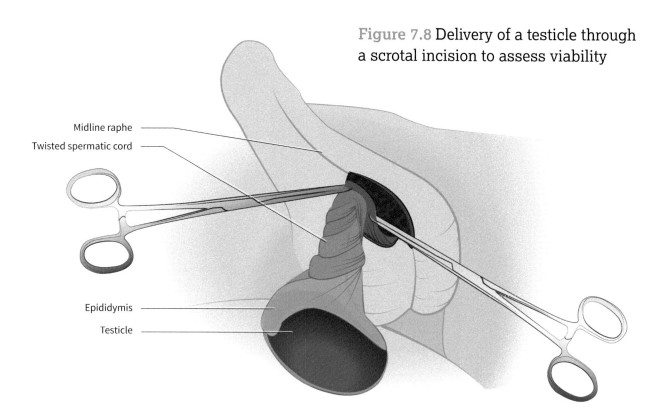

Figure 7.8 Delivery of a testicle through a scrotal incision to assess viability

Midline raphe

Twisted spermatic cord

Epididymis

Testicle

COMPLICATIONS

Early

> Scrotal oedema or haematoma.
> Wound infection.
> Testicular infarction—this is a rare complication that has a similar clinical presentation to testicular torsion but occurs in the postoperative period.

Intermediate and late

> Infertility—a consequence of both the disease process requiring surgery and the surgery itself.
> Testicular atrophy—rare.

POSTOPERATIVE CARE

Inpatient

> Patients are typically discharged after 1–2 days.

Outpatient

> Follow-up appointment at 6–8 weeks.
> Testicular prosthesis may be requested at a later stage if orchidectomy performed.

 SURGEON'S FAVOURITE QUESTION

How does testicular torsion present?

Signs and symptoms of torsion include sudden-onset, severe testicular pain radiating to the lower abdomen, scrotal erythema/swelling, nausea/vomiting, high-riding testis with a transverse lie, and absent cremasteric reflex.

VASECTOMY

Louis Hainsworth

DEFINITION

The surgical interruption of the vas deferens.

✓ INDICATIONS

> Surgical male sterilization as a means of contraception in men who are certain that they do not want to have further children.

✗ CONTRAINDICATIONS

> Patients who are uncertain they no longer want to father children.

> Presence of hydrocoeles/varicocoeles that may interfere with the procedure.
> Anatomic variations that preclude the safe identification/isolation of the vas deferens.
> Scrotal skin infections.
> Scrotal scarring/previous trauma.
> Untreated coagulopathy.

ANATOMY

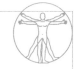

Gross anatomy

> The vas is a paired fibromuscular structure that travels within the spermatic cord.
> It transports spermatozoa from the epididymis to the ejaculatory ducts.
> When the vas reaches the seminal vesicles, it enlarges, terminating as the ampulla of the ductus, which then merges with the duct of the seminal vesicles, forming the ejaculatory ducts.
> The ejaculatory ducts enter at base of the prostate and terminate at the verumontanum.

Neurovasculature

> The vas receives sympathetic innervation from the pelvic plexus.
> The vas receives its arterial supply via the artery of the vas deferens (deferential artery), which is derived from the superior vesical artery (a branch of the internal iliac artery).
> The vas drains into the pelvic venous plexus.

Histology

> The vas is comprised of three histological layers:
> 1 Outer layer.
> 2 Middle muscular layer—this layer of contractile smooth muscle wall of the vas propels semen during ejaculation through peristaltic motion.
> 3 Internal mucosal layer—a layer of pseudostratified columnar epithelium containing apical stereocilia that enable forward propagation of sperm within the vas.

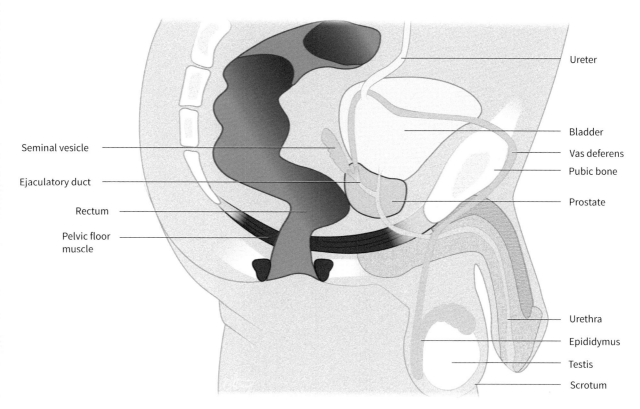

Figure 7.9 Course of the vas deferens

STEP-BY-STEP OPERATION

Anaesthesia: local.

Position: supine.

Considerations: The ambient temperature of the theatre should be checked to ensure it is adequately warm to prevent the cremasteric reflex.

1 The external genitalia are examined, and the vas deferens is palpated. The penis is retracted superiorly to ensure an adequate view of the operative field.

2 Each vas deferens is identified and held by a three-point fixation technique using the thumb and the index and middle fingers.

3 A small bleb of local anaesthetic is used to numb the scrotal skin at the site of instrumentation/incision, and a deeper anaesthetic block is achieved by infiltrating along the spermatic cord to the level of the external ring bilaterally.

4 A small puncture incision is made through the median raphe of the scrotum, and vasectomy ringed forceps are used to retrieve the spermatic cord.

5 A portion of vas is carefully dissected from its surrounding fascia within the spermatic cord, with care being taken to ensure the surrounding blood vessels are not stretched/ruptured.

6 The freed length of vas is cut.

7 The lumen of vas is occluded using electrocautery, and a 'barrier' of fascia is placed between the cut ends of the vas (fascial interposition). These steps reduce the risk of recanalization.

8 In the 'open-ended' technique, the cut ends of the vas are left to retract to their natural positions (reduces epididymal congestion, vas granuloma formation, and development of post-vasectomy pain syndrome).

9 The procedure is then repeated for the other vas using the same incision.

10 The wound edges rarely require closure with sutures, and antibacterial ointment and gauze are used as a dressing.

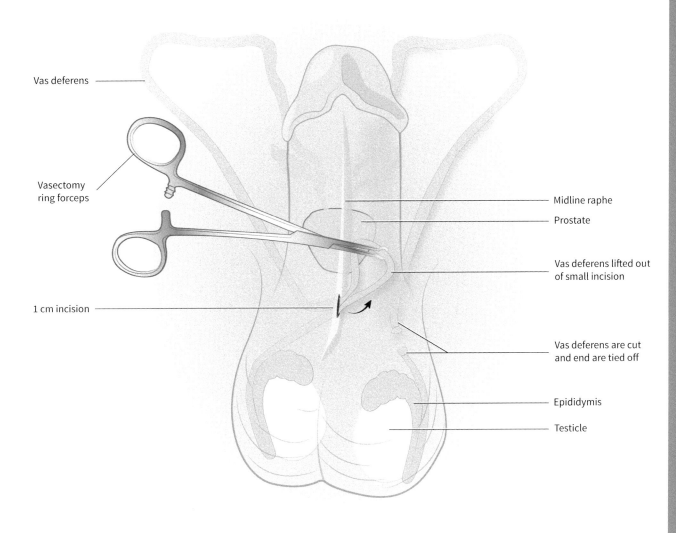

Vas deferens

Vasectomy
ring forceps

1 cm incision

Midline raphe

Prostate

Vas deferens lifted out
of small incision

Vas deferens are cut
and end are tied off

Epididymis

Testicle

Figure 7.10 Cutting of a freed loop of vas deferens

COMPLICATIONS

Early

› Bruising/haematoma.
› Iatrogenic damage to the spermatic vessels that compromises blood supply to the testicles.

Intermediate and late

› Epididymal congestion causing pain and swelling.
› Infection.
› Sperm granuloma formation—usually occurs 2–3 weeks postoperatively and consists of a small nodule secondary to sperm leaking from the vas.

› Post-vasectomy pain syndrome—occurs due to nerve damage and can occur immediately or later on.
› Persisting fertility—in the early period, this is usually due to unprotected sex before azoospermia is established; in the late period, failure can be due to spontaneous recanalization of the vas.

UROLOGY

POSTOPERATIVE CARE

Inpatient

> Day-case procedure.
> Application of ice packs or support garments to the scrotum help reduce swelling and pain.

Outpatient

> Patients are advised to lie supine as much as possible in the first 1–2 days post-procedure and limit themselves to light activities for the first week.

> Before patients can be certified as sterile, they need to have two negative sperm samples (azoospermia) obtained at least 3 months post-vasectomy and at least one month apart. In the meantime, advise patients to use a second form of birth control.

SURGEON'S FAVOURITE QUESTION

Can a vasectomy be reversed?

Yes. This can be achieved through vasovasostomy (anastomosing the cut segments of the vas) or vasoepididymostomy (anastomosing the vas to the epididymis).

CIRCUMCISION

Katrina Mason

DEFINITION
Surgical removal of the foreskin (prepuce) that covers the glans of the penis.

✓ INDICATIONS

> Foreskin malignancy.

> Unsalvageable traumatic foreskin injury.

> Balanitis Xerotica Obliterans (BXO)—inflammatory condition causing scarring of the foreskin and adherence to the glans.

> Phimosis—severe narrowing of the foreskin orifice; can be congenital (rare) or a result of trauma, scarring, or infection.

> Paraphimosis—resulting from a tight foreskin and causing a tight constriction and resultant swelling of the glans.

> Recurrent balanitis and balanoposthitis—infection of the glans and foreskin (circumcision may be indicated in refractory cases where medical management has failed).

> Risk-reducing procedure for HIV transmission in men living in high-prevalence, high-risk populations.

✗ CONTRAINDICATIONS

Relative

> Chordee—deficient ventral skin causing angulation of the penile shaft (the foreskin may be required at a later stage for reconstruction in these instances).

> Untreated coagulopathy.

> Normal physiological phimosis in infants and toddlers.

Absolute

> Hypospadias.

> Buried penis.

> Ambiguous genitalia.

ANATOMY

Gross anatomy

> The penile shaft is composed of three columns of erectile tissue:
  > Corpus cavernosa x 2.
  > Corpus spongiosum x 1—within which the urethra runs. The distal extension of the corpus spongiosum covers the tips of the cavernosa and forms the glans of the penis.

> The three erectile structures are surrounded by deep penile (Buck) fascia, the dartos fascia, and the penile skin.

> The glans has a raised proximal rim called the corona. The sagittal slit, through which the urethra exits, sits at the tip of the glans.

> The foreskin, or penile prepuce, is a continuation of the penile skin, which at the corona becomes double-sided, and therefore retractable, and covers the glans of the penis.

> The frenulum is a Y-shaped band of connective tissue on the underside of the glans that tethers the foreskin to the glans.

Neurovasculature

> The dorsal nerve of the penis supplies the glans and foreskin (it is a terminal branch of the pudendal nerve S2–S4).

> Arterial supply is via the dorsal artery of the penis (a branch of the internal pudendal artery).

> The penis is drained via the superficial dorsal vein of the penis.

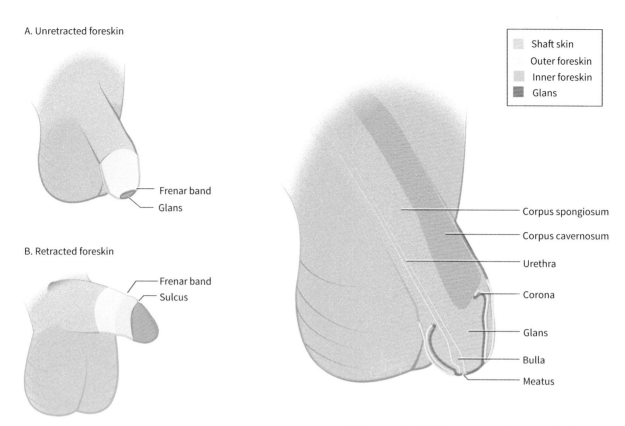

A. Unretracted foreskin

Frenar band
Glans

B. Retracted foreskin

Frenar band
Sulcus

Shaft skin
Outer foreskin
Inner foreskin
Glans

Corpus spongiosum
Corpus cavernosum
Urethra
Corona
Glans
Bulla
Meatus

Figure 7.11 Gross anatomy of the penis

STEP-BY-STEP OPERATION

Anaesthesia: A dorsal penile nerve block (DPNB) is commonly used in conjunction with a general anaesthetic.

Position: supine.

Considerations: Various well-established surgical techniques are used: dorsal slit, sleeve, guillotine technique, or with aid of devices such as Plastibell®, Mogen® clamp, Gomco® clamp, and The Shang Ring®. The various devices are used in accordance with age and size of penis.

1. The preputial orifice is dilated and any adhesions between the foreskin and glans are separated (especially necessary in infants where the foreskin has not spontaneously separated).
2. A device is used to create a circumferential incision, leaving a cuff of penile skin roughly 2–5 mm proximal to the corona.
3. Bipolar diathermy is used for haemostasis to prevent damage to the penile blood supply.
4. The larger ventral vessels are ligated with sutures.
5. The proximal penile skin is sutured to the coronal preputial sleeve (mucosa) with an absorbable suture.
6. Petroleum-based jelly is applied to the wound as a dressing.

Figure 7.12 Surgical cirumcision

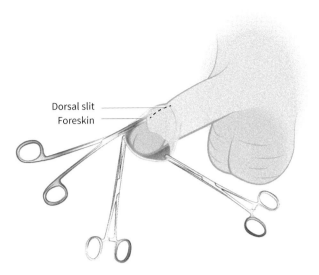

Dorsal slit
Foreskin

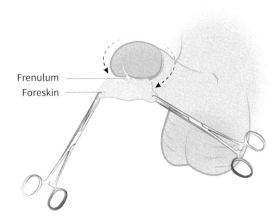

Frenulum
Foreskin

COMPLICATIONS

Early

> Haemorrhage.
> Pain and discomfort.
> Damage to skin of penis and glans from diathermy.

Intermediate and late

> Meatal stenosis.
> Removal of too much or too little skin with resulting unsatisfactory cosmetic result.
> Amputation of glans.
> Inclusion cysts.
> Infection.

POSTOPERATIVE CARE

Inpatient

> Circumcision is performed as a day-case procedure; patients are discharged once they have passed urine.

Outpatient

> Petroleum-based ointments (e.g., Vaseline®) can be applied regularly to the wound and glans to avoid irritation.

> Parents are advised that children should remain home from school for one week.
> Adults are advised to avoid sexual intercourse until fully healed (commonly 4–6 weeks).

 ## SURGEON'S FAVOURITE QUESTION

When does the foreskin separate from the glans during normal development?

The foreskin is normally adherent to the glans in infancy and up to the first 3 years of life. It gradually spontaneously separates during this time, and by 3 years, 90% of boys will have a retractable foreskin.

8 CARDIOTHORACICS

LAY PING ONG

CORONARY ARTERY BYPASS GRAFTING (CABG)

Nick Wroe

DEFINITION

The use of a venous or arterial graft to bypass significant coronary artery stenosis to restore blood flow to the myocardium. Can be done open or with minimally invasive techniques such as robotic surgery.

✓ INDICATIONS

- Multivessel disease is the main indication for CABG over PCI (percutaneous coronary intervention), particularly in the context of complex anatomy or diabetic patients (more diffuse/progressive disease).
- Single vessel disease where:
  › PCI has failed.
  › Patients are unsuitable for long-term dual antiplatelet therapy.
  › There is a large amount of ischaemic myocardium.
  › There is significant left main coronary artery disease.
- Unstable angina or angina that severely limits activity and that cannot be controlled medically.

- Ischaemia in a non-ST elevation myocardial infarction (NSTEMI) that is refractory to medication.
- An emergency CABG is indicated in ST elevation myocardial infarction (STEMI) where PCI is not possible.
- Where PCI has failed.

✗ CONTRAINDICATIONS

- Patients who are asymptomatic.
- Patients with coronary artery disease who carry a low risk of myocardial infarction (MI), whereby PCI may be indicated.

ANATOMY

The coronary arteries

- The left and right coronary arteries arise from the left and right aortic sinuses, distal to the aortic valve.
- Left coronary artery (LCA):
  › The LCA branches to yield the circumflex artery, which wraps around to the posterior aspect of the left atrium, and the left anterior descending (LAD), which produces a series of diagonal arteries to supply the left ventricle.
  › The left marginal artery branches from the circumflex artery.
- Right coronary artery (RCA):
  › The RCA runs in the groove between the right atrium and ventricle.
  › Along its path, the RCA gives rise to the acute marginal artery.
- 70% of individuals have a right dominant coronary circulation where the RCA continues as the posterior interventricular artery. In a left dominant circulation, this artery comes from the circumflex.
- Stenosis can occur at any site, but the most significant stenoses occur along the LAD and the LCA, as these supply the majority of the left ventricular tissue.

Graft anatomy

- A section of blood vessel taken from one of three sites
- The internal mammary artery/internal thoracic artery (the most commonly used graft):
  › Branches from the subclavian artery proximal to the vertebral arteries.
  › The artery descends along the internal anterior chest wall parallel to edges of the sternum, where it branches into the musculophrenic and superior epigastric arteries.
- The saphenous veins:
  › The long saphenous vein ascends the anteromedial thigh and drains into the femoral vein at the sapheno-femoral junction.
  › The short saphenous vein ascends the posterior calf to drain into the popliteal vein.
- The radial artery:
  › Arises from the bifurcation of the brachial artery to then run distally along the anterior forearm.

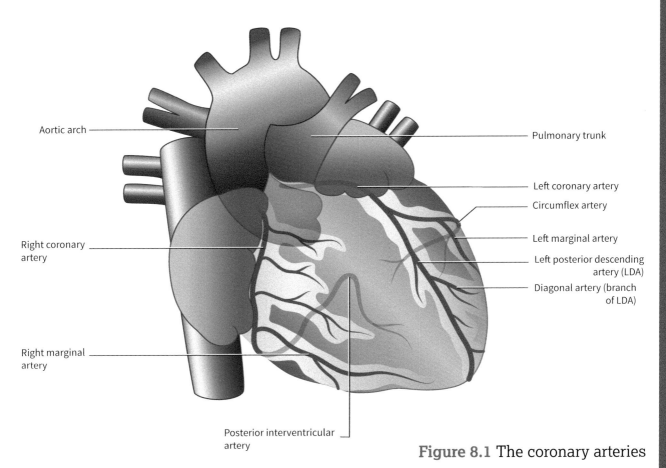

Aortic arch

Pulmonary trunk

Left coronary artery

Circumflex artery

Left marginal artery

Left posterior descending artery (LDA)

Diagonal artery (branch of LDA)

Right coronary artery

Right marginal artery

Posterior interventricular artery

Figure 8.1 The coronary arteries

STEP-BY-STEP OPERATION

Anaesthesia: general.

Position: supine.

Considerations: Two teams work simultaneously, with one exposing the heart and the second focusing on harvesting the graft. Minimally invasive techniques and 'off-pump' or 'beating heart' surgery can be used, often reserved for elderly patients with multiple comorbidities or patients with calcified aortas who may not tolerate the aortic manipulation required for cardiopulmonary bypass. Intraoperative transoesophageal ECHO (TOE) is often used

1 A median sternotomy incision is made, and the sternum is split using a sternal saw.

2 The bypass graft is harvested from either the chest wall, the wrist, or the leg.

3 Cardiopulmonary bypass is then established by delivering cardioplegia (potassium-enriched solution) into the heart, causing the heart to stop beating.

4 Circulation is then directed through the cardiopulmonary bypass (CPB) machine, which includes an oxygenation and heat exchanging pump. Anticoagulation is achieved with heparin to prevent clot formation within the CPB machine.

5 Once bypass has been achieved, the left internal mammary artery is anastomosed beyond the point of stenosis.

6 When the saphenous vein or radial artery grafts are used, the distal portion is anastomosed with the diseased coronary artery at a point beyond the stenosed section of the vessel, and the proximal portion is most commonly anastomosed to the ascending aorta.

7 The graft patency is then commonly checked with TOE.

8 The patient is slowly weaned off bypass by gradually warming the patient and by reversing cardioplegia.

9 The sternum is commonly closed using sternal wires, and then the chest wall is closed in layers.

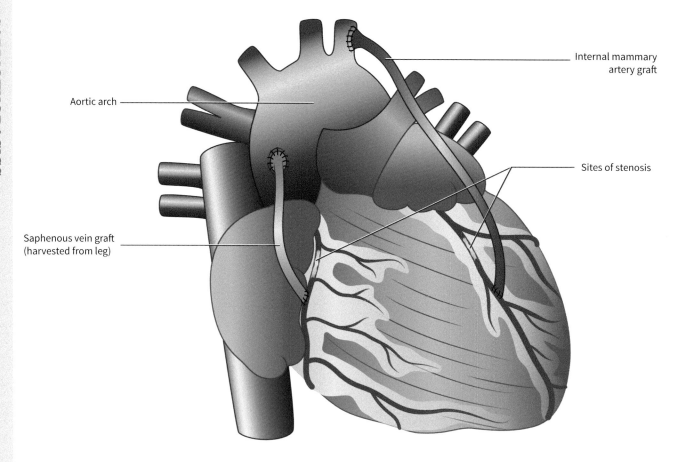

Internal mammary artery graft

Aortic arch

Sites of stenosis

Saphenous vein graft (harvested from leg)

Figure 8.2 Internal mammary artery bypass graft for stenosis of the LAD and a saphenous vein bypass graft for stenosis of the RCA.

COMPLICATIONS

Early

- Acute kidney injury, requiring dialysis in 1–2%.
- Bleeding, which may warrant reoperation or transfusion (common in 30%).
- Neurological complications—stroke or transient ischaemic attack, delirium, cognitive decline, neuropsychiatric abnormalities, peripheral neuropathy (uncommon).
- MI (uncommon).
- Pleural effusion—often small and treated with medication.
- Arrhythmia, including atrial fibrillation (common in 15–40%).

- Aortic dissection.
- Pericardial effusion and tamponade.
- Death (1%).

Intermediate and late

- Deep sternal wound infection and mediastinitis (1%).
- Leg wound complications—dermatitis, cellulitis, ulcers, greater saphenous neuropathy.
- Radial artery harvest can result in a self-limiting numbness and tingling in the distal forearm.
- Graft restenosis—more common in venous grafts.

POSTOPERATIVE CARE

Inpatient

▸ The patient usually spends less than 24 hours on intensive care if no complications occur.

▸ The patient will be started on lifelong antiplatelets, statins, and blood pressure therapy to prevent the progression of ischaemic heart disease.

Outpatient

▸ Cardiac rehabilitation—exercise, reducing risk factors, and dealing with emotional sequelae.

▸ Regular cardiology outpatient appointments with transthoracic echocardiograms.

💬 SURGEON'S FAVOURITE QUESTION

Why does aortic manipulation during the institution of CPB result in complications?

Patients requiring CABG have atherosclerotic disease that also affects major vessels such as the aorta. Any underlying atheroma (calcified/non-calcified) along the ascending aorta has the potential when manipulated to lead to stroke or distal embolization.

AORTIC VALVE REPAIR/REPLACEMENT

Nick Wroe

CARDIOTHORACICS

DEFINITION

Surgical repair of a stenosed or regurgitating aortic valve or replacement with either a prosthetic or a biological valve.

✓ INDICATIONS

- Symptomatic severe aortic stenosis (AS) or severe aortic regurgitation (AR).
- Asymptomatic patients with severe AS or AR and:
  - Require cardiac artery bypass graft surgery.
  - Having surgery on the aorta or other heart valves.
  - A left ventricular ejection fraction <50%.
  - An abnormal exercise test showing symptoms/signs attributed to AS.
- Severe AR with progressive left ventricular (LV) dilatation.
- Infective endocarditis resulting in a non-functioning valve—repair versus replacement depends on extent of valve disease.
- Indications for mechanical versus biological:

- A bioprosthetic valve is made from either bovine or porcine heart valves. These do not last as long as their mechanical counterparts and do not require anticoagulation, so they are often preferred in the elderly.

✗ CONTRAINDICATIONS

- Asymptomatic patients with normal left ventricular function.
- Patients who are unfit for surgery should be considered for:
  - Transcatheter Aortic Valve Implantation (TAVI)—an endovascular technique used to replace aortic valves.
  - Aortic valve balloon angioplasty, where a balloon is blown up to open a stenosed aortic valve.

ANATOMY

- The heart consists of four valves. The mitral (bicuspid) and tricuspid valves are atrioventricular valves. The aortic and pulmonary valves are classed as semilunar valves.

The atrioventricular valves

- Consist of two or three leaflets that open during diastole to allow blood flow into the ventricle and close to prevent the backflow of blood during systole.
- Papillary muscles are anchored to the ventricular walls. Chordae tendineae (fibrous cords) connect the papillary muscles to the valve leaflets. During systole, contraction of the ventricle and the papillary muscles pulls the atrioventricular valves shut.

The semilunar valves

- The semilunar valves sit at the base of the aorta and the pulmonary trunk. They open during systole to allow the flow of blood from the ventricles into their

respective vessels; during diastole, the cusps meet to prevent the backflow of blood.
- The semilunar valves comprise three half-moon (hence 'semilunar') cusps known as the right, left, and posterior cusps.

The aortic valve

- The left and right cusps contain the left and right aortic sinuses from which the coronary arteries derive, and the posterior cusp contains a non-coronary sinus with no derivations.
- At the base of the aortic valve is a fibrous ring (a continuation of the cardiac skeleton). This structure calcifies with age, resulting in a sclerotic noose around the lumen of the aorta that limits blood flow in senile AS.
- Around 2% of the population have a bicuspid (two-cusp) aortic valve, which has an increased risk of becoming stenosed at a much younger age.

Figure 8.3 Valves of the heart

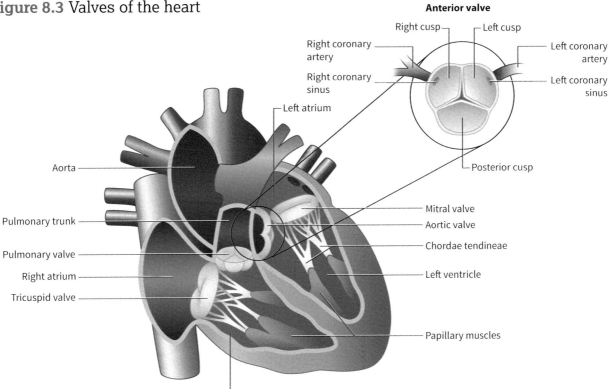

STEP-BY-STEP OPERATION

Anaesthesia: general.

Position: supine.

Considerations: The use of intraoperative transoesophageal ECHO (TOE) is commonplace.

1 The chest wall is opened using a median sternotomy incision.

2 Cardiopulmonary bypass is then established by delivering cardioplegia (potassium-enriched solution) into the heart, causing the heart to stop beating.

3 Circulation is then directed through the cardiopulmonary bypass (CPB) machine, which includes an oxygenation and heat exchanging pump. Anticoagulation is achieved with heparin to prevent clot formation within the CPB machine.

4 The aorta is cross-clamped. Using a transverse incision from its root, the aorta is dissected, and the diseased valve is excised.

5 For replacement of the aortic valve due to calcification, the valve annulus is first decalcified and then the replacement valve is sewn in the annulus using a parachute technique.

6 In a minority of cases, a repair can be performed:

   a Uneven leaflet heights can be corrected by resection of the offending leaflet to match the height of the other leaflets.

   b An oversized valve can be plicated; this involves folding an oversized cusp back on itself so that it matches the others. Once in position, it is sutured into place.

   c A pathologically fused bicuspid valve can be corrected by separating the diseased cusps.

7 In cases of a weakened or heavily stenosed valve, a complete or incomplete annuloplasty can be performed where a stiff prosthetic ring is sutured into part of or the full circumference of the annulus.

8 Once the replacement or repair is complete, the aorta is closed using a non-absorbable suture. TOE is commonly used to ensure no paravalvular leak.

9 The patient is slowly weaned off bypass by gradually warming the patient and by reversing cardioplegia.

10 Drains are placed, and the chest wall is closed using sternal wires. The soft tissue is then closed in in layers.

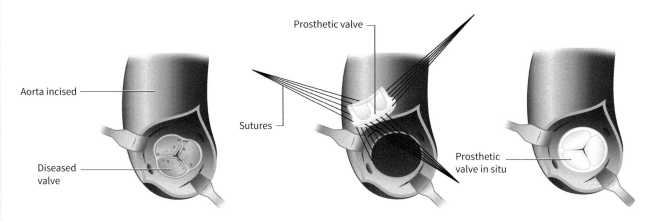

Figure 8.4 Replacement of a stenosed aortic valve

COMPLICATIONS

Early

> Bleeding.
> Myocardial infarction.
> Stroke or transient ischaemic attack.
> Atrial fibrillation.
> Heart block due to the proximity of the conducting system, which may require a permanent pacemaker.

Intermediate and late

> Endocarditis—fever and a new murmur in a patient who has undergone valve replacement surgery is endocarditis until proven otherwise.
> Embolism or haemolysis—more common with prosthetic valves.
> Deep sternal wound infections.
> Paravalvular leak.
> Graft failure—biological valves are prone to 'wearing out', especially in younger patients.
> Mortality (2%).

POSTOPERATIVE CARE

Inpatient

> Intensive care for 24 hours if no other complications arise.
> Total hospital stay of 5–7 days.

Outpatient

> Strenuous activities, including driving and full-time work, should be delayed until 4–6 weeks postoperatively to allow for the sternum to heal.
> Patients with mechanical valves will need lifelong anticoagulation with warfarin and aspirin.

> Patients with biological heart valve replacements do not need lifelong anticoagulation and should be provided with warfarin for 3 months, then aspirin 75mg once daily alone lifelong.
> Follow-up appointment at 6 weeks with echocardiogram and/or TOE (transoesophageal echocardiography).
> Yearly follow-up appointments if asymptomatic and have normal cardiac function.
> Antibiotic prophylaxis is required should the patient require dental treatment.
> A temporary or permanent pacemaker may be required.

SURGEON'S FAVOURITE QUESTION

What is a commonly associated pathology with a bicuspid aortic valve?

Ascending aorta dilatation as part of bicuspid aortic valve aortopathy. This can occur due to either a biomechanical or connective tissue disorder mechanism. In certain patients in whom the diameter of the ascending aorta reaches a threshold >55mm, an aortic root replacement will be performed.

MITRAL VALVE REPAIR/REPLACEMENT

Nick Wroe

DEFINITION

Surgical repair or replacement of the mitral valve due to severe stenosis (MS) or regurgitation (MR).

✓ INDICATIONS

- Severe mitral valve disease (mitral valve area ≤1.5cm³) AND:
  - Symptomatic patient—e.g. congestive cardiac failure not responsive to medical management or left atrial dilatation with arrhythmias e.g. atrial fibrillation.
  - Patient undergoing other cardiac surgery or cardiopulmonary bypass for other indications.
- Indications for mechanical versus biological replacement:
  - A bioprosthetic valve is made from either bovine (cow) or porcine (pig) heart valves. These do not last as long as their mechanical counterparts, so they are often chosen in the elderly or in active individuals for whom lifelong anticoagulation is not an option for their lifestyle.
  - Modern mechanical valves consist of a metal ring and are either monoleaflet or bileaflet discs that rotate to open or close with the flow of blood.
- In severe rheumatic disease or calcified valve leaflets, replacement is preferred over repair.

✗ CONTRAINDICATION

- In rheumatic mitral stenosis, percutaneous mitral balloon valvotomy is preferred when there is favourable valve morphology, mild regurgitation, and no left atrial thrombosis.

ANATOMY

- The heart consists of four valves. The mitral (bicuspid) and tricuspid valves are atrioventricular valves. The aortic and pulmonary valves are classed as semilunar valves.

The semilunar valves

- The semilunar valves sit at the base of the aorta and the pulmonary trunk. During systole, they allow the flow of blood from the ventricles into their respective vessels; during diastole, the cusps meet to prevent the backflow of blood.
- The semilunar valves comprise three half-moon (hence "semilunar") cusps known as the right, left, and posterior cusps.

The mitral valve

- The mitral valve serves as the conduit for blood flowing from the left atrium to the left ventricle.

- The valve has two leaflets that are anchored to a fibrous annulus, and there is a commissure on each side between the leaflets. During diastole, the valves allow the free flow of blood in one direction. During systole, the two leaflets come together to prevent the backflow of blood into the left atrium.
- Papillary muscles anchored to the ventricular walls are connected to chordae tendineae, which pull the atrioventricular valves shut during systole. The high tensile strength of the chordae tendineae means that the valves remain shut against the flow of blood.

Pathology

- Mitral regurgitation is where the mitral valve prolapses up into the left atrium during systole. This regurgitation occurs with necrosis of the papillary muscles and often is due to myocardial infarction.

Figure 8.5 Anatomy of the mitral valve

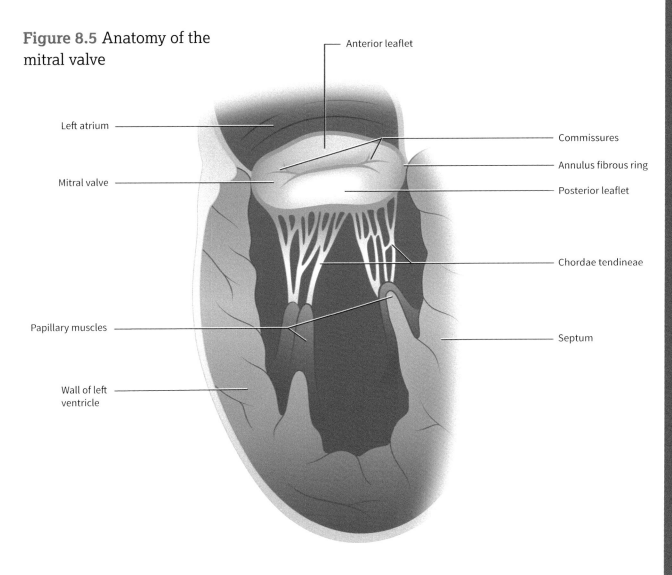

- Anterior leaflet
- Left atrium
- Mitral valve
- Commissures
- Annulus fibrous ring
- Posterior leaflet
- Chordae tendineae
- Papillary muscles
- Septum
- Wall of left ventricle

STEP-BY-STEP OPERATION

Anaesthesia: general.

Position: supine.

Considerations: The use of intraoperative transoesophageal ECHO (TOE) is commonplace.

1 Using either a median sternotomy or a minimally invasive approach (right-sided parasternal incision through the third and fourth costal cartilages), the thoracic cavity is opened.

2 Cardiopulmonary bypass is then established by delivering cardioplegia (potassium-enriched solution) into the heart causing the heart to stop beating.

3 Circulation is then directed through the cardiopulmonary bypass (CPB) machine, which includes an oxygenation and heat exchanging pump. Anticoagulation is achieved with heparin to prevent clot formation within the CPB machine.

4 An incision is made into either the left or right atrial groove (between the atrium and ventricle). If using the latter approach, the interatrial septum must first be dissected to allow access.

5 Where feasible, the valve is repaired:

a Excess leaflet tissue resulting in prolapse—resected with a subsequent annuloplasty (a stiff prosthetic ring is sutured into the circumference of the annulus).

b Loss of leaflet volume—corrected using a patch of pericardium.

c Fusion of leaflets—a commissurotomy is performed where the junctions between leaflets are incised or the diseased valve is resected or plicated into a more natural shape.

6 Once the leaflets of the valve have been assessed and, where applicable, repaired, the integrity of the chordae

tendineae is assessed and, if required, replaced with synthetic substitutes.

7 Where repair of the valve is not possible, it is replaced with a prosthetic or biological valve. TOE is commonly used to ensure no paravalvular leak.

8 Once the repair or replacement is achieved, the patient is slowly weaned off bypass by gradually warming the patient and by reversing cardioplegia.

9 Drains are placed, the chest wall is closed using sternal wires, and the soft tissue is closed in layers.

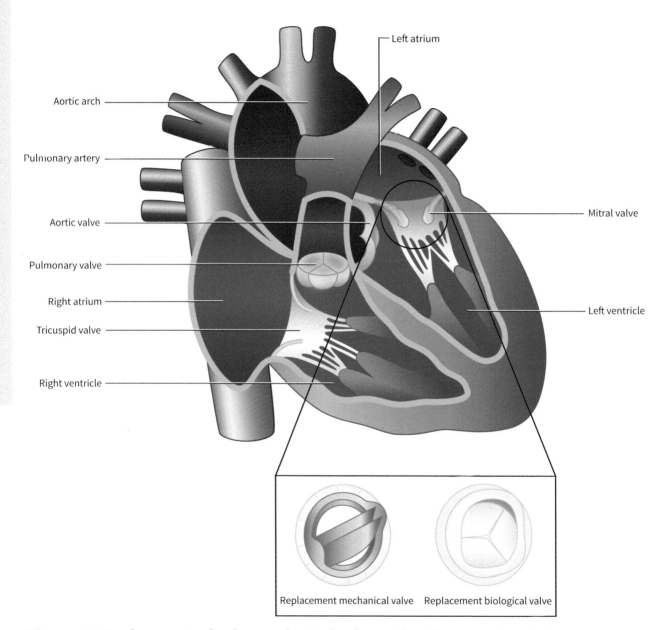

Figure 8.6 Replacement of a diseased mitral valve with either a mechanical or biological valve

COMPLICATIONS

Early

> Bleeding.
> Myocardial infarction.
> Stroke or transient ischaemic attack.
> Atrial fibrillation.
> Heart block, due to the proximity of the conducting system, which may require a permanent pacemaker.
> Left ventricular rupture.
> Systolic anterior motion (SAM), the dynamic anterior movement of the mitral valve towards the interventricular system that creates left ventricular outflow obstruction. This can lead to haemodynamic instability and intractable hypotension (requires medical therapy or prompt surgical revision).

Intermediate and late

> Endocarditis—fever and a new murmur in a patient having undergone valve replacement surgery is endocarditis until proven otherwise.
> Embolism or haemolysis—more common with prosthetic valves.
> Deep sternal wound infections.
> Paravalvular leak.
> Graft failure—biological valves are prone to 'wearing out', especially in younger patients.
> Mortality (2%).

POSTOPERATIVE CARE

Inpatient

> Intensive care for 24 hours if no other complications arise.
> Total hospital stay of 5–7 days.

Outpatient

> Strenuous activities, including driving and full-time work, should be delayed until 4–6 weeks postoperatively to allow for the sternum to heal.
> Patients with mechanical valves will need lifelong anticoagulation with warfarin and International Normalised Ratio (INR) monitoring.

> Patients with biological heart valve replacements do not need lifelong anticoagulation and should be provided with warfarin and aspirin 75mg daily for 3 months, then aspirin alone.
> First outpatient review is usually at 6 weeks with echocardiogram and/or TOE (transoesophageal echocardiography), then yearly if asymptomatic and have normal cardiac function.
> Antibiotic prophylaxis is required should the patient require dental treatment.
> A temporary or permanent pacemaker may be required.

💬 SURGEON'S FAVOURITE QUESTIONS

What is the functional classification of mitral valve regurgitation?

Carpentier's Classification:

Type 1: Normal Leaflet Motion but with Annular Dilatation.

Type 2: Excess Leaflet Motion (Prolapse).

Type 3: Restricted Leaflet Motion (either restricted opening or closing motion).

This classification is important in identifying the exact pathology to help plan the surgery.

THORACOSCOPIC PULMONARY LOBECTOMY

Nick Leaver

DEFINITION

The surgical removal of a lobe of a lung.

✓ INDICATIONS

- Lung cancer—primary (non-small cell lung cancer, large cell lung cancer, carcinoid) or metastatic, which is confined to one lobe.
- Bronchiectasis, chronic obstructive pulmonary disease (COPD), or a fungal infection, which is confined to a single lobe and is not responding to initial medical management.
- Rare indications:
  - Congenital cystic adenomatoid malformation (CCAM).
  - Uncontrollable bleeding (e.g., trauma).
  - Infarction.
  - Abscess.

✗ CONTRAINDICATIONS

Relative

- Inadequate cardiopulmonary reserve—e.g., an FEV_1 <2 litres or reduced diffusing capacity of the lung for carbon monoxide.

Absolute

- Tumours invading the chest wall or mediastinum (T3 or T4).
- Tumours crossing lobes—pneumonectomy may be considered.
- Tumours with lymph node involvement beyond N2 nodal disease.
- Tumours with brain metastasis—palliative treatment only.

ANATOMY

Gross anatomy

- The right lung is composed of upper, middle, and lower lobes, while the left lung only consists of upper and lower lobes.
- The middle and lower lobes of the right lung are separated by the oblique fissure, which begins anteriorly in the sixth intercostal space at the costochondral junction and curves to end at the fifth thoracic vertebra.
- The upper and middle lobes of the right lung are separated by the horizontal fissure, which is at the level of the fourth intercostal space and meets the oblique fissure at the mid-clavicular line.
- The left lung is divided into the upper and lower lobes by the oblique fissure.

Neurovasculature

- The phrenic nerve descends through the thoracic cavity, immediately anterior to the hilum of the lung, to reach the diaphragm.
- Each lobe contains a hilum, the point of entry for the blood vessels and bronchus.
- Each lung has one pulmonary artery that branches to give one lobar artery per lobe. These lobar arteries then divide further into segmental arteries.
- Capillaries converge to form progressively larger veins. These eventually form the four pulmonary veins that drain back to the left atrium.
- The lung drains into the superficial and deep lymphatic plexuses. These plexuses converge to the bronchopulmonary nodes, located in the hilum, which then continue to the bronchomediastinal trunks and into the junction of the internal jugular and subclavian veins.

Figure 8.7 Lobes of the lungs

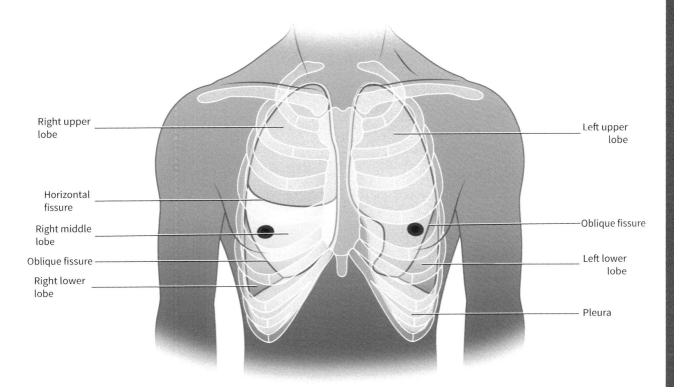

Right upper lobe

Horizontal fissure

Right middle lobe

Oblique fissure

Right lower lobe

Left upper lobe

Oblique fissure

Left lower lobe

Pleura

STEP-BY-STEP OPERATION

Anaesthesia: general, with single-lung ventilation, using a double lumen endotracheal tube, which allows for one lung to be deflated.

Position: either the left or right lateral decubitus position.

Considerations: Lobectomy can be performed as either an open approach or through video-assisted thoracoscopic approach (VATS), as described below.

1 A large incision is made for the 'utility port'. When removing the lower lobes, the port is above the inferior pulmonary vein. For upper and middle lobes, the incision is above the superior pulmonary vein.

2 The thoracoscope is inserted through an incision into the seventh intercostal space in the mid-clavicular line. Anterior and posterior ports are created for instruments.

3 The hilar lymph nodes are then either completely dissected with a complete mediastinal lymph node dissection (CMLND) or the sentinel lymph node is biopsied.

4 The operated lung is deflated, and the upper lobe is retracted posteriorly to expose the hilum. The pleura within the fissure is then dissected so that the pulmonary veins are exposed. Care is taken to identify the phrenic nerve.

5 The pulmonary vein is dissected and stapled, and the fissure is then further dissected until the pulmonary artery and bronchus are identified. The artery is then freed and stapled, allowing for greater visualisation of the bronchus.

6 The bronchus is stapled closed.

7 Staples are placed along the line of the fissure until the lobe is completely freed.

8 The lobe is then placed in a drawstring bag and removed through the utility port.

9 An 'air' test is performed by the anaesthetist, wherein the remaining lung is inflated to check for air leaks. To prevent further bleeding and air leaking, a fibrin sealant is sprayed onto any areas of bleeding, along the staple lines, and over the end of the closed bronchus.

10 To complete the procedure, chest drains are inserted, the muscle layers are approximated, and the incision is closed in layers.

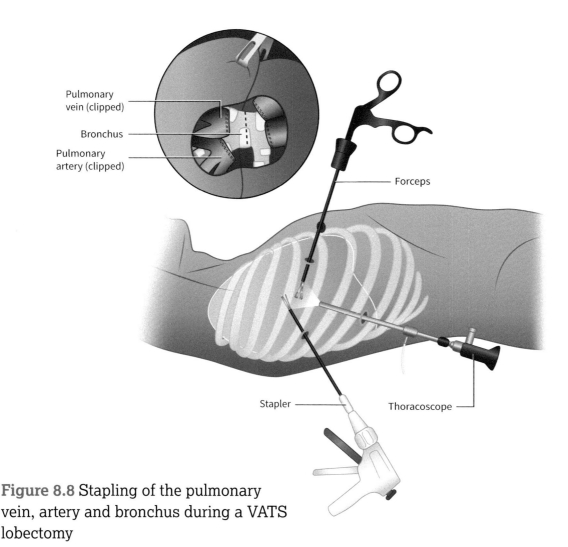

Pulmonary
vein (clipped)

Bronchus

Pulmonary
artery (clipped)

Forceps

Stapler

Thoracoscope

Figure 8.8 Stapling of the pulmonary vein, artery and bronchus during a VATS lobectomy

COMPLICATIONS

Early

> Arrhythmias—atrial fibrillation/flutter (common 10%).
> Chyle leak.
> Atelectasis.
> Respiratory failure.
> Intercostal nerve damage may occur if the ribs are spread using the thoracotomy approach.
> The superficial cutaneous nerves can be damaged, leading to reduced sensation of the anterior chest.
> Conversion to pneumonectomy may occur if the lung cancer spread is too great and the cancer resection margins involve the major vessels of the heart.

Intermediate and late

> Lobar torsion (0.4%) is a rare complication and occurs because of the increased space within the thorax. The remaining lobe(s) twists causing decreased air entry and blood flow, requiring an emergency thoracotomy to untwist the lobe.
> Prolonged, >7 days, postoperative air leak.
> Pneumonia.
> Empyema.
> Surgical site infection.
> Bronchopleural fistula (1%). This presents the same symptoms as a pneumothorax and results in prolonged chest drain insertion.

POSTOPERATIVE CARE

Inpatient

- ▸ Pain control can be administered by an epidural catheter or patient-controlled analgesia.
- ▸ Postoperative chest X-ray is used to confirm that there is no pneumothorax.
- ▸ The chest drain should be removed 24–48 hours postoperatively.
- ▸ The patient is usually discharged 3–5 days postoperatively.

Outpatient

- ▸ Follow-up depends upon the indication for resection, but for cancers, surveillance follow-up with history, examination, chest X-ray (CXR), and/or CT are usually every 3–6 months for the first 2–3 years, then annually.

💬 SURGEON'S FAVOURITE QUESTIONS

Is a rising fluid level within the pleural space of the resected lobe, as seen on a postoperative CXR, acceptable?

This is not acceptable within the context of a lobectomy, as it may suggest the development of an empyema (infection within the pleural spaces) and will require further treatment with antibiotics or decortication.

THORACOSCOPIC PULMONARY LOBECTOMY

PERCUTANEOUS PATENT FORAMEN OVALE REPAIR

Nick Leaver

DEFINITION

The closure of a patent foramen ovale (PFO) by a percutaneous approach.

✓ INDICATIONS

- Cyanosis in a newborn caused by a PFO.
- Stroke risk reduction secondary to a PFO.
- Migraines caused by a PFO.

✗ CONTRAINDICATIONS

- Eisenmenger's syndrome—a PFO enlarges over time, leading to pulmonary hypertension that causes the reversal of flow of blood through the shunt and subsequent cyanosis. Closure of the PFO is not curative.
- In patients >60 years old with stroke due to PFO (antiplatelet therapy is preferred).
- Presence of inferior vena cava (IVC) filter.
- Coagulopathy.
- Use of long-term anticoagulants for other reasons.
- Vascular, cardiac, or PFO anatomy unsuitable for device placement.

ANATOMY

- An atrial septal defect (ASD) is a congenital malformation where the tissue that forms the interatrial septum fails to properly form and thus allows for blood to pass between the left and right atria.
- A (PFO) is the failure of closure of the foramen ovale after birth.
- In utero, the foramen ovale is an important shunt that is formed during the fourth week of gestation. Its function is to divert semi-oxygenated blood away from the pulmonary circulation (right atrium) into the systemic circulation (left atrium).
- Following birth, due to the increasing pressure in the left atrium overcoming the pressure in right atrium, the foramen ovale closes.
- Progressively, the septum fuses. Within one year, a rounded depression (fossa ovalis) is the only remaining remnant of the foramen ovale.
- In up to 20% of the population, the foramen ovale remains patent throughout life and remains asymptomatic during normal physiological activities.

Figure 8.9 Physiological cardiac shunts

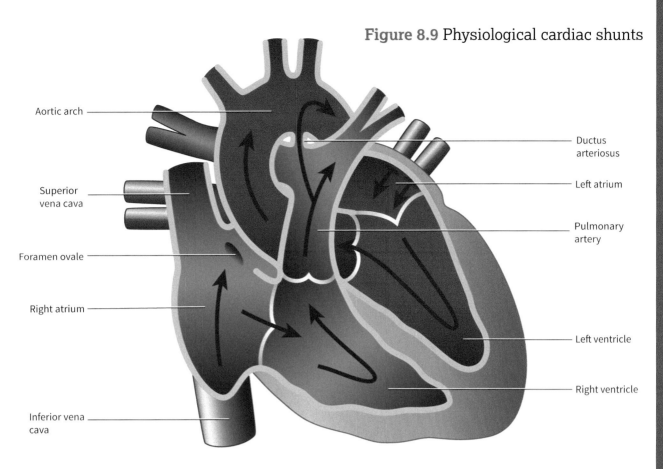

Aortic arch

Superior vena cava

Foramen ovale

Right atrium

Inferior vena cava

Ductus arteriosus

Left atrium

Pulmonary artery

Left ventricle

Right ventricle

STEP-BY-STEP OPERATION

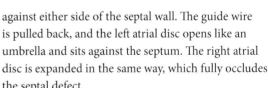

Anaesthesia: sedation or general anaesthetic.

Position: supine.

Considerations: Transoesophageal ECHO (TOE) is used to guide the catheter into position. In the presence of pulmonary hypertension, a second catheter, containing a camera, is passed into the right atrium; it monitors cardiac pressures and aids in guiding the catheter.

1 An incision into the femoral vein is made, and IV heparin is administered.

2 A catheter is inserted into the femoral vein and passed upwards to the inferior vena cava.

3 The catheter is then passed into the right atrium and through the PFO into the left atrium.

4 Under ultrasound guidance, a balloon is inflated to grade the size of the PFO.

5 A correctly sized closure device is selected.

6 A guide wire with a large sheath is used to position the occlusion device and is passed up and positioned in the left upper pulmonary vein.

7 The occlusion device contains two self-expandable discs (made from Nitinol wire mesh), which will sit against either side of the septal wall. The guide wire is pulled back, and the left atrial disc opens like an umbrella and sits against the septum. The right atrial disc is expanded in the same way, which fully occludes the septal defect.

8 Throughout the procedure, air must be continuously removed from the catheter to prevent air embolisation.

9 An echocardiogram confirms that the device is positioned correctly. The occlusion device can then be released from the guide wire.

10 The guide wire is removed, and the wound is dressed.

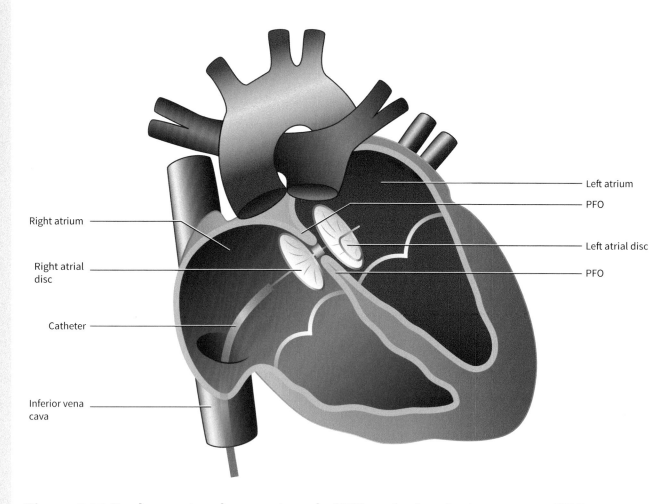

Right atrium

Right atrial disc

Catheter

Inferior vena cava

Left atrium

PFO

Left atrial disc

PFO

Figure 8.10 Deployment and expansion of a PFO occlusion device across a PFO

COMPLICATIONS

Early

- Air embolism (<5%) can be caused by introduction of air from the catheter and can be identified by ST elevation on ECG.
- Arrhythmias—new onset atrial fibrillation is most common (4%).
- Cardiac perforation—rare but potentially fatal complication (through tamponade).

Intermediate and late

- Thrombus formation.
- Device migration, erosion, embolisation or thrombosis causing recurrent ischaemic stroke.
- Residual shunt on echo (20% of cases), which require further monitoring and follow-up.

POSTOPERATIVE CARE

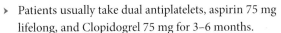

Inpatient

➤ PFO closure can be day-case surgery, but patients usually stay overnight for cardiac monitoring and to have a postoperative ECHO.

Outpatient

➤ Patients usually take dual antiplatelets, aspirin 75 mg lifelong, and Clopidogrel 75 mg for 3–6 months.

➤ An echocardiogram is performed after 4 weeks and again after a further 6 months.

 SURGEON'S FAVOURITE QUESTIONS

What is the difference between an ASD and a PFO?

An ASD is a congenital defect, while a PFO is failure of the foramen ovale to close (i.e., it is not a congenital defect of the heart and is confined to the fossa ovalis). ASDs can be larger and may affect the atrio-ventricular fibrous skeleton.

PLEURODESIS

Nick Leaver

DEFINITION

› Surgical adhesion of the parietal and visceral lung pleura to obliterate the pleural space.

✓ INDICATIONS

› Massive pleural effusions:
  › Malignant (e.g., breast, ovarian, lymphoma).
  › Benign (e.g., congestive heart failure, cirrhosis refractory to treatment).
› Recurrent pneumothoraces.
› Broncho-pleural fistula.

✗ CONTRAINDICATIONS

› Pleurodesis will fail if the lung cannot fully expand to the chest wall, e.g.:
  › Endobronchial obstruction.
  › Fibrotic inelastic pleura 'trapped lung'.
  › Entrapped lung—inflammatory or malignant process restricting expansion.

ANATOMY

› The pleura is composed of two layers: the parietal pleura and the visceral pleura.
› The lung is covered by the visceral pleura, whilst the chest wall is covered by a layer of parietal pleura.
› The parietal pleura is continuous with the visceral pleura and so creates a potential space between the two layers, called the pleural cavity, which is filled with pleural fluid.
› The left and right pleural cavities are not connected, and hence a pneumothorax or effusion is one sided.
› The pleural fluid is produced by the parietal pleura and is reabsorbed by the lymphatic vessels in the pleural cavity. If production exceeds absorption, or if drainage is blocked, a pleural effusion occurs.
› As the visceral pleura coats the lung, it receives its blood supply from the bronchial circulation.
› The parietal pleura receives its blood supply via the intercostal arteries lying under each rib.
› The visceral pleura receives innervation via the autonomic nervous system.
› The parietal pleura is innervated by the intercostal nerves and branches of the phrenic nerve.

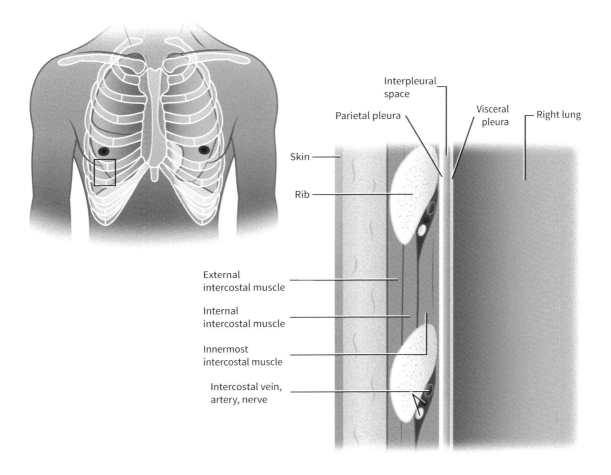

Interpleural space

Parietal pleura

Visceral pleura

Right lung

Skin

Rib

External intercostal muscle

Internal intercostal muscle

Innermost intercostal muscle

Intercostal vein, artery, nerve

Figure 8.11 Layers and structures of the thoracic wall

STEP-BY-STEP OPERATION

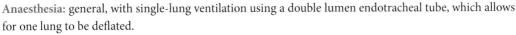

Anaesthesia: general, with single-lung ventilation using a double lumen endotracheal tube, which allows for one lung to be deflated.

Position: either the left or right lateral decubitus position.

Considerations: Pleurodesis can be performed as either an open approach or through video-assisted thoracoscopic approach (VATS), as described below.

1 Two to three incisions are made, typically in the seventh intercostal space, in the mid-axillary line, and working ports are inserted in the lateral chest wall.

2 The camera is inserted into a port (usually in the seventh intercostal space), and the pleural fluid is drained from the pleural cavity.

3 The surgeon may take biopsies with forceps from the lung or pleura if deemed macroscopically abnormal.

4 Talc (hydrated magnesium silicate) is powdered onto the surface of the lung, and any excess talc is suctioned out of the pleural space. The talc causes an inflammatory response, resulting in adhesions between the parietal and visceral pleura that obliterate the pleural space. Other chemical agents can be used, such as tetracycline or iodopovidone.

5 Mechanical pleurodesis involves 'roughing up' the parietal pleura by irritating it with a gauze. This irritation causes a similar inflammatory response as to the talc, causing adhesions to form between the visceral and parietal pleura.

6 A pleurectomy can be performed where the parietal pleura is stripped from the thoracic wall, causing the same inflammatory that which results in adhesions and obliteration of the pleural cavity.

7 Once the pleurodesis is complete, the lung is re-expanded and the incision sites closed.

8 A chest drain is inserted and clamped for 1–2 hours.

CARDIOTHORACICS

Figure 8.12 Mechanical pleurodesis

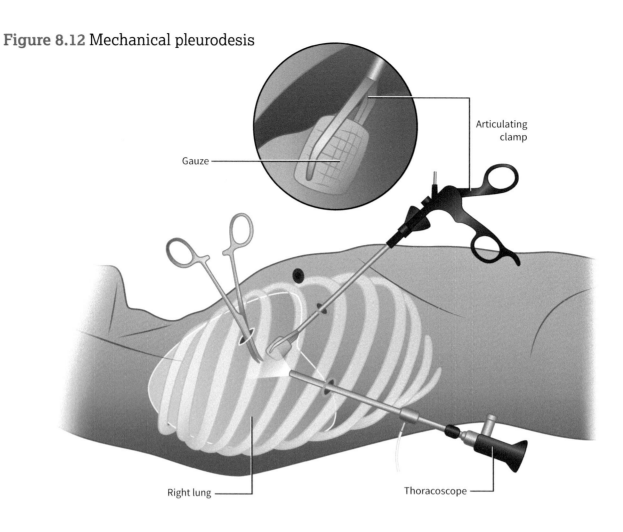

Gauze

Articulating clamp

Right lung

Thoracoscope

COMPLICATIONS

Early

› Chest pain.
› Fever through mild systemic inflammatory response.
› Tachycardia.
› Hypoxaemia rarely progressing to respiratory failure/ Acute Respiratory Distress Syndrome.

Intermediate and late

› Infection (e.g., empyema).

› Cardiac: hypotension, arrhythmias, myocardial infarction.
› Pneumothorax.
› Empyema.
› The pleura can take from a few weeks to a few months to become fully adherent.
› Failure requiring repeat pleurodesis.

POSTOPERATIVE CARE

Inpatient

- The chest drain is kept in place until drainage is less than 150 ml in 24 hours in order to maintain apposition of pleural surfaces.
- Patients are encouraged to mobilise early, as this will lead to higher chances of an adherent lung and reduced incidence of chest infections.

- Early discharge is important for patients with malignant pleural effusion, as this group of patients usually have a limited life expectancy, and this therapeutic procedure's main aim is to improve quality of life.

Outpatient

- Outpatient follow-up is not required if procedure is successful.

SURGEON'S FAVOURITE QUESTION

What other procedure could be done concurrently with a VATS pleurodesis for a patient with recurrent pneumothoraces?

A bullectomy, which involves stapling off any areas of the lung surface with 'blebs', which are a source of recurrent pneumothoraces, as these are areas of lung wall weakness.

THORACOTOMY

Christina Cheng

DEFINITION

A surgical procedure to gain access to the pleural space, or structures within the chest: heart, lungs, oesophagus, thoracic aorta, or anterior thoracic spine.

✔ INDICATION

- Any pulmonary resections, mediastinal operations, or oesophageal operations that are unsuitable to a minimally invasive approach.
- Surgical approach to the posterior mediastinum and vertebral column (e.g., scoliosis surgery or descending thoracic aorta surgery).
- Emergency trauma surgery to manage correctable causes of shock: decompressing cardiac tamponade, managing exsanguinating cardiac or vascular injuries, and evacuating air embolism.
- As a conversion from failure of video-assisted thoracoscopic surgery (VATS).

✖ CONTRAINDICATIONS

- In the context of trauma, thoracotomy is likely to be futile if, >10 mins pre-hospital CPR, there are no signs of life or massive non-survivable injuries.
- Where smaller access is suitable (e.g., thoracostomy or VATS).

ANATOMY

Gross anatomy

- Thoracotomy can be divided into three different approaches; the choice of approach is based on the aim of surgery being performed:
  - Posterolateral thoracotomy is used to access the posterior mediastinum, lung, and oesophagus.
  - Anterolateral thoracotomy is used for unilateral lung transplant and an open-chest massage.
  - Transverse thoracosternotomy is used to access the superior mediastinum and for excision of large mediastinal masses.
- Layers of the thoracic wall: subcutaneous tissue, external intercostal muscle, internal intercostal muscle, innermost intercostal muscle, parietal pleura, interpleural space, visceral pleura, and the lung.

Neurovasculature

- The intercostal neurovascular bundle runs in the costal groove on the inferior border of the rib and contains, from top to bottom: vein, artery, nerve ('VAN'). These structures run deep to the intercostal muscles and are covered by the parietal pleura.
- Muscles of the chest wall
  - Lateral: latissimus dorsi and serratus anterior.
  - Anterior: pectoralis major and minor.
  - Posterior: trapezius, rhomboid major and minor.

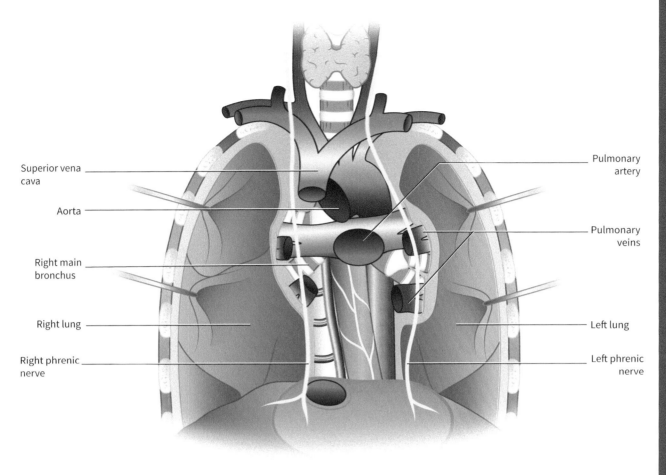

Superior vena cava

Aorta

Right main bronchus

Right lung

Right phrenic nerve

Pulmonary artery

Pulmonary veins

Left lung

Left phrenic nerve

Figure 8.13 Gross anatomy of the thorax

STEP-BY-STEP OPERATION

Anaesthesia: general, with a double lumen endotracheal tube that allows for one lung to be deflated.

Position: The most common approach is the posterolateral approach, which requires the lateral decubitus position.

1. A skin incision is made from the fifth intercostal space (just below level of nipple) and runs from the anterior axillary line and extends posteriorly to below the tip of the scapula.

2. The incision is continued cranially between the medial border of the scapula and the vertebral spinous processes and continues to the level of the spine of scapula.

3. The latissimus dorsi is divided, and serratus anterior is identified and retracted.

4. To avoid damage to the underlying intercostal neurovascular bundle, the intercostal muscles just above the sixth rib are divided.

5. Prior to entering the pleural cavity, the lung is deflated.

6. The intrathoracic procedure of choice is then undertaken.

7. Chest drains are inserted.

8. Muscle layers are approximated, and the wound is closed in layers.

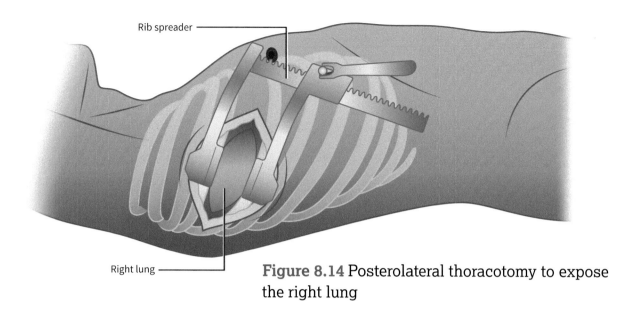

Figure 8.14 Posterolateral thoracotomy to expose the right lung

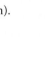

COMPLICATIONS

Early

> Atelectasis.
> Respiratory failure.
> Bleeding.

Intermediate and late

> Pneumothorax (made less common with the placement of a chest drain).

> Infection.
> Arrhythmias.
> Pulmonary oedema.
> Bronchopleural fistula.
> Thoracotomy pain syndrome (chronic pain).
> Cardiac herniation (if pericardium disrupted).
> Right heart failure (with extensive lung resection).

POSTOPERATIVE CARE

Inpatient

> Inpatient course is largely dependent upon indication for thoracotomy and postoperative complications, but generally chest tube management and removal as guided by serial chest X-rays.
> Regular physiotherapy and early mobility are recommended.

Outpatient

> Specific follow-up and typical duration of hospital stay will be guided based on the indication and type of surgery performed.

💬 SURGEON'S FAVOURITE QUESTION

In the lateral decubitus position, poor positioning may lead to shoulder displacement. What are the structures that may be at risk if this occurs?

The brachial plexus (lower four cervical nerves and first thoracic nerve, C5, C6, C7, C8, T1). Injury can cause pain, numbness, weakness, and/or loss of movement in the shoulder, arm, or hand.

9 NEUROSURGERY

WILLIAM B LO, MATHEW GALLAGHER

BURR HOLE

James Brooks and Mathew Gallagher

DEFINITION

The creation of one or two small openings through the cranium and dura.

✓ INDICATIONS

- Chronic subdural haematoma causing mass effect or resulting in symptoms such as headache, reduced level of consciousness, or focal neurological deficit (e.g., hemiparesis or dysphasia).
- Access for:
  - Hydrocephalus: placement of a temporary or permanent cerebrospinal fluid diversion device (external ventricular drain or ventricular catheter in shunt operation).
- Infection: aspiration of an abscess.
- Tumour: for biopsy of tumour.
- Functional neurosurgery: electrode placement in deep brain stimulator insertion (e.g., for Parkinson's disease) or electroencephalogram (EEG) electrode insertion for recording in patients with epilepsy.

✗ CONTRAINDICATIONS

- Uncorrected coagulopathy.

ANATOMY

- The scalp is composed of the skin, the connective tissues, the galea aponeurosis, the loose connective tissue, and the periosteum.
- Deep to the skull bones are the meninges, which cover the brain and continue inferiorly in the spinal canal to cover the spinal cord and nerve roots.
- The meninges are composed of (from superficial to deep): the dura mater, the arachnoid mater, and the pia mater.
- There are *real* and *potential* spaces between the meninges:
  - The dura is adherent to the cranium, but in between is the *potential* extradural space where an extradural haematoma can form, usually from middle meningeal artery injury.
- Between the dura and the arachnoid mater is the *real* subdural space where acute and chronic subdural haematomas can form, usually from tearing of bridging veins.
- Between the arachnoid and the pia mater is the real subarachnoid space filled with cerebrospinal fluid, where subarachnoid haemorrhages occur after rupture of an arterial aneurysm or arteriovenous malformation.
- A chronic subdural haematoma most commonly forms following the tearing of bridging veins between the dura and the pia mater, often secondary to minor head injuries in elderly patients with cerebral atrophy.

Figure 9.1 Layers of the scalp and the meninges

Subdural hematoma

Skin

Subcutaneous connective tissue

Galea aponeurosis

SCALP

Loose connective tissue

Periosteum

Dura mater

Bone

Arachnoid space

Pia mater

Arachnoid mater

STEP-BY-STEP OPERATION

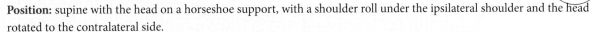

Anaesthesia: general or local.

Position: supine with the head on a horseshoe support, with a shoulder roll under the ipsilateral shoulder and the head rotated to the contralateral side.

Considerations: Where there is hair, the scalp should be shaved.

1 Two 3 cm incisions are marked over the anterior and posterior parts of the haematoma, which are frequently in the frontal or parietal region. The two incisions should be along the incision of a potential trauma craniotomy flap in case a conversion is required. Alternatively, a single incision can be marked over the thickest part of the haematoma.

2 An incision straight down to bone is made with a scalpel, and self-retainers are used to open the incision.

3 The periosteum is displaced off the bone with a periosteal elevator.

4 A high-speed pneumatic drill with a 14 mm diameter perforator clutch drill bit is used to create a burr hole perpendicular to the cranium at each opening. The perforator stops automatically when the inner table of the cranium is breached, preventing 'plunging' and injury to the underlying brain.

5 Thin bone fragments are removed using a blunt hook and artery clip. The dura is coagulated with bipolar diathermy and then opened in a cruciate fashion with a finer scalpel.

6 The liquefied haematoma is released from the burr hole(s) under pressure.

7 The haematoma is irrigated with warm normal saline or Ringer's solution (an isotonic solution) until clear.

8 A drain is left in the subdural space if the brain does not re-expand.

9 The galea aponeurosis is closed with an absorbable suture and the skin with a non-absorbable suture.

NEUROSURGERY

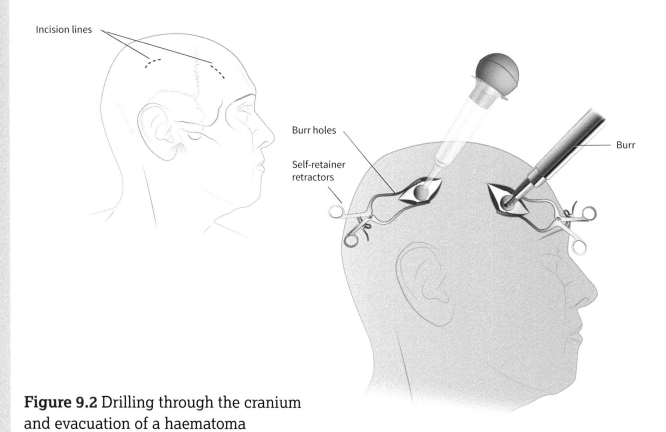

Figure 9.2 Drilling through the cranium and evacuation of a haematoma

COMPLICATIONS

Early

> Cerebral haematoma.
> Cerebral vascular accident (<5%).
> Seizure (<10%).

Intermediate and late

> Haematoma re-accumulation (<10%—risk reduced by the use of a drain for 48 hours).

> Tension pneumocephalus (<5%—air in the subdural space causing pressure effect.)
> Infection (<5%—superficial skin or subdural empyema).

POSTOPERATIVE CARE

Inpatient

> Hourly neurological observations.
> Gradual mobilisation.
> Removal of the drain at 24–48 hours.
> If there are residual symptoms, repeat CT of the head to exclude recurrence.

Outpatient

> Removal of sutures after 7 days.
> 6-week review after discharge.
> Future haemorrhage and thromboembolism risks should be assessed before recommencement of antiplatelet/ anticoagulant.

SURGEON'S FAVOURITE QUESTION

What scale do we use to describe adult conscious level?

The Glasgow Coma Scale (GCS). This is formed from the patient's eye opening, verbal, and motor responses and is scored out of 15. The lowest score is 3.

Eye opening (E)	Verbal response (V)	Motor response (M)
4 – Spontaneously	5 – Orientated	6 – Obey commands
3 – To voice	4 – Confused	5 – Localise to pain
2 – To pain	3 – Inappropriate words	4 – Normal flexion/withdraw from pain
1 – None	2 – Incomprehensible sounds	3 – Abnormal flexion to pain
	1 – None	2 – Extension to pain
	(T – Intubated)	1 – None

It is important to give a breakdown of the GCS in the form of E, V, and M because motor response is the most useful predictor of neurological status and is less affected by confounding conditions (e.g., inability to open eyes due to peri-orbital haematoma in an intubated patient who has sustained a head injury).

CRANIOTOMY

James Brooks and Mathew Gallagher

NEUROSURGERY

DEFINITION

The creation and temporary removal of a bone flap from the cranium to access the intracranial compartment.

✓ INDICATIONS

For removing an intracranial tumour

- Histological diagnosis.
- Improvement in quality of life—relief or control of focal neurological deficit or symptoms secondary to raised intracranial pressure (headache, vomiting, visual disturbance, and reduced conscious level).
- Improving life expectancy and prognosis.

Other

- Evacuation of traumatic or spontaneous intracranial haematoma (extradural, acute subdural, or intracerebral).

- Treatment of vascular abnormality (e.g., clipping of aneurysm).
- Removal of abscess or empyema.
- Insertion of subdural grid or strip electrode for investigation of epilepsy or resection of epileptogenic lesion or brain tissue.

✗ CONTRAINDICATIONS

- Uncorrected coagulopathy.
- Short life expectancy or poor performance status that cannot be improved by surgery.

ANATOMY

- The scalp is composed of the **s**kin, the **c**onnective tissue, the galea **a**poneurosis, the **l**oose connective tissue, and the **p**eriosteum.
- The cranial vault comprises the frontal, sphenoid, temporal, parietal, and occipital bones. Where two bones join is called a suture.
- The meninges (dura mater, arachnoid mater, and pia mater) cover the brain.
- The cranial cavity is divided into the supratentorial and infratentorial compartments by the tentorium cerebelli. The supratentorial compartment contains the cerebrum, which is divided into two hemispheres by the falx cerebri. Each hemisphere is divided into the frontal, temporal, parietal, occipital, and insular lobes. The infratentorial compartment contains the brain stem and the cerebellum.
- Each lobe contains important functional areas:
  - The prefrontal cortex is responsible for thought, cognition, and personality; the inferior frontal region in the dominant hemisphere (usually left)

  is Broca's area, responsible for expressive speech function.
  - The pre-central gyrus of the posterior frontal lobe contains the primary motor cortex.
  - The post-central gyrus of the parietal lobe contains the primary sensory cortex.
  - The dominant posterior superior temporal gyrus contains the Wernicke's area for receptive speech function.
  - The temporal lobe contains the primary olfactory cortex, primary and secondary auditory cortex, and visual memory cortex. The hippocampus in the temporal lobe is involved in new memory formation.
  - The occipital lobe contains the primary, secondary, and tertiary visual cortex.
- Intracranial tumours in order of incidence:
  1. Metastasis.
  2. Meningioma.
  3. Glioma.
  4. Others.

264

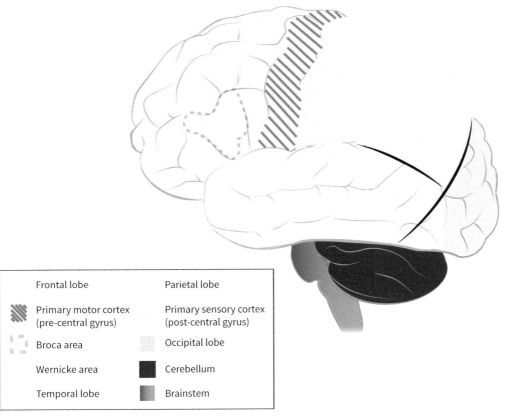

Figure 9.3 Functional areas of the brain

Frontal lobe   Parietal lobe

Primary motor cortex (pre-central gyrus)   Primary sensory cortex (post-central gyrus)

Broca area   Occipital lobe

Wernicke area   Cerebellum

Temporal lobe   Brainstem

STEP-BY-STEP OPERATION

Anaesthesia: general or local for awake tumour resection in eloquent areas (e.g., primary motor cortex and speech areas). Dexamethasone is often given preoperatively to reduce cerebral oedema.

Position: The patient's head is secured with a Mayfield three-pin head frame attached to the operating table.

Considerations: Neuronavigation is often used to plan the craniotomy site. 'Neuronavigation' is the use of computer software to map preoperative imaging to the patient's head in theatre in order to guide surgery. The surgeon watches a screen combining the preoperative imaging and the real-time position of an instrument (stereotactic probe), enabling them to both locate the tumour and appreciate their location in the brain.

1 The scalp is incised and reflected off the cranium. Raney clips are placed along the scalp edge to reduce blood loss.

2 Burr holes are fashioned in the skull, and the bone flap is created with a craniotome (drill tip with a foot plate that protects the dura) attached to the pneumatic drill to connect the burr holes.

3 Hitch stitches are used to attach the dura to the skull or soft tissue to prevent extradural haematomas forming.

4 The dura is coagulated and then opened using a scalpel or scissors to create a flap.

5 An extrinsic tumour (e.g., meningioma) can be resected by dissecting the tissue plane between the cortex and the tumour.

6 For an intrinsic tumour that does not extend to the brain surface, the brain cortex is opened (a 'corticotomy') in order to access the tumour. The resection can be performed with bipolar diathermy, suction, cavitron ultrasonic surgical aspirator (CUSA), pituitary rongeurs, and microinstruments. A microscope is often used.

7 The dura is closed with absorbable sutures.

8 After haemostasis, the bone flap is replaced if the brain is not too oedematous. The bone flap is secured with titanium plates and screws or sutures.

9 The scalp is closed in two layers: absorbable suture to the galea aponeurosis and non-absorbable suture or clips to the skin.

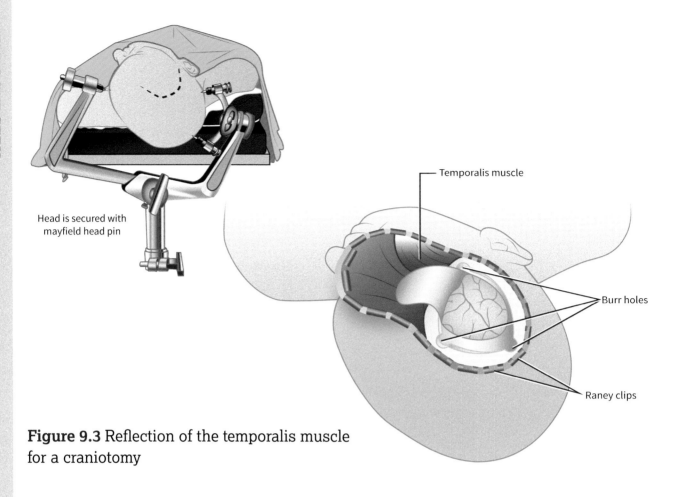

Head is secured with
mayfield head pin

Temporalis muscle

Burr holes

Raney clips

Figure 9.3 Reflection of the temporalis muscle
for a craniotomy

COMPLICATIONS

Early

> Intracranial haematoma (<5%).
> Focal cerebral oedema (<5%).
> Neurological deficit (including hemiparesis and dysphasia) (<10%).

Intermediate and late

> Electrolyte imbalance <5% (typically syndrome of inappropriate ADH secretion).

> Cerebrospinal fluid leak (<5%).
> Hydrocephalus (<5%).
> Infection <5% (wound or bone flap).
> Seizures (10–20%).
> Tumour recurrence.
> Death (<1%).

POSTOPERATIVE CARE

Inpatient

> Hourly neurological observations for 6 hours, postoperative fluid balance and bloods. If the patient is not recovering appropriately, an urgent postoperative CT of the head should be performed to exclude haemorrhage.
> MRI of the head within 3 days to assess residual tumour (for intrinsic tumours).
> Reducing dexamethasone course.

> Thromboembolic prophylaxis from 24 hours if no haemorrhage.

Outpatient

> Guided by diagnosis.
> Removal of sutures at 7 days.
> Oncology review for adjuvant therapy (e.g., stereotactic radiosurgery, radiotherapy, or chemotherapy if appropriate).
> Regular MRI brain to exclude recurrence.

SURGEON'S FAVOURITE QUESTION

Which drug is commonly used to treat cerebral oedema?

Dexamethasone, with a dose up to 16 mg daily in divided doses. Normally given with gastric protection medication such as a proton pump inhibitor to prevent gastric ulcers.

LUMBAR LAMINECTOMY

Alexander Dando and Mathew Gallagher

DEFINITION

Removal of the lumbar lamina in order to decompress and access the contents of the spinal canal.

✓ INDICATIONS

- Decompression of the lumbar spinal canal and nerves +/- treatment of an intraspinal lesion. These can be divided into emergency or elective:
  - Emergency—cauda equina syndrome or severe pain secondary to intervertebral disc herniation, trauma, epidural haematoma, abscess, and neoplasm causing neurological deficit.
  - Elective—lumbar stenosis, lateral recess stenosis, lumbar disc herniation, extradural compressive lesions, intradural tumours.

✗ CONTRAINDICATIONS

- Uncorrected coagulopathy or antiplatelet/coagulation drugs.
- Local skin infection.
- Spinal deformity or instability—can be worsened by laminectomy.

ANATOMY

Vertebral column

- The vertebral column consists of 33 vertebrae: 7 cervical, 12 thoracic, 5 lumbar, 5 sacral, which are fused together, and 3 coccygeal vertebrae, which are also fused together.
- Vertebrae are separated by intervertebral discs.
- The spinal cord runs within the vertebral canal, from the foramen magnum to vertebral level L1/2 (in adults). Below this is the cauda equina, which comprises the remaining nerve roots on the way to their exit levels.
- The vertebral column is supported by several ligaments: the anterior and posterior longitudinal ligaments, the ligamenta flava, the interspinous ligaments, and the supraspinous ligament.
- Running parallel to the vertebral column are the erector spinae muscles.

Vertebrae

- Each vertebra can be divided into two sections. The anterior vertebral body takes most of the load-bearing function. The posterior vertebral arch protects and allows the spinal cord, nerve roots, and central vessels to pass through it.
- The posterior vertebral arch consists of laminae, pedicles, and a spinous process, as well as transverse processes in the thoracic vertebrae.
- At each vertebral level, there is an associated intervertebral foramina, formed between the inferior vertebral notch of the vertebra above and the superior vertebral notch of the vertebra below. Spinal nerves travel out of these foramina.
- Between the vertebrae lie the intervertebral discs, consisting of an outer annulus fibrosis and an inner nucleus pulposus. The intervertebral discs are avascular in adults.

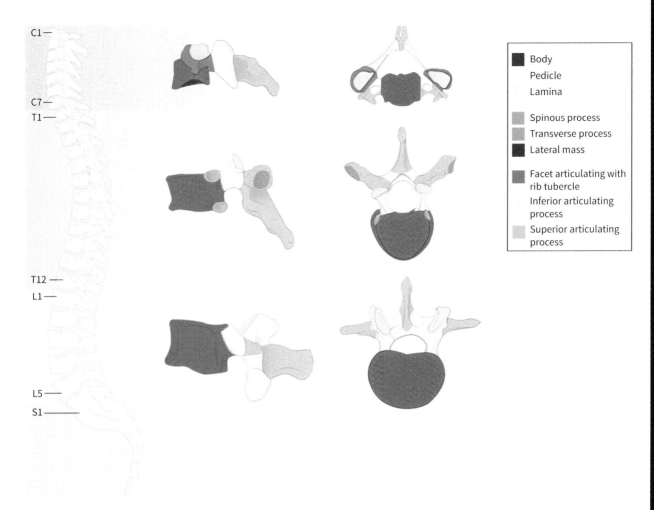

C1 —
C7 —
T1 —
T12 —
L1 —
L5 —
S1 —

	Body
	Pedicle
	Lamina
	Spinous process
	Transverse process
	Lateral mass
	Facet articulating with rib tubercle
	Inferior articulating process
	Superior articulating process

Figure 9.5 Structure of vertebrae from all sections of the vertebral column

STEP-BY-STEP OPERATION

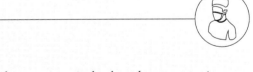

Anaesthesia: general.

Position: prone on a Wilson's or Montreal frame.

1 Using fluoroscopy and a spinal needle, the correct vertebral level is identified and marked.
2 A midline incision is made, and the subcutaneous tissue is dissected in the midline with monopolar diathermy.
3 The thoracolumbar fascia is identified and dissected in order to access the spinous processes.
4 The paraspinal muscles are dissected off the spinous processes and the laminae, and the level is confirmed again with fluoroscopy.
5 Retractors are placed to maintain the surgical field. The spinous process and the supraspinous and interspinous ligaments superior and inferior to the operated level are removed.
6 Using Kerrison up cuts, the lamina is removed bilaterally. The ligamentum flavum is also removed. The dura is carefully exposed.

7 For degenerative spinal or lateral recess stenosis, any remaining hypertrophied or calcified ligament or degenerative tissue is removed. The intervertebral foramen, narrowed by the hypertrophic facet joint, may need to be undercut. The dura and nerve roots are confirmed to be adequately decompressed.
8 For disc herniation, the dura is retracted away from the affected side with a nerve root retractor, and a discectomy is performed.
9 Following decompression, the retractor is removed and the wound is closed. The fascia and subcutaneous tissues are closed with absorbable sutures, and the skin is closed with non-absorbable sutures.

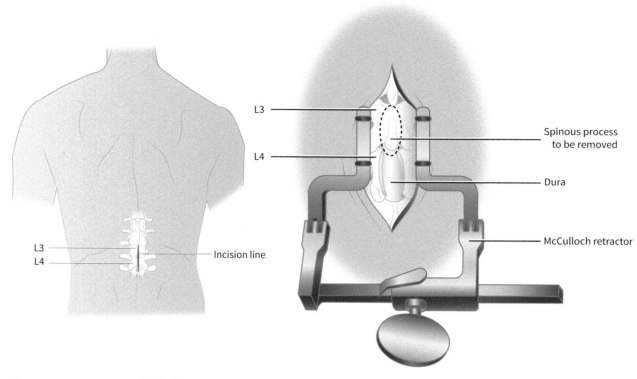

Figure 9.6 Removal of the spinous process at L4 to aid decompression

COMPLICATIONS

Immediate

> Dural tear and cerebrospinal fluid (CSF) leak (<10%).
> Nerve root injury causing neurological deficit (<1%).
> Postoperative haematoma requiring evacuation (<1%).

Intermediate and late

> Pseudomeningocele (a collection of CSF in the soft tissue from an iatrogenic CSF leak).
> Infection (5%—usually superficial but can potentially cause meningitis if deep).
> Inadequate decompression, recurrence of symptoms.
> Spinal instability requiring further surgery (<5%).

POSTOPERATIVE CARE

Inpatient

> Hourly neurological observations.
> Analgesia with early mobilisation.

Outpatient

> Removal of sutures at 7 days.

> Routine 3-month review, no further imaging required unless ongoing unresolved symptoms at 6 months.

SURGEON'S FAVOURITE QUESTION

What clinical signs are seen in cauda equina syndrome?

Saddle anaesthesia—partial or complete.

Sphincter disturbance—urinary retention, urinary or faecal incontinence, decreased anal tone.

Acute motor weakness.

VENTRICULOPERITONEAL (VP) SHUNT INSERTION

James Brooks and Mathew Gallagher

DEFINITION

The placement of a permanent cerebrospinal fluid (CSF) diversion device from the lateral ventricle to the peritoneal cavity.

✔ INDICATIONS

- Hydrocephalus—excessive intracranial CSF accumulation, as a result of disordered or imbalanced CSF production, circulation, and absorption, leading to raised intracranial pressure (headache, vomiting, visual impairment, and decreased consciousness).
- Can be classified as:
  - *Communicating*—there is communication between the ventricles and the subarachnoid space and is characterised by panventricular dilatation.
  - *Non-communicating or obstructive* —an obstruction within the ventricular system or at the outlets of the fourth ventricle.

✘ CONTRAINDICATIONS

- Concurrent infection of the CSF, or systemically.
- Concurrent moderate to severe intraventricular haemorrhage.
- Uncorrected coagulopathy.
- High CSF cell count, including concurrent intraventricular haemorrhage (increased risk of shunt obstruction).

ANATOMY

- CSF is produced in the choroid plexus, which is present in the lateral, third, and fourth ventricles.
- From the lateral ventricles, CSF flows through the foramina of Monro bilaterally into the midline third ventricle. This connects to the fourth ventricle via the cerebral aqueduct. From the fourth ventricle, CSF circulates through the bilateral foramina of Luschka and the foramen of Magendie in the midline into the spinal and cerebral convexity subarachnoid space.
- CSF is absorbed from the subarachnoid space into the dural venous sinuses through arachnoid granulations.
- Normal CSF pressure is <15mm Hg.

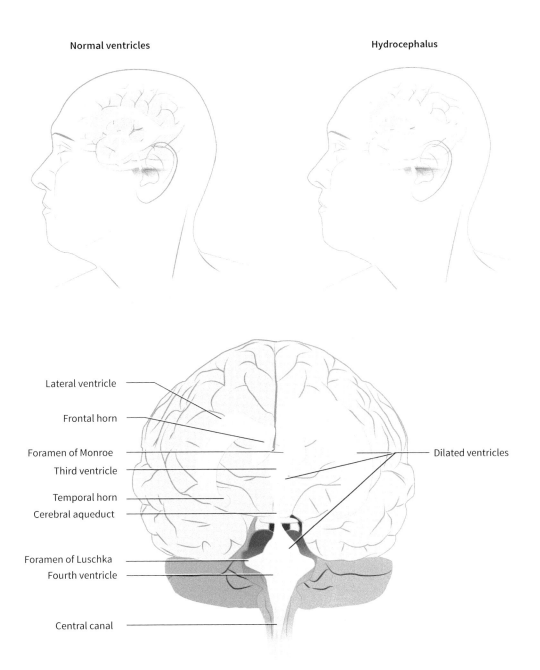

Normal ventricles

Hydrocephalus

Lateral ventricle

Frontal horn

Foramen of Monroe

Third ventricle

Temporal horn

Cerebral aqueduct

Foramen of Luschka

Fourth ventricle

Central canal

Dilated ventricles

Figure 9.7 Cerebral ventricular system and changes associated with hydrocephalus

STEP-BY-STEP OPERATION

Anaesthesia: general.

Position: supine with the head turned to the left on a horseshoe support and a sandbag/shoulder roll under the right shoulder. Shunts are commonly inserted on the right side, as most patients are left-side dominant.

Considerations: Neuronavigation is often used to plan the craniotomy site. 'Neuronavigation' is the use of computer software that maps preoperative imaging to the patient's head in theatre in order to guide surgery. The surgeon watches a screen combining the pre-op imaging and the real-time position of an instrument (stereotactic probe), enabling them to both locate the tumour and appreciate their location in the brain.

1 Cranial site: An inverted hockey stick or inverted U incision is made 3cm superior and posterior to the superior tip of the pinna, ensuring that the incision does not overlie any shunt component. A pocket is created in the soft tissue for the placement of the valve. A burr hole is fashioned.

2 Abdominal site: A right subcostal (5 cm) paramedian transverse incision is made over the right rectus abdominis. The anterior rectus sheath is opened transversely and the rectus muscle split vertically in a muscle-sparing fashion. The posterior rectus sheath and the peritoneum, which are sometimes adherent, are opened. Peristalsing bowel must be visualised to confirm that the peritoneal cavity is entered.

3 A metal tunnelling device is advanced from the cranial to the abdominal site (or vice versa) to recreate a passage in the subcutaneous fat layer, superficial to the clavicle and vascular structures in the neck.

4 The shunt valve and the distal (peritoneal) catheter are assembled, and the catheter is passed through the tunneller.

5 The tunneller is removed. The valve and distal catheter are placed in the optimal position. The valve and distal catheter are primed by filling with saline.

6 The dura is coagulated and opened with a small cruciate incision. The ventricular catheter is passed into the occipital horn of the right lateral ventricle. Once the catheter enters the ventricle. The stylet can be removed, and the catheter is 'soft passed' to a predetermined length (commonly 7cm in adults). CSF should be observed dripping out of the catheter.

7 The ventricular catheter is connected to the valve and secured with a tie.

8 After confirmation of free CSF dripping from the distal end, the distal catheter is inserted into the peritoneal cavity.

9 The cranial site and abdominal sites are closed. The abdomen is closed in layers—the posterior rectus sheath, anterior rectus sheath, dermis, and skin—to prevent migration of the catheter and incisional hernia.

Figure 9.8 Positioning and tunneling of a ventricular catheter from the occipital horn of the lateral ventricle into the peritoneal cavity

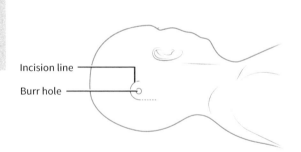

Incision line
Burr hole

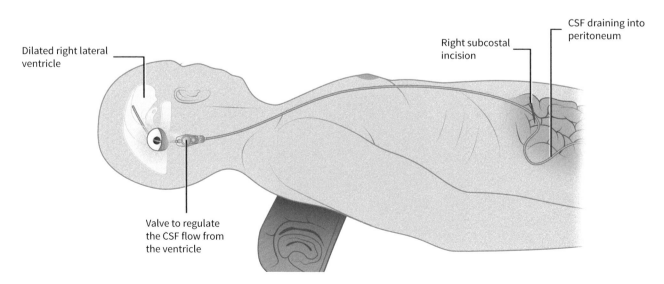

Dilated right lateral ventricle

Right subcostal incision

CSF draining into peritoneum

Valve to regulate the CSF flow from the ventricle

COMPLICATIONS

Early

> Failure – 40%.
> Cerebral haemorrhage.
> Seizure(s) (<1%).
> Bowel perforation.
> Injury to neck vascular structures.
> Pneumothorax.

Intermediate and late

> Over-drainage of CSF.
> Subdural haematoma.
> Under-drainage or shunt obstruction caused by debris, choroid plexus, or blood clot.
> Shunt disconnection or shunt fracture (most commonly in the neck).
> Catheter migration out of peritoneal cavity.
> Infection (10%—superficial and CSF).

POSTOPERATIVE CARE

Inpatient

> Hourly neurological observations.
> Some surgeons perform postoperative CT head and abdominal X-ray to confirm catheter position.

Outpatient

> Removal of sutures at 7 days.
> Routine review between 6–8 weeks.
> No regular imaging unless patient symptomatic of shunt malfunction (e.g., headaches, vomiting, visual symptoms).

 SURGEON'S FAVOURITE QUESTION

How much CSF is produced per day?

CSF is produced by the choroid plexus at a rate of 0.35ml/min, equivalent to approximately 500ml/day.

ENDOSCOPIC TRANSSPHENOIDAL PITUITARY SURGERY

Mathew Gallagher

DEFINITION

A minimally invasive transnasal and sphenoid sinus approach using an endoscope to excise or biopsy a tumour in the pituitary sellar region.

✓ INDICATIONS

Can be used for any sella turcica space-occupying lesion, with the aim of tissue diagnosis, control of symptoms, removal of mass effect, and treatment of pituitary apoplexy.

- Pituitary adenomas (functioning and non-functioning)—most common.
- Meningioma.
- Craniopharyngioma.
- Rathke cleft cyst.
- Metastasis.

✗ CONTRAINDICATIONS

- Prolactinoma—this responds to medical treatment effectively (dopamine agonists). Therefore, it is mandatory to check prolactin level in patients with a suspected pituitary adenoma.
- Tumour anatomy:
  - A tumour with a large suprasellar (superior to the sella turcica).
  - A tumour with a small sella.
  - Ectatic or tortuous carotid arteries protruding medially and obstructing the transsphenoidal access.
- Active sinusitis.

ANATOMY

Gross anatomy

- The pituitary gland resides in the sella turcica, a bony fossa formed by part of the sphenoid bone.
- The gland is attached to the hypothalamus superiorly through the pituitary stalk.
- The gland is overlain by a dural fold called the diaphragm sella.
- The sphenoid sinus is located anteroinferiorly, the clivus posteroinferiorly, and the cavernous sinuses laterally on either side.
- The pituitary gland is composed of anterior and posterior lobes:
  - The anterior pituitary produces adrenocorticotrophic hormone (ACTH), growth hormone (GH), thyroid-stimulating hormone (TSH), follicle-stimulating hormone (FSH), luteinising hormone (LH), and prolactin.
  - The posterior pituitary produces oxytocin and anti-diuretic hormone (ADH).
- The sphenoid sinus is a mucous membrane-lined nasal sinus located at the superior posterior aspect of the nasal cavity in the midline. It is separated from the nasal cavity by a thin shelf of bone. Frequently, a thin bony septum divides the sinus, although the position of the septum is variable.

Neurovasculature

- Within each cavernous sinus lies the internal carotid artery and the following cranial nerves: oculomotor (III), trochlear (IV), ophthalmic (V1), and maxillary (V2) branches of trigeminal (V) and abducent (VI).
- The blood supply of the pituitary gland is derived from the paired superior and inferior hypophyseal arteries, which arise bilaterally from the internal carotid arteries.
  - The superior hypophyseal arteries supply the anterior lobe and the pituitary stalk.
  - The inferior hypophyseal arteries supply the posterior lobe.
- Venous drainage is via the hypophyseal vein.

Figure 9.9 Anatomical relations of the pituitary glands

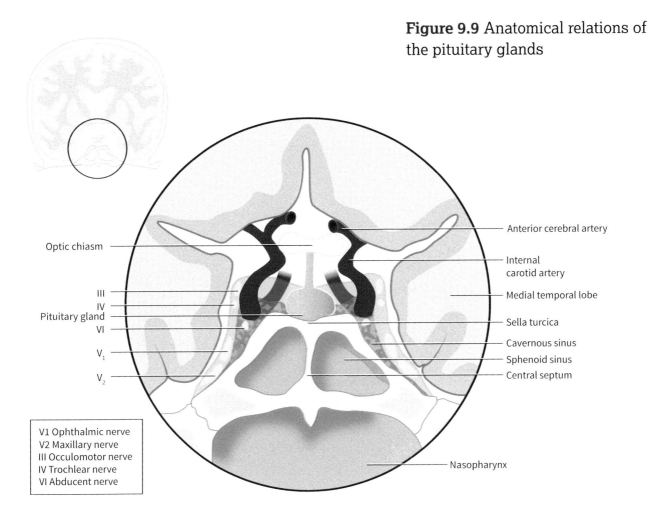

Optic chiasm

III
IV
Pituitary gland
VI

V₁

V₂

Anterior cerebral artery

Internal
carotid artery

Medial temporal lobe

Sella turcica

Cavernous sinus

Sphenoid sinus

Central septum

Nasopharynx

V1 Ophthalmic nerve
V2 Maxillary nerve
III Occulomotor nerve
IV Trochlear nerve
VI Abducent nerve

STEP-BY-STEP OPERATION

Anaesthesia: general.

Position: supine with the head on a soft head ring.

Considerations: During induction anaesthesia, the nasal cavities are prepared using neuropatties soaked with adrenaline and cocaine ('Moffett's solution'), which results in local vasoconstriction.

1   Using the endoscope, the right nasal cavity is entered and the middle turbinate is lateralised (fractured) to create more access. This can be done bilaterally if required.

2   A mucosal flap from the nasal septum may be created to help seal the sphenoid sinus at the end of the operation.

3   The sphenoid ostium, which marks the entry into the sphenoid sinus, is identified at the posterior aspect of the nasal cavity.

4   The anterior sphenoid wall is fractured and removed; excess sphenoidal mucosa is then removed.

5   The superior posterior sella bone is then opened, and the endoscope and instruments can be passed through *both* nostrils.

6   The dura is coagulated in an 'X' pattern and opened with a scalpel.

7   The tumour is removed using curettes and suction (Neuronavigation can be used).

8   To avoid cerebrospinal fluid (CSF) leak, the sellar and the sphenoid sinus can be packed or sealed by various materials following tumour excision. Options include fat graft harvested from the abdomen/fascia lata, fibrin or hydrogel sealant, and collagen-based dura substitute. A nasal septal mucosal flap (if prepared earlier) can be transposed to cover the sphenoid sinus.

9   The nasal cavity is packed with synthetic biodegradable foam.

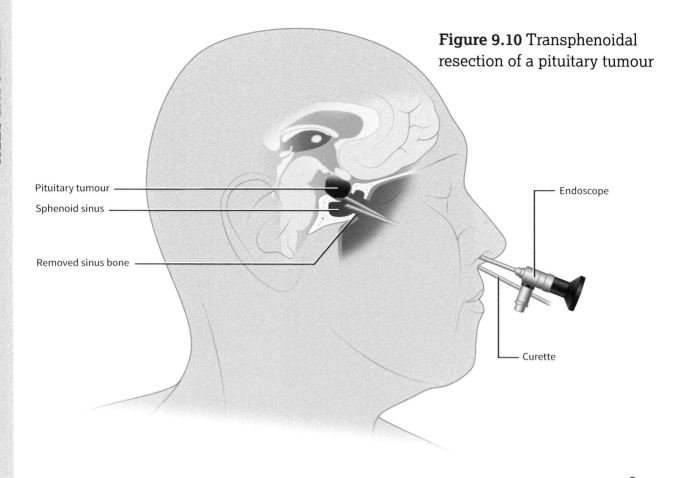

Figure 9.10 Transphenoidal resection of a pituitary tumour

Pituitary tumour

Sphenoid sinus

Removed sinus bone

Endoscope

Curette

COMPLICATIONS

Early

> Carotid artery injury (<1%).
> Visual loss from optic chiasm damage/compression (<1%).

Intermediate and late

> Hormonal disturbance (~15%)—diabetes insipidus caused by reduced ADH, panhypopituitarism.

> CSF rhinorrhoea (~2%)—this may require repair surgery or lumbar drain insertion.
> Infection and nasal crusting (1%).

POSTOPERATIVE CARE

Inpatient

> Monitoring and correction of electrolyte and fluid balance: if urine output is >250 ml/hr for 3 consecutive hours, serum sodium is >145 mmol/l, and urine specific gravity is <1.005, the patient has developed diabetes insipidus. Subcutaneous Desmopressin 1 microgram should be given.
> Oral hydrocortisone replacement should be given until hormonal status is established.

> The 'sick day rule' should be followed: double hydrocortisone dose in case of intercurrent illness and seek medical attention if the patient has persistent vomiting and acute severe illness.
> MRI pituitary.
> Endocrine review.
> Ophthalmology review.

Outpatient

> A steroid record card should be given to the patient to help manage steroid replacement and alert future healthcare professionals to the specific risks of the patient.

SURGEON'S FAVOURITE QUESTION

What is the most common form of visual field loss found with pituitary pathology?

A superior temporal quadrantanopia, progressing to a bitemporal hemianopia due to compression on the inferior aspect of the optic chiasm.

10 ORTHOPAEDICS

GANESH DEVARAJAN, GARETH ROGERS

DUPUYTREN'S CONTRACTURE RELEASE

Yashashwi Sinha

ORTHOPAEDICS

DEFINITION

The release of flexion contractures resulting from proliferation of the palmar and digital fascia.

✓ INDICATIONS

- Functional problems resulting from flexion deformity, including decreased range of motion and loss of dexterity.
- Metacarpal-phalangeal (MCP) joint fixed flexion contracture ≥30 degrees.
- Proximal interphalangeal (PIP) joint flexion >20 degrees.
- Maceration of the palmar skin folds.

✗ CONTRAINDICATIONS

- Multiple previous surgical releases of contractures with subsequent recurrence.
- Inability to undertake hand therapy postoperatively.

ANATOMY

Gross anatomy

- The palmar aponeurosis consists of pretendinous bands, the lateral digital sheet, and the natatory, spiral, and Grayson's ligaments.
- The four pretendinous bands of the aponeurosis begin at the wrist and fan across the palm, extending to the bases of each digit before bifurcating to form the spiral bands.
- Each pretendinous band aligns with one finger; disease along here causes central cords to form, producing the classically described contractures.
- Lateral digital sheets are thickened areas of superficial fascia on the lateral aspects of the fingers, lateral to the neurovascular bundles (NVB) of the digits.
- The natatory (superficial palmar transverse) ligament passes transversely across the hand at the base of the fingers.
- Spiral ligaments pass deep to NVBs to reach the lateral digital sheets. Spiral cords distort the NVBs, particularly at the level of the MCP joint.

- Grayson's ligaments are thin and attach the tendon sheath to skin (holding its position during digit movement).

Pathology

- In a non-diseased hand, the individual elements and layers of the palmar aponeurosis are separate entities. In Dupuytren's disease, however, these become incorporated into a single thick cord.
- Fingers affected by Dupuytren's contractures in order of incidence:
  - Ring (most common).
  - Little.
  - Middle.
  - Index.
  - Thumb (least common).

Figure 10.1 **Components of the palmar aponeurosis**

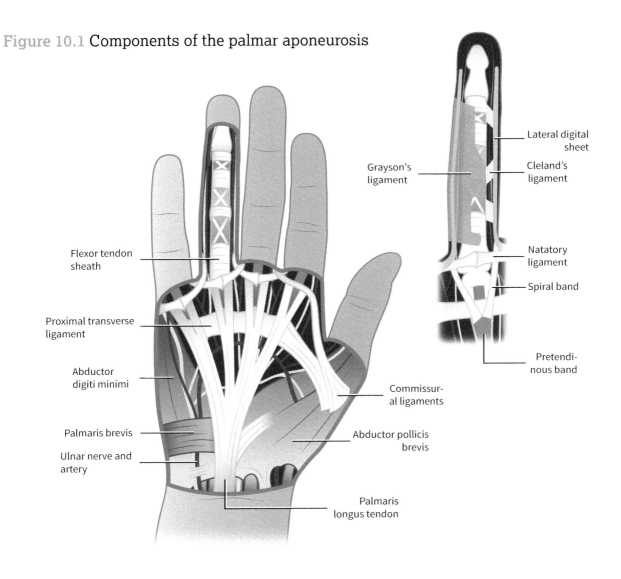

Flexor tendon sheath

Proximal transverse ligament

Abductor digiti minimi

Palmaris brevis

Ulnar nerve and artery

Palmaris longus tendon

Commissural ligaments

Abductor pollicis brevis

Grayson's ligament

Lateral digital sheet

Cleland's ligament

Natatory ligament

Spiral band

Pretendinous band

STEP-BY-STEP OPERATION

Anaesthesia: general or regional.

Position: supine with arm on board with tourniquet.

1 Make either a Z-plasty or Brunner incision running down the affected digit and, if affected, into the webspace.
2 Elevate the skin flaps above the central cords; these should be slightly thicker than sub-dermal.
3 Excise any longitudinal cord tissue.
4 Blunt dissect the neurovascular bundle away from the central cords all the way to the extent of the distal interphalangeal joint.
5 Now that the cords have been freely dissected, reassess for any further flexion deformity:
    a Boutonniere deformity of the proximal interphalangeal joint—splint in full extension for 6 weeks.
    b Volar plate contracture—release the tough ligament tissue with sharp dissection.

6 Assess the perfusion of fingers by releasing the tourniquet. If the finger fails to perfuse:
    a Blunt dissect away tissue to directly observe the arteries supplying the affected digits.
    b Flex the finger to the original position and reassess blood flow.
    c Bathe the vessel in verapamil or glyceryl trinitrate (GTN) solution and reassess blood flow.
7 Close the Z-plasty or Brunner incision with either absorbable interrupted or continuous sutures.
8 If the wound is unable to be closed, a skin graft is considered or the wound is left open to heal by secondary intention.

Figure 10.2 Excision of longitudinal cord tissue

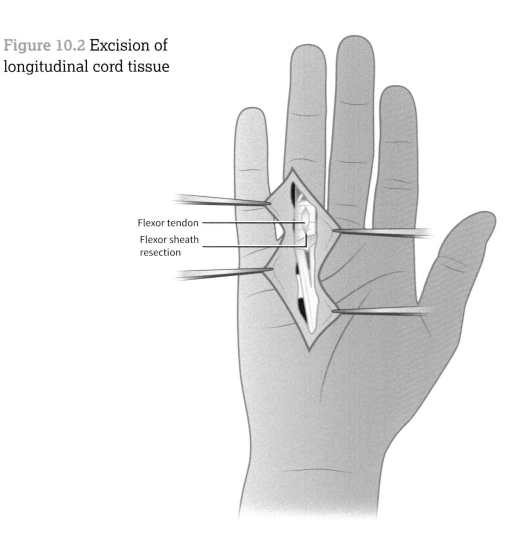

Flexor tendon

Flexor sheath resection

COMPLICATIONS

Early

> Vascular injury (including those related to the use of a tourniquet).
> Digital nerve injury—paraesthesia of the affected digit.
> Skin loss or failure of flap resulting in requiring a skin graft.
> Local pain (due to digital nerve injury and neuromas).
> Wound infection.

Intermediate and late

> Recurrence (25%, repeat surgery is often less successful).
> Complex regional pain syndrome (nociceptive sensitisation causing allodynia and vasomotor dysfunction).
> Stiffness and incomplete correction.

POSTOPERATIVE CARE

Outpatient

› Hand should be splinted in full extension for 1 week. Dressings are then removed and hand therapy commenced.

› The affected digit should be splinted in full extension, at night, for 3 months.

› Outpatient follow-up appointment in 6–8 weeks or via hand physiotherapists.

SURGEON'S FAVOURITE QUESTION

What patient demographic is commonly affected by idiopathic Dupuytren's?

Dupuytren's disease typically affects elderly men of northern European descent.

ARTHROSCOPIC ROTATOR CUFF TENDON REPAIR

Stephanie Arrigo

DEFINITION

Repair of one or more of the four rotator cuff tendons surrounding and supporting the shoulder.

✓ INDICATIONS

- Tears that:
  - Do not improve with conservative treatments.
  - Affect patient's activities of daily living.
  - Are traumatic (early surgery leads to better prognosis).

✗ CONTRAINDICATIONS

- Large tears of longstanding duration, since repairs to these injuries are unlikely to be successful or provide clinical benefit.
- Atraumatic tears with cuff degeneration in patients for whom conservative measures are effective.

ANATOMY

Gross anatomy

- The glenohumeral joint (GHJ):
  - The bony articulations of the scapula and the proximal humerus combine to form a highly mobile ball-and-socket joint.
  - The GHJ is stabilised by its capsule, the rotator cuff muscles, and the long head of biceps brachii muscle.
  - The GHJ is further stabilised by the superior, middle, and inferior glenohumeral ligaments, the coracohumeral ligament, the transverse humeral ligament, and the coraco-acromial ligament.
  - The proximal humerus has two tubercles: the greater tubercle, found laterally on the humerus, and the lesser tubercle, located anteriorly. They are separated by an intertubercular sulcus, through which the tendon of the long head of biceps brachii runs.
- Rotator cuff muscles:
  - The rotator cuff comprises four muscles originating from the scapula, whose tendons merge to form a common tendon over the posterior, superior, and anterior aspects of the GHJ.
  - The rotator cuff muscles are the supraspinatus, the infraspinatus, the teres minor, and the subscapularis.
  - The primary function of the rotator cuff muscles is to provide dynamic stability of the GHJ.
  - Each muscle is also responsible for a specific active movement that can be clinically tested for weakness when trying to determine if a tear is present.

Neurovascular

- The supraspinatus and infraspinatus are innervated by the suprascapular nerve.
- The teres minor is innervated by the axillary nerve.
- The subscapularis is innervated by the subscapular nerve.
- The GHJ receives its arterial supply from the anterior and posterior circumflex humeral arteries (branches of the axillary artery).

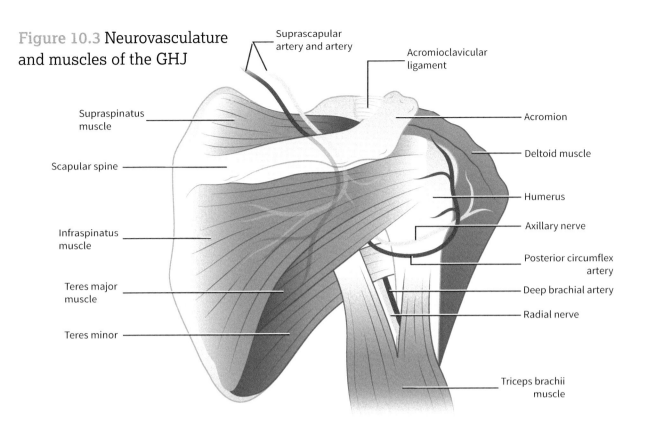

Figure 10.3 Neurovasculature and muscles of the GHJ

Suprascapular artery and artery

Acromioclavicular ligament

Supraspinatus muscle

Scapular spine

Infraspinatus muscle

Teres major muscle

Teres minor

Acromion

Deltoid muscle

Humerus

Axillary nerve

Posterior circumflex artery

Deep brachial artery

Radial nerve

Triceps brachii muscle

STEP-BY-STEP OPERATION

Anaesthesia: general.

Position: lateral position (with the affected shoulder uppermost) or in the 'beach chair' position with light traction applied to the arm.

Considerations: antibiotics are administered at induction.

1   First, the posterior portal incision is made 1–2 cm medial to the postero-lateral tip of the acromion. The joint is then flushed with normal saline.

2   Through the posterior port, the arthroscope is inserted to assess the GHJ and the surface of the rotator cuff. The rotator cuff tear is assessed for muscle involvement, size, location, and retraction.

3   A lateral portal is made in line with the mid-clavicle and 2–3 cm lateral to its lateral edge. This port allows for the removal of anterior bursal adhesions, the release of coracohumeral and coracoacromial ligaments, and assessment of the mobility of the tear using a grasper.

4   The tear is mobilised and debrided through the lateral port. The footprint of the tuberosity is then debrided using a high-speed burr.

5   Still using the posterior port, the arthroscope is repositioned into the subacromial bursa to assess the bursal surface of the rotator cuff.

6   The arthroscope is then transferred to the lateral port.

7   The tear is repaired using a combination of sutures and suture-anchors approximating the tendon to the tuberosity footprint.

8   Posterior adhesions are released through the posterior port.

9   An anterior portal is created halfway between the acromioclavicular joint and the lateral aspect of the coracoid to aid with suture passing.

10 Once the repair is complete, the joint is flushed with normal saline. The skin is closed in a deep layer with absorbable sutures and a superficial layer with non-resorbable sutures.

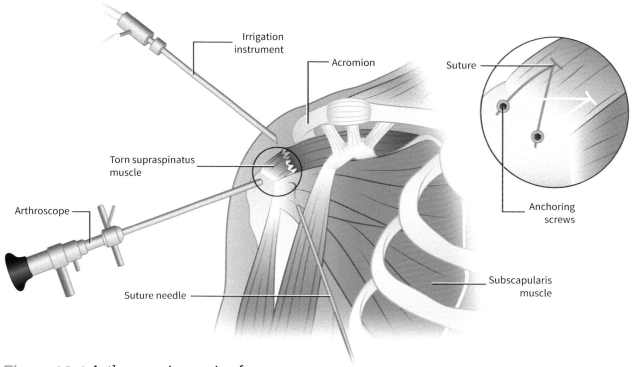

Figure 10.4 Arthroscopic repair of a tear in supraspinatus

COMPLICATIONS

Early

> Bleeding.
> Damage to the musculocutaneous, axillary, or subscapular nerves during port incision. This damage can result in neuralgia, paraesthesia, and paralysis of the innervated muscle.
> Shoulder and arm swelling whilst the saline flush is absorbed.

Intermediate and late

> Infection (superficial or deep).
> Recurrence or failure of complete healing—the risk of which is increased with the size and age of the tear.
> Chronic pain.
> Shoulder stiffness with frozen shoulder in 5–10%.

POSTOPERATIVE CARE

Inpatient

> Physiotherapy should be started immediately postoperatively, starting with passive movement and progressing to active movements.

Outpatient

> The arm is placed in a polysling for a minimum of 4 weeks to immobilise the shoulder joint.

> Closed chain pendulum exercises where the distal aspect of the extremity is fixed to an object that is stationary and force is transferred through the extremity.

> Wound check and sutures removal at 2 weeks.

> Follow-up appointment in 6 and 12 weeks with physiotherapy from 2 weeks.

 ## SURGEON'S FAVOURITE QUESTION

Which muscle is most commonly involved in a degenerative rotator cuff tear?

The supraspinatus, though when the tear is larger, it is not uncommon for it to also involve the infraspinatus and the teres minor (SIT tear).

LUMBAR SPINAL FUSION

Carly Bisset

DEFINITION

Spinal surgery that permanently arthrodeses two or more vertebrae with either metal rods or cages filled with bone graft.

✓ INDICATIONS

- Unstable vertebral fracture.
- Correction of spinal deformities, such as scoliosis or kyphosis.
- Spondylolisthesis.
- Severe osteoarthritis causing excessive vertebral movement and pain.
- Localised neoplastic diseases (limited use).
- Post-infection instability.

✗ CONTRAINDICATIONS

Relative

- Established osteomyelitis.

Absolute

- Severe osteoporosis
- Diffuse multi-level neoplastic disease.
- Multiple-level diffuse degenerative disease.

ANATOMY

Vertebral column

- The vertebral column consists of 33 vertebrae: 7 cervical, 12 thoracic, 5 lumbar, 5 sacral (fused together), and 4 coccygeal (fused together). Vertebrae are separated by intervertebral discs.
- The spinal cord runs within the vertebral canal, from the foramen magnum to vertebral level L1/2 (in adults). Below this is the cauda equina, which comprises the remaining nerve roots that descend the vertebral canal before exiting at the appropriate level.
- The vertebral column is supported by several ligaments: the anterior and posterior longitudinal ligaments, the ligamenta flava, the interspinous ligaments, and the supraspinous ligament. Running along the vertebral column are the erector spinae muscles.

Vertebrae

- Each vertebra can be divided into two sections. The anterior vertebral body functions to bear most of the load. The posterior vertebral arch protects and allows the spinal cord and nerve roots, along with the central vessels, to pass through it.
- The posterior vertebral arch consists of laminae, pedicles, and a spinous process, as well as transverse processes in thoracic vertebrae.
- At each vertebral level, there is an intervertebral foramen located between the inferior vertebral notch of the vertebra above and the superior vertebral notch of the vertebra below. Spinal nerves travel out of these foramina to innervate peripheral structures.
- Between the vertebrae lie the intervertebral discs, consisting of an outer annulus fibrosus and an inner nucleus pulposus. The intervertebral discs are avascular in adults.

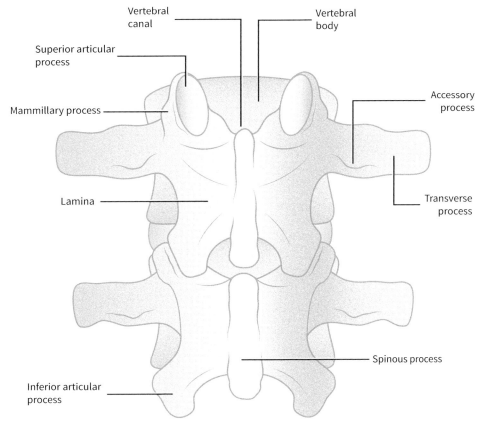

Figure 10.5 Gross structure of the thoracic vertebra

STEP-BY-STEP OPERATION

Anaesthesia: general.

Position: prone.

1 A 3–4 cm midline incision is made directly over the spinous process running between the paraspinal muscles.

2 The large muscles of the back are retracted, and the lumbar dorsal fascia overlying the spinous processes is cauterised.

3 To create more space to visualise nerve roots, a high-speed burr is used to create a laminectomy.

4 If needed, a discectomy can be performed to allow for nerve root decompression.

5 For an instrumented fusion, metal plates, screws, or rods can be used to hold two vertebrae until they fuse. Bone grafts may still be inserted into the intervertebral space to further promote fusion.

6 For a non-instrumented fusion, a bone graft is prepared, either allografted (donor bone) or autografted from the patient's iliac crest. This requires a second incision over the site of bone grafting.

7 The prepared bone graft fragments are then packed into the anterior and lateral aspects of the disc space. An inter-body spacer is inserted, and the posterior aspect of the space is sealed with bone graft fragments.

8 Using Floseal™ (a liquid coagulant), complete haemostasis of the operative site is confirmed. It is vital that this is achieved in order to prevent epidural haematoma formation.

9 The operative site is closed with absorbable sutures—first the lumbar dorsal fascia, then the subcutaneous tissues, followed by the skin.

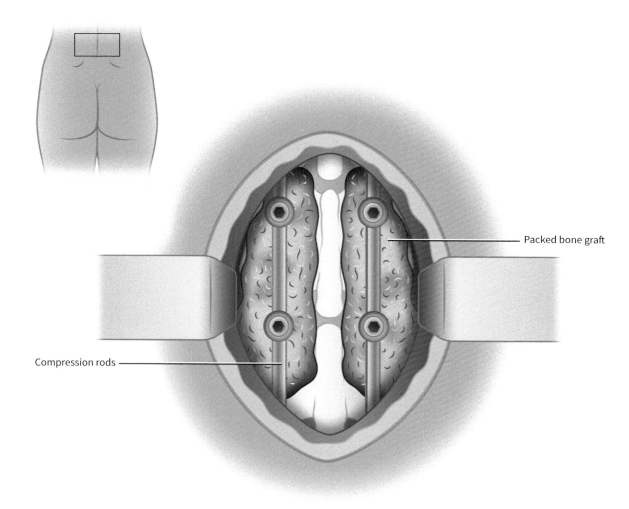

Figure 10.6 Compression rods and bone graft for lumbar spinal fusion

COMPLICATIONS

Early

> Bleeding and epidural haematoma formation.
> Nerve injury, which may cause leg pain and weakness, saddle anaesthesia, and bladder or bowel dysfunction.
> Paralysis.
> Dural tear and cerebrospinal fluid (CSF) leakage causing orthostatic headache.

Intermediate and late

> Infection.
> Chronic pain at graft site (10%).
> Osteoarthritis at vertebral joints on either side of fusion due to altered movement and stress.
> Failure to relieve symptoms.
> Mortality (1 in 350).

POSTOPERATIVE CARE

Inpatient

▸ The patient remains in hospital for 2–3 days.

▸ Full weight-bearing is encouraged with physiotherapy, which continues for many months.

▸ Patients need to be counselled about preventing the risks of Deep Vein Thrombosis (DVT), as pharmaceutical thromboprophylaxis is avoided due to the risk of epidural haematoma formation.

Outpatient

▸ Follow-up appointment 6–8 weeks postoperatively.

 SURGEON'S FAVOURITE QUESTION

How many vertebrae are there?

The vertebral column consists of 33 vertebrae: 7 cervical, 12 thoracic, 5 lumbar, 5 sacral (fused together), and 4 coccygeal (fused together).

INTERVERTEBRAL SPINAL DISCECTOMY

Stephanie Arrigo

DEFINITION

Debridement and excision of a symptomatic extruded intervertebral disc.

✓ INDICATIONS

> Cauda equina syndrome (a surgical emergency).
> Symptomatic intervertebral disc prolapse potentially stenosing the spinal canal/compressing the spinal nerve root.

✗ CONTRAINDICATIONS

Relative

> Clinical signs and radiological findings discrepancy.
> Mechanical (rather than sciatic) back pain.
> Inadequate conservative treatment.

ANATOMY

Vertebral column

> The vertebral column consists of 33 vertebrae: 7 cervical, 12 thoracic, 5 lumbar, 5 sacral (fused together), and 4 coccygeal (fused together). Vertebrae are separated by intervertebral discs.
> The spinal cord runs within the vertebral canal, from the foramen magnum to vertebral level L1/2 (in adults). Below this is the cauda equina, comprising the remaining nerve roots and descending the vertebral canal before exiting at the appropriate level.
> The vertebral column is supported by several ligaments: the anterior and posterior longitudinal ligaments, the ligamenta flava, the interspinous ligaments, and the supraspinous ligament. Running along the vertebral column are the erector spinae muscles.

Vertebrae

> Each vertebra can be divided into two sections. The anterior vertebral body functions to bear most of the load. The posterior vertebral arch protects and allows the spinal cord and nerve roots, along with the central vessels, to pass through it.
> The posterior vertebral arch consists of laminae, pedicles, and a spinous process, as well as transverse processes in thoracic vertebrae.
> At each vertebral level, there is an intervertebral foramen located between the inferior vertebral notch of the vertebra above and the superior vertebral notch of the vertebra below. Spinal nerves travel out of these foramina to innervate peripheral structures.
> Between the vertebrae lie the intervertebral discs, consisting of an outer annulus fibrosus and an inner nucleus pulposus. The intervertebral discs are avascular in adults.

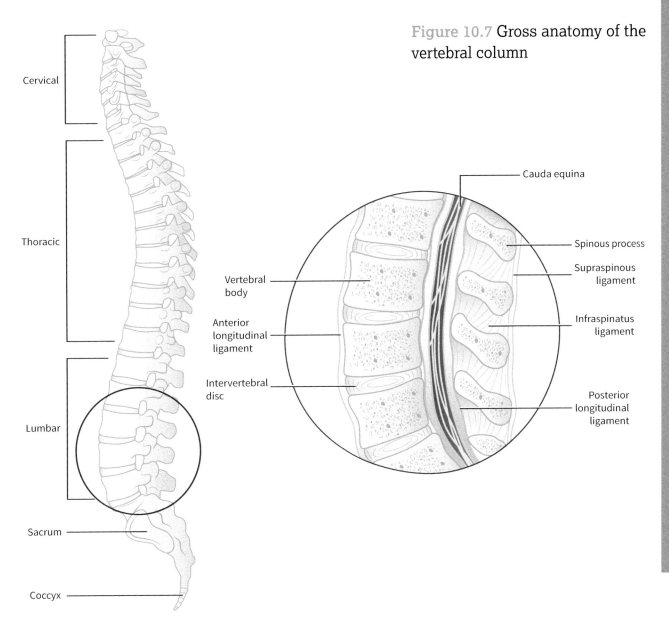

Figure 10.7 **Gross anatomy of the vertebral column**

Cervical

Thoracic

Lumbar

Sacrum

Coccyx

Cauda equina

Spinous process

Supraspinous ligament

Infraspinatus ligament

Posterior longitudinal ligament

Vertebral body

Anterior longitudinal ligament

Intervertebral disc

STEP-BY-STEP OPERATION

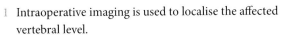

Anaesthesia: general. Hypotensive anaesthetic techniques create less venous ooze during the procedure.

Position: knee-to-chest position.

1 Intraoperative imaging is used to localise the affected vertebral level.

2 A 6–9 cm incision is made along the line of the spinous processes, through skin, followed by fascia.

3 The spinal muscles running beside the spinous processes are retracted.

4 A high-speed burr is used to create a laminotomy. This is where the inferior part of the lamina of the vertebra above, and the superior part of the lamina of the vertebra below, are removed.

5 The ligamentum flavum is removed.

6 The cauda equina/spinal cord need to be carefully retracted out of the field of view.

7 Through the widened intervertebral foramen, the protruding disc is identified, dissected, and removed using a micrograsper or forceps. It is important that the prolapsed part of the disc is removed completely to avoid recurrence.

8 Absolute haemostasis must be achieved.

9 The wound is washed and closed in layers.

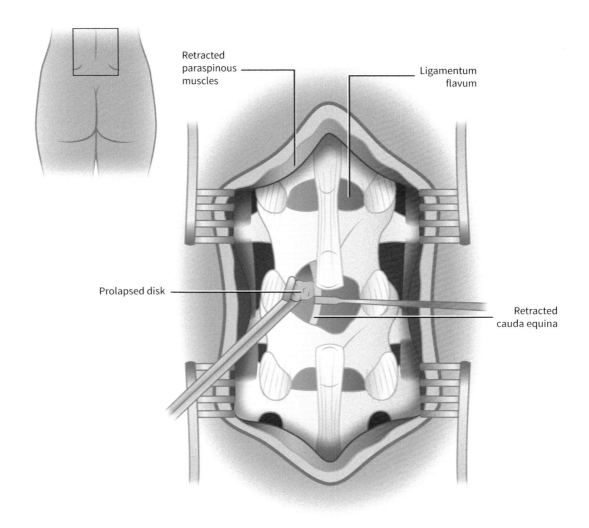

Figure 10.8 Excision of a prolapsed intervertebral disk

COMPLICATIONS

Early

> Bleeding, which may lead to an epidural haematoma.
> Fracture.
> Nerve root damage, which may result in leg pain and weakness, saddle anaesthesia, and bladder or bowel dysfunction.
> Paralysis.
> Posterior longitudinal ligament injury.

> Wrong level surgery.
> Dural tear and cerebrospinal fluid (CSF) leakage causing orthostatic headache.

Intermediate and late

> Residual disc prolapse.
> Infection.
> Fibrotic scar tissue formation.
> Recurrent prolapse (5–15%).

POSTOPERATIVE CARE

Inpatient

▸ Pain control via patient-controlled analgesia (PCA).

Outpatient

▸ Early mobilisation with a specific exercise programme via physiotherapy.

▸ Dressing change and/or suture removal after 7 days by general practice nurse.

▸ Follow-up appointment in 4–6 weeks.

 SURGEON'S FAVOURITE QUESTION

What are the symptoms of cauda equina syndrome (CES)?

Classically presents with worsening low back and leg pain, leg weakness, saddle anaesthesia (decreased sensation on the inner thighs and buttocks), altered function of the bladder and bowel, and sexual dysfunction.

TOTAL HIP REPLACEMENT (THR) ANTEROLATERAL APPROACH

Stephanie Arrigo

DEFINITION
Replacement of the femoral head and acetabulum with a surgical prosthesis.

✓ INDICATIONS

> End-stage arthritis (inflammatory or degenerative) following failure of conservative and medical interventions.
> Avascular necrosis of the femoral head.
> Femoral neck fracture in patients with good mobility.

✗ CONTRAINDICATIONS

Absolute
> Severe dementia or psychiatric disease—unable to comply with hip precautions (any movement putting excessive strain on the hip joint).
> Systemic infection.

Relative
> Age.
> Obesity.

ANATOMY

Gross anatomy
> The hip joint comprises two articulating surfaces: the head of the femur and the acetabulum of the pelvis, which form a stable ball-and-socket synovial joint.
> The articular surfaces are lined by hyaline cartilage.
> The acetabulum:
> The acetabulum comprises the acetabular fossa, the location for attachment of the ligamentum teres, and the lunate surface, which surrounds the fossa and articulates with the femur.
> The lunate surface is crescent shaped and open at the inferior aspect, forming the acetabular notch, which houses the transverse acetabular ligament.
> The ligamentum teres connects the acetabular fossa to the head of femur at the fovea.
> The acetabular labrum deepens the acetabulum, enhancing the stability of the joint.
> The joint capsule attaches to the pelvis via the margins of the acetabulum, the transverse ligament, and the margin of the obturator foramen, and to the femur via the intertrochanteric line anteriorly and the intertrochanteric crest posteriorly.

Neurovasculature
> The hip joint is innervated by branches from the femoral, obturator, and superior gluteal nerves, as well as the nerve to the quadratus femoris.
> Vascular supply to the hip joint arises from the obturator artery via the medial and lateral femoral circumflex arteries (the main supply travelling beneath the capsule).
> The femoral head receives minimal blood supply from the artery of the ligamentum teres, which is not clinically significant.
> Additional arteries supplying the hip joint include the superior and inferior gluteal arteries and the first perforating branch of the deep artery of the thigh.

Figure 10.9 Structures forming the acetabulum

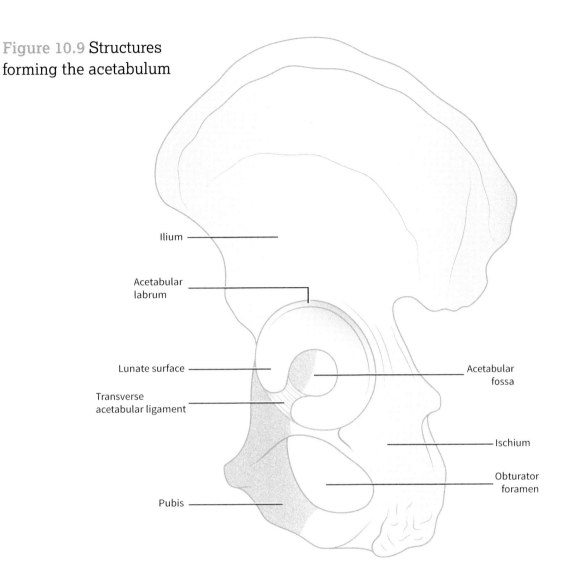

- Ilium
- Acetabular labrum
- Lunate surface
- Transverse acetabular ligament
- Pubis
- Acetabular fossa
- Ischium
- Obturator foramen

STEP-BY-STEP OPERATION

Anaesthesia: general or spinal.

Position: lateral position with the affected leg flexed to 90°.

1. A 10–12 cm longitudinal incision is made over the tip of the greater trochanter extending in line with the femur. The subcutaneous tissue is incised.
2. A small incision is made into the tensor fascia lata, and the leg is abducted. Using blunt dissection, the fibres of the gluteus maximus are parted.
3. The leg is then externally rotated, the tip of the greater trochanter is identified and the fibres of the gluteus medius split. The insertion of the gluteus medius into the greater trochanter is freed.
4. Blunt dissection is used to expose the joint capsule, which is then incised. The limb is then rotated externally and the hip dislocated.
5. An osteotomy is performed to separate the femoral head from the neck of the femur; a cork screw is then used to remove the femoral head.

6. The acetabulum is prepared with clearance of soft tissue and reaming of the bone.
7. The femur is prepared by creating an entry point in the postero-lateral aspect of the femoral canal. The femur is then sequentially reamed and the canal rasped to fit the shape of the implant.
8. A trial is performed with a 'dummy' acetabular and stem prosthesis to assess stability, range of movement, and leg length. The appropriate size implant is then cemented in.
9. The wound is washed. The deep layer of the external rotators and joint capsule is closed with non-absorbable sutures, and the superficial subcutaneous tissue is closed with absorbable sutures.

ORTHOPAEDICS

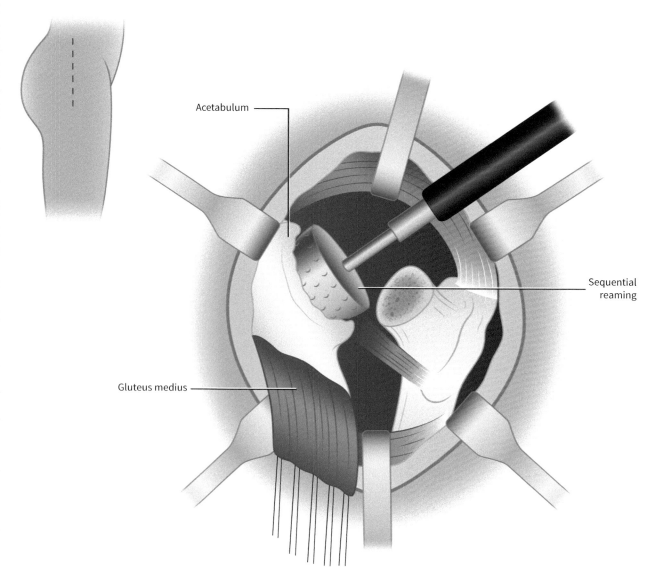

Acetabulum

Sequential reaming

Gluteus medius

Figure 10.10 Sequential reaming of the acetabulum

COMPLICATIONS

Early

> Bleeding and haematoma.
> Damage to the sciatic nerve and, less commonly, the femoral nerve.
> Fracturing of the femoral shaft during insertion of the femoral component.
> Urinary retention.

Immediate and late

> Dislocation (usually within the first six weeks).
> Infection of the prosthetic joint or superficial tissues.
> Loosening (may be due to infection or wear particles).
> Periprosthetic fracture—often due to trauma in elderly patients with osteoporosis.
> Leg length discrepancy.

POSTOPERATIVE CARE

Inpatient

- Check AP pelvis and lateral of hip X-rays.
- Early mobilisation with weight-bearing status determined by the prosthesis used.
- Hip precautions—avoid crossing legs or excessive flexion of the hips.

Outpatient

- Venous thromboembolic (VTE) prophylaxis for 1 month.
- Follow-up appointment in 6 weeks.

 SURGEON'S FAVOURITE QUESTION

What are the classifications of hip replacement?

- Hemiarthroplasties:
  - Cemented
  - Uncemented
- Total hip replacements:
  - Cemented
  - Uncemented
  - Hybrid
  - Reverse hybrid

WEDGE RESECTION OF INGROWN TOENAIL

Katrina Mason

DEFINITION

Marginal excision of the nail plate and nail fold to treat an ingrown toenail (onychocryptosis).

✓ INDICATIONS

> Failure of conservative management.

✗ CONTRAINDICATIONS

> Ingrown toenail on both the lateral and medial sides. Excision on both sides will leave the toenail too thin,

and therefore it may be more appropriate to completely remove the toenail (total nail avulsion).

> Active local infection or abscess.

ANATOMY

Gross anatomy

> The nail plate is composed of hard, keratinised squamous cells attached to the nail bed inferiorly.

> The nail fold is where the nail plate proximally attaches to the underlying tissues and consists of the dorsal roof superiorly and the ventral floor inferiorly. The ventral floor is the site of the germinal matrix. The germinal matrix is responsible for the majority of nail production.

> The eponychium (cuticle) is the distal portion of the nail fold.

> The paronychium is the soft tissue along the lateral borders of the nail plate.

> The sterile matrix is the distal portion of the nail bed and is tightly adherent to both the overlying nail plate

and the underlying periosteum. Along with the dorsal roof, it is a secondary site of nail production.

> The nail plate is loosely attached to the germinal matrix but is densely attached to the sterile matrix.

> Nails grow at roughly 3–4 mm per month (0.1 mm/ day).

Pathology

> Onychocryptosis involves an abnormally wide or incurved nail plate, classically affecting the lateral aspect of the big toe.

> Onychocryptosis causes trauma to the surrounding soft tissue, resulting in pain, inflammation, and/or chronic infection.

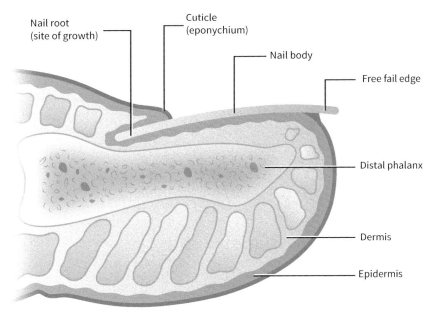

Figure 10.11 Anatomy of the nail bed

STEP-BY-STEP OPERATION

Anaesthesia: Regional is achieved using a ring block at the base of the toe with 1% lidocaine. Local anaesthetic should not contain adrenaline due to the risk of avascular necrosis.

Position: supine/sitting.

1   A tourniquet is wrapped around the base of toe to ensure a bloodless field for optimal visualisation of structures.

2   Blunt dissection is used to separate the nail plate from the surrounding soft tissues.

3   Scissors cut vertically along the depth of the nail plate roughly 3–5 mm parallel to the affected lateral border.

4   The nail plate and the underlying germinal centre are avulsed.

5   An oblique 0.5 cm incision at the base of the nail is made to expose and excise the germinal matrix.

6   Two one-minute applications of 90% liquid phenol are applied to the exposed nail bed (sterile matrix) and nail fold (germinal matrix). This causes cellular destruction, which prevents nail regrowth (matrixectomy).

7   The operative site is washed with normal saline.

8   The site is dressed with a non-adherent dressing, then gauze, and is secured with tape.

ORTHOPAEDICS

Figure 10.12 Incision to expose
and excise the germinal matrix

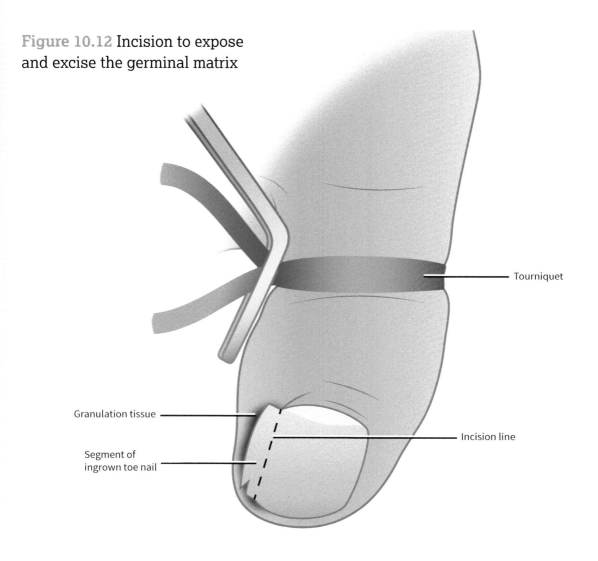

Tourniquet

Granulation tissue

Incision line

Segment of
ingrown toe nail

COMPLICATIONS

Early

> Bleeding.
> Pain and discomfort.
> Local skin burns from phenol.

Intermediate and late

> Recurrence of ingrown toenail (1–2%).
> Narrower nail.
> Infection.

POSTOPERATIVE CARE

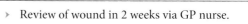

Outpatient

> Dressing removed after 48 hours in clinic. Redressed with
simple dressing.

> Review of wound in 2 weeks via GP nurse.

SURGEON'S FAVOURITE QUESTION

What are the surgical techniques for treatment of ingrown toenails?

Wedge nail resection or total nail avulsion. These can be performed in combination with matrixectomy (removal/destruction of sterile and germinal matrix to prevent nail regrowth).

CARPAL TUNNEL DECOMPRESSION SURGERY

Richard Bartlett

DEFINITION

Decompression of the median nerve as it passes through the carpal tunnel of the wrist, by transecting the flexor retinaculum.

✔ INDICATIONS

▸ Symptoms of carpal tunnel syndrome (CTS) for >6 months, with failure of conservative management.

▸ Functional weakness or atrophy of the muscles supplied by the median nerve in the hand.

✘ CONTRAINDICATIONS

▸ Pregnancy—CTS often resolves spontaneously following delivery.

ANATOMY

Gross anatomy

▸ Borders of the carpal tunnel:
  › Radial aspect—trapezium, scaphoid, and flexor carpi radialis.
  › Ulnar aspect—hook of hamate, triquetrum, and pisiform.
  › Dorsally—concave arch of carpal bones and central metacarpal rays.
  › Ventrally—the flexor retinaculum, which is anchored to the scaphoid tuberosity and trapezium on the radial side; it then transverses the carpal tunnel to attach to the pisiform bone and hook of hamate on the ulnar side.

▸ Contents of the carpal tunnel:
  › Four tendons of flexor digitorum superficialis.
  › Four tendons of flexor digitorum profundus.
  › Tendon of flexor pollicis longus.
  › The median nerve.

▸ Structures surrounding the carpal tunnel:
  › Superficial to the flexor retinaculum and on the ulnar side of the ventral wrist runs the ulnar artery and nerve.
  › Superficial to the flexor retinaculum and running down the midline of the ventral wrist is the tendon of palmaris longus (absent in 14% of the population).

Neurovasculature

▸ The recurrent branch of the median nerve (RBMN) supplies motor innervation to the thenar eminence (opponens pollicis, abductor pollicis brevis, and flexor pollicis brevis) and two lumbrical muscles.

▸ The RBMN runs a variable course at risk of damage during surgery and therefore should always be identified prior to the transection of the flexor retinaculum.

Cardinal lines

▸ Kaplan's line runs from the apex of the first web space to the ulnar side of the ventral surface of the hand.

▸ An innominate line runs from the radial border of the ring finger to the wrist crease.

Figure 10.13 Carpal tunnel contents

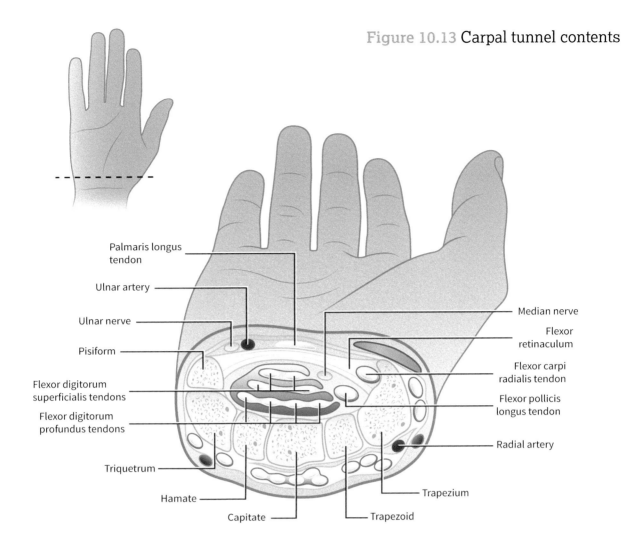

- Palmaris longus tendon
- Ulnar artery
- Ulnar nerve
- Pisiform
- Flexor digitorum superficialis tendons
- Flexor digitorum profundus tendons
- Triquetrum
- Hamate
- Capitate
- Median nerve
- Flexor retinaculum
- Flexor carpi radialis tendon
- Flexor pollicis longus tendon
- Radial artery
- Trapezium
- Trapezoid

STEP-BY-STEP OPERATION

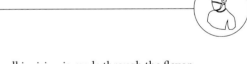

Anaesthesia: regional.

Position: supine with the arm rested on a hand table.

1 The cardinal lines are marked.
2 A longitudinal incision is made from the intersection of the cardinal lines and on the medial side of the thenar eminence. This site of incision minimises the risk of damage or scarring of the underlying median nerve.
3 The subcutaneous tissue is retracted to expose the underlying longitudinal fibres of the palmar fascia.
4 A self-retaining retractor is inserted for exposure, and a scalpel is used to incise the palmar fascia along the full length of the skin incision site.
5 The flexor retinaculum is identified, and the incision site is inspected for any anatomical variations in the RBMN.

6 A small incision is made through the flexor retinaculum, through which a McDonald retractor is inserted and is used to elevate the flexor retinaculum, separating it from the underlying structures.
7 With the retractor in place, a scalpel is used to dissect the distal segment of the ulnar aspect of the flexor retinaculum.
8 Tissue scissors are then used to dissect the more proximal segment of the ulnar aspect of the flexor retinaculum.
9 The contents of the carpal tunnel are inspected, and the release of the median nerve is confirmed.
10 The wound is closed in layers with non-absorbable and absorbable skin sutures. A pressure dressing is applied.

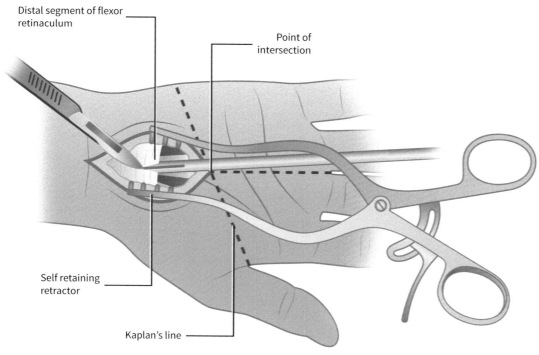

Distal segment of flexor retinaculum

Point of intersection

Self retaining retractor

Kaplan's line

Figure 10.14 Dissection of the flexor retinaculum

COMPLICATIONS

Early

> Bleeding.
> Palmar discomfort.

Intermediate and late

> Infection.
> Excessive fibrosis leading to movement restriction.
> Nerve damage: most commonly affecting the RBMN (which results in thenar wasting), the median nerve itself (loss of flexor grip strength), or, in very rare cases, the ulnar nerve.
> Recurrence of CTS symptoms, either from failure to sufficiently expand the volume of the carpal tunnel or recurrence of pathology.
> Complex regional pain syndrome due to nociceptive sensitisation, resulting in allodynia and vasomotor dysfunction.

POSTOPERATIVE CARE

Outpatient

> Simple analgesia for pain relief.
> Gentle exercises to reduce stiffness.
> Remove pressure dressing at 2 days.
> Wound review at 2 weeks in the community by GP nurse.
> No routine outpatient appointment required.

SURGEON'S FAVOURITE QUESTIONS

Which structure is compressed in CTS, and how does this relate to the typical clinical presentation?

Median nerve—sensory changes in median nerve distribution (thumb, index, and half of the middle finger) and weakness of the LOAF muscles (lateral lumbricals, opponens pollicis, abductor pollicis brevis, and flexor pollicis brevis).

ARTHROSCOPIC ACL RECONSTRUCTION

Shahab Shahid

DEFINITION

Surgical repair of the anterior cruciate ligament (ACL) of the knee, usually following traumatic rupture.

✓ INDICATIONS

- Unstable knee with ACL tear.
- Multiligament injury to knee +/- meniscal tear.

✗ CONTRAINDICATIONS

- ACL tear with no symptomatic instability.

- Low demand or elderly patient.
- Significant arthritis of knee.
- Partial tear of ACL.
- Lack of motivation to complete the long rehabilitation programme.

ANATOMY

Gross anatomy

- The knee joint is a hinge-type synovial joint composed of three compartments: the patellofemoral compartment and the medial and lateral femorotibial compartments.
- Ligaments:
  - The knee has four main stabilising ligaments: the anterior and posterior cruciates (ACL and PCL) and the medial and lateral collateral ligaments.
  - The ACL runs from the posterolateral intercondylar eminence of the femur to just anterior to the intercondyloid eminence of the tibia, blending in with the anterior horn of the medial meniscus.
  - The ACL consists of three bundles: an anteromedial, an intermediate, and a posterolateral. It functions to limit anterior translation and medial rotation of the tibia and posterior translation and lateral rotation of the femur. The overall ligament is fully taut in knee extension. However, some bundles are taut in intermediate and flexed positions.

Neurovasculature

- The knee receives sensory and motor innervation from the femoral, sciatic, and obturator nerves.
- The femoral nerve provides musculocutaneous branches to the quadriceps muscles and, distal to the knee, gives off the saphenous nerve.
- The sciatic nerve descends in the posterior compartment of the upper leg, innervating the hamstring muscles. It enters the popliteal fossa and divides into the tibial nerve and the common peroneal nerve.
- The vascular supply to the knee joint is from genicular arteries and branches of the femoral and popliteal arteries.

Tendon graft types

- Autografts: harvested from the patient.
  - Bone-Patellar Tendon-Bone (B-PT-B) graft.
  - Hamstring tendon graft—the tendons of gracilis and semitendinosis.
- Allografts: harvested from a deceased donor:
  - Quadriceps tendon.
  - Achilles tendon.
  - Synthetic grafts.

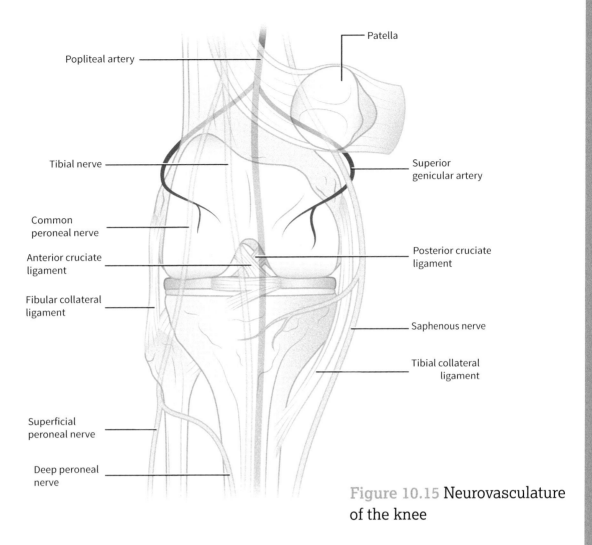

Popliteal artery

Patella

Tibial nerve

Superior genicular artery

Common peroneal nerve

Anterior cruciate ligament

Posterior cruciate ligament

Fibular collateral ligament

Saphenous nerve

Tibial collateral ligament

Superficial peroneal nerve

Deep peroneal nerve

Figure 10.15 Neurovasculature of the knee

STEP-BY-STEP OPERATION

Anaesthesia: general.
Position: supine with a thigh tourniquet and leg held in the flexed position.
Considerations: intravenous antibiotics.

1 Standard arthroscopic portals established anteromedially and anterolaterally. The scope is then inserted with a saline flush.

2 After an evaluation of surrounding structures, a motorised shaver is used to completely remove the damaged ACL.

3 For graft harvesting, a 4 cm incision is made either into the posteromedial aspect of the knee (hamstring graft) or anteriorly below the patella (patellar tendon graft). Once harvested, the graft is trimmed to size.

4 Using appropriate instrumentation, tunnels are made in the tibia and femur in the line of the ACL. The tunnel begins in the upper part of the external tibia and exits in the intercondylar eminence at the site of the ACL attachment.

5 To widen the tunnel, a guide pin is inserted and drilled over with a cannulated drill. A guide pin is then drilled into the femoral ACL attachment site. A cannulated drill is used to widen the tunnel.

6 Sutures are passed through the tunnels and are used to pull the prepared graft through the tibial tunnel and the femoral tunnel.

7 The graft is anchored to the femur first and then the tibia under physiological tension with interference screws.

8 The wounds are closed with absorbable sutures with the knee in flexion.

9 A pressure cuff is applied proximal to the operation site for 3 days.

10 A Bledsoe brace is applied for 14 days to control the range of movements.

Figure 10.16 Anchoring of an ACL graft

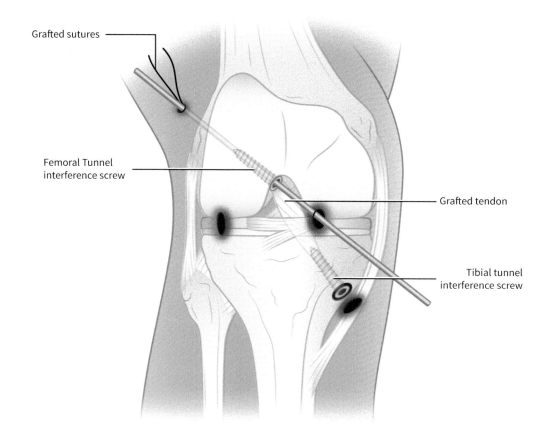

Grafted sutures

Femoral Tunnel interference screw

Grafted tendon

Tibial tunnel interference screw

COMPLICATIONS

Early

> Swelling and stiffness.
> Common fibular and saphenous nerve injury resulting in hypoaesthesia and foot drop. These occur especially if a hamstring from the medial side of the thigh is harvested.
> Numbness.

Intermediate and late

> Deep Vein Thrombosis (DVT) or Pulmonary Embolism (PE).

> Infection.
> The graft tendon may stretch or loosen, which can progressively result in an unstable knee.
> The graft may fail, resulting in an unstable knee (less than 10%) requiring surgical revision.
> Limited range of movement.
> Pain (18% suffer from pain, especially when crouching or kneeling).

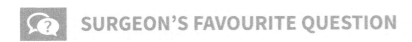

POSTOPERATIVE CARE

Inpatient

- Pain control, elevation, and mobilise full weight-bearing in a brace.

Outpatient

- Dressing change at 2 weeks in general practice.
- Follow-up appointment in 6 weeks.

- A week after surgery, the initial rehabilitation begins (6 weeks). The patient is encouraged to weight bear as much as tolerated. It can take 4–6 months for normal activity to resume.

SURGEON'S FAVOURITE QUESTION

Which tendons are commonly used as grafts for this surgery?

Gracilis, semitendinosus, and patellar tendons.

TOTAL KNEE REPLACEMENT (TKR)

Yashashwi Sinha

DEFINITION

Replacement of the knee joint with a surgical prosthesis.

✓ INDICATIONS

- End-stage arthritis (inflammatory or degenerative) following failure of conservative and medical interventions.
- Knee pain and stiffness interfering with quality of life.
- Distal femur fracture in patients with good mobility.

✗ CONTRAINDICATIONS

Absolute

- Systemic infection.
- Septic arthritis.

Relative contraindications:

- Age.
- Obesity.
- Comorbidities.

ANATOMY

Gross anatomy

- The knee joint is a hinge-type synovial joint composed of three compartments: the patellofemoral compartment and the medial and lateral femorotibial compartments.
- Ligaments:
  - The knee has four main stabilising ligaments: the anterior and posterior cruciates (ACL and PCL) and the medial and lateral collateral ligaments.
  - The ACL runs from the posterolateral intercondylar eminence of the femur to just anterior to the intercondyloid eminence of the tibia, blending in with the anterior horn of the medial meniscus.
  - The ACL consists of three bundles: an anteromedial, an intermediate, and a posterolateral. It functions to limit anterior translation and medial rotation of the tibia and posterior translation and lateral rotation of the femur. The overall ligament is fully taut in knee extension. However, some bundles are taut in intermediate and flexed positions.

Neurovasculature

- The knee receives sensory and motor innervation from the femoral, sciatic, and obturator nerves.
- The femoral nerve provides musculocutaneous branches to the quadriceps muscles and distal to the knee gives off the saphenous nerve.
- The sciatic nerve descends in the posterior compartment of the upper leg, innervating the hamstring muscles. It enters the popliteal fossa and divides into the tibial nerve and the common peroneal nerve.
- The vascular supply to the knee joint is from genicular arteries and branches of the femoral and popliteal arteries. The knee receives sensory and motor innervation from the femoral, sciatic, and obturator nerves.

Pathology

- It is the wear of articular surfaces and subsequent loss of joint space, osteophyte formation, subchondral cysts, and sclerosis that demonstrate osteoarthritis on weight-bearing radiographs of the knee.

Figure 10.17 Articulating components of the knee joint

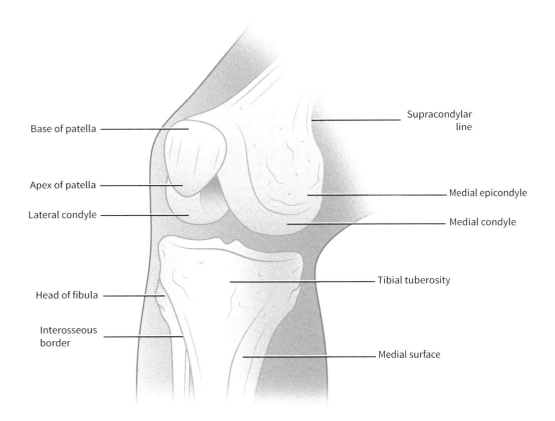

Base of patella

Apex of patella

Lateral condyle

Head of fibula

Interosseous border

Supracondylar line

Medial epicondyle

Medial condyle

Tibial tuberosity

Medial surface

STEP-BY-STEP OPERATION

Anaesthesia: general or spinal.

Position: supine position with the knee flexed, foot bolster and side support.

1   A tourniquet is applied, and a midline incision is made through the skin from the distal quadriceps to the tibial tuberosity. The medial parapatellar approach to the knee joint is used.

2   The knee is extended, and the patella is dislocated laterally. The knee is then flexed, and the fat pad and the medial and lateral meniscus are excised.

3   An intramedullary alignment rod is inserted through a drill hole at the apex of the intercondylar notch and the femoral sizing jig applied. The femur is then measured.

4   The femoral cutting jig is applied, and the anterior, medial, and lateral condyles are cut.

5   The tibia is prepared by drilling at the footprint of the ACL, through which an intramedullary rod is inserted.

The tibial cutting jig is applied 2 mm from the side with the least wear. A bone saw is then used to cut 2 mm from the tibial plateau.

6   The patella is resurfaced, trialled with a patella button, and tracking is assessed.

7   Trial femur and tibia components are positioned with various sizes inserted, and stability in flexion and extension is assessed.

8   Once satisfied, the appropriate component sizes are cemented into the prepared surfaces.

9   The wound is washed and closed in layers—first the capsule, followed by the fat and skin. The wound is dressed with a simple dressing and a crepe bandage.

Figure 10.18 Cutting of the tibial plateau

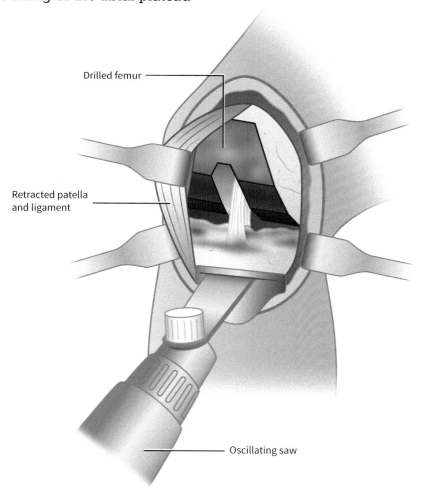

Drilled femur

Retracted patella and ligament

Oscillating saw

COMPLICATIONS

Early

> Bleeding and haematoma.
> Popliteal artery injury.
> Fracture of the tibia or femur.
> Rupture of patellar tendon.

Intermediate and late

> Deep vein thrombosis and pulmonary embolus.
> Infection—superficial or deep.

> Loosening, which may be due to infection or wear particles.
> Periprosthetic fracture—often due to trauma in elderly patients with osteoporosis.
> Failure of prosthesis.

POSTOPERATIVE CARE

Inpatient

- Check antero-posterior and lateral knee radiographs day one postoperatively.
- VTE prophylaxis (normally extended for 1 month).
- Early mobilisation.

Outpatient

- Follow-up appointment in 6 weeks.

 SURGEON'S FAVOURITE QUESTION

What artery can be damaged during the tibial cut?

Popliteal artery.

ARTHROSCOPIC MENISCECTOMY

Shahab Shahid and Stephanie Arrigo

DEFINITION
Arthroscopic-guided trimming or repair of the medial or lateral meniscus of the knee.

✓ INDICATIONS

> Large or moderate tear in the outer zone of the meniscus.
> Symptomatic meniscal tears causing pain, locking, limited function, or reduced range of movement.

✗ CONTRAINDICATIONS

> Asymptomatic tears.
> Knee joint infection.

ANATOMY

Gross anatomy
> Key articulations:
>> The tibio-femoral articulation is between the medial and lateral femoral condyles with the corresponding tibial plateaus.
>> The patellofemoral joint is between the triangular-shaped patella and the anterior femur.
>> The surfaces of the patella and tibia are entirely covered by hyaline cartilage and unite to form a synovial hinge joint.
>> Movements at the knee are flexion, extension, and rotation (the femur medially rotates on the tibia, locking the joint in extension).
> Femur:
>> The femoral condyles are separated by an intercondylar fossa—the area of attachment for the anterior and posterior cruciate ligaments.
>> Superior to the femoral condyles, on the medial and lateral aspects of the femur—are the proximal attachments of the knee's collateral ligaments.
> Tibia:
>> The tibial plateau consists of medial and lateral condyles separated by an intercondylar fossa.
>> The intercondylar region is the site of the menisci and distal attachment of the anterior and posterior cruciate ligaments.

> Patella:
>> A triangular-shaped sesamoid bone located on the anterior aspect of the knee joint and articulating with the femur.
>> The patella is connected to the tibial tuberosity via the patellar tendon.
> Menisci:
>> The menisci are crescent-shaped fibrocartilaginous structures that improve congruency of the articular surfaces whilst functioning as shock absorbers; they are connected anteriorly by the transverse ligament.
>> The medial meniscus is also attached to the medial collateral ligament and to the capsule of the knee joint, decreasing its mobility and increasing its vulnerability to injury.

Neurovasculature
> The joint is innervated by the obturator, femoral, tibial, and common fibular nerves.
> The blood supply to the knee joint arises from an anastomosis created by branches of the descending genicular artery (from the femoral artery), popliteal artery, and anterior and posterior tibial arteries.

Figure 10.19 Anatomy of the tibio-femoral joint surface

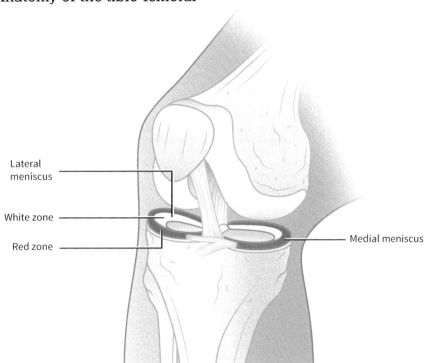

Lateral meniscus

White zone

Red zone

Medial meniscus

STEP-BY-STEP OPERATION

Anaesthesia: general or spinal anaesthesia.

Position: supine with the thigh and knee flexed.

1 A tourniquet can be placed around the thigh to restrict blood flow and improve the surgeon's view of the surgical field.

2 Two stab incisions are made on either side of the patellar tendon below the patella. An accessory portal may be made in the suprapatellar area.

3 With the knee flexed, the arthroscope with a blunt trochar is inserted into the inferior lateral incision.

4 The trochar is then passed under the patella whilst extending the knee to access the suprapatellar pouch.

5 A full arthroscopy is performed to inspect for damage to all structures, with special attention being paid to the medial and lateral menisci and the anterior and posterior cruciate ligaments.

6 Arthroscopic punches and graspers are used through the other portals to trim and remove or repair the meniscus.

7 The edges of the trimmed cartilage are smoothed with a shaver.

8 The knee is flushed with saline at the end of the procedure. The portals can be left open or closed with absorbable sutures with the knee in flexion.

Figure 10.20 Arthroscopic shaving of the medial femoral condyle

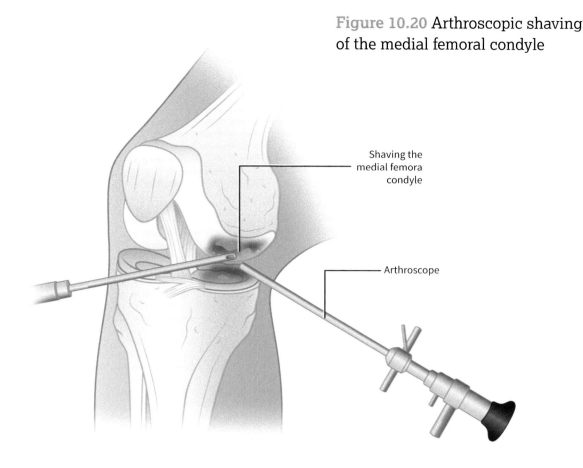

Shaving the medial femora condyle

Arthroscope

COMPLICATIONS

Early

> Common peroneal nerve injury, which may result in numbness below the knee or foot drop.
> Haemarthrosis.
> Cartilage or meniscal damage.

> Retained meniscal remnants, which may cause the knee to lock.

Intermediate and late

> Infection.

POSTOPERATIVE CARE

Inpatient

> Analgesia.
> Early mobilisation with the use of crutches.
> Elevation when immobile to reduce swelling and risk of Deep Vein Thrombosis (DVT).

Outpatient

> Progressive weight-bearing exercises, with a return to everyday activities at 2 weeks.
> Return to active sports at 4–6 weeks.
> Outpatient follow-up appointment at 6 weeks.

SURGEON'S FAVOURITE QUESTION

What is 'O'Donoghue's unhappy triad'?

O'Donoghue's unhappy triad comprises anterior cruciate ligament (ACL) tear and medial collateral ligament (MCL) injury (tear or sprain) with a medial meniscal tear. It often results from valgus stress with rotation of the knee in contact sports trauma.

CEPHALOMEDULLARY FEMORAL NAIL

Gareth Rogers

DEFINITION

Fixation of a femoral fracture with an intramedullary nail and a head screw.

✓ INDICATIONS

> Subtrochanteric fractures.
>> Reverse oblique trochanteric fractures.
>> Diaphyseal femoral fractures.
>> Painful pathological lesions prone to fractures where most of the femur needs to be stabilised.

✗ CONTRAINDICATIONS

> Completely bed bound.
> Sclerotic bone conditions resulting in dense bone where entry into and reaming the canal are difficult.

ANATOMY

Gross anatomy

> The proximal femur is composed of the head, neck, and proximal shaft.
> The intertrochanteric ridge runs from superior-lateral to inferior-medial between the greater and lesser trochanters.
> The neck-shaft angle is 130 +/-7° in adults, with approximately 10° of anteversion.
> Muscular attachments of the femur:
>> The vastus lateralis originates from the greater trochanter and inserts into the patella as part of the quadriceps tendon, a common tendon formed by the rectus femoris, vastus medialis, intermedius, and lateralis.
>> The obturator internus, the superior and inferior gemelli, the piriformis, and the gluteus medius and minimus muscles all insert into the greater trochanter.
>> The iliopsoas originates from the iliac fossa and the lumbar spine and inserts into the lesser trochanter.

Neurovasculature

> The sciatic nerve originates from L4–S3 and descends in the leg, innervating the hamstring muscles. Within the popliteal fossa, it divides into the common peroneal nerve and the tibial nerve.
> The femoral nerve derives from the rootlets of L2–L4 and divides within the thigh into anterior and posterior branches. The anterior branch supplies the anterior cutaneous surface and the sartorius. The posterior branch is responsible for the innervation of the quadriceps muscles.
> The arterial supply to the femoral head is distal to proximal via the medial (predominantly) and lateral circumflex arteries.
> The vascular supply to the femoral head from the artery of the ligamentum teres is insignificant.
> Lying in close proximity with the proximal femur are the sciatic, femoral, and pudendal nerves.

Figure 10.21 **Gross anatomy of the hip**

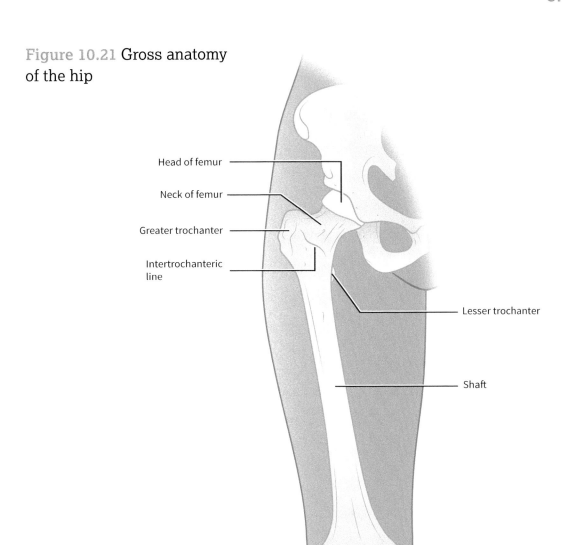

Head of femur

Neck of femur

Greater trochanter

Intertrochanteric line

Lesser trochanter

Shaft

Lateral condyle

Medial epicondyle

Patellar groove

STEP-BY-STEP OPERATION

Anaesthesia: general or spinal.

Position: supine on a traction table with the fractured leg in traction and the contralateral hip in stirrup.

Considerations: Cephalomedullary nails are inserted with the aid of a portable image intensifier (II). Antibiotics are administered at induction.

1   Using appropriate traction, the fracture is first reduced by closed technique using the II.

2   The entry point of the nail is identified using fluoroscopy, and a lateral incision is made proximal to the tip of the greater trochanter (GT). Sharp dissection is then used through the fascia lata and blunt dissection through the gluteus medius to expose the GT.

3   A guide wire is then inserted 2–3 mm medial to the tip of the GT on anteroposterior (AP) view and at the centre of the GT on lateral view. Once position is confirmed, the guide wire is inserted down to the level of the lesser trochanter.

4   An entry reamer is passed over the guide wire, which is then exchanged for a long ball tip guide wire that is manually pushed across the fracture to the knee (confirmed with II).

5 The wire is measured to identify the size of the nail.

6 Sequential reamers are passed down the cortex to allow for the passage of the nail (ream until the passage width is 1–1.5 mm greater than the size of the nail to be used).

7 The nail and a locking jig are built and inserted under II. The guide wire is then removed.

8 The head screw guide wire is inserted through the proximal locking jig into the centre of the femoral head under II to ensure adequate tip-apex distance. The guide wire is then measured and the head screw inserted.

9 The nail is distally locked freehand using II.

10 The wound is irrigated and closed in layers.

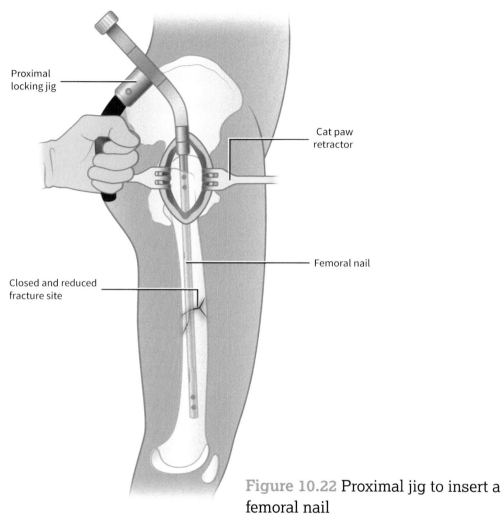

Figure 10.22 Proximal jig to insert a femoral nail

COMPLICATIONS

Early

- ▸ Peripheral neuropathy (direct or tractional) affecting the pudendal, sciatic, or femoral nerves, which can result in paralysis of the supplied muscles and neuralgia or paraesthesia of the innervated cutaneous surfaces.

- ▸ Myocardial infarction and stroke at time of surgery due to fat embolism or thrombosis.

Intermediate and late

- ▸ Infection.

- ▸ Implant failure.

- ▸ Deep Vein Thrombosis (DVT) and Pulmonary Embolism (PE).

- ▸ Non-union—15–20% in multifragmentary subtrochanteric fractures.

- ▸ Mortality—average one-year mortality rates are 10–20%, highly dependent on comorbidities.

POSTOPERATIVE CARE

Inpatient

> Physiotherapy—most patients should be mobilising and fully weight-bearing from day 1 postoperatively unless there are concerns regarding the strength of the construct.

Outpatient

> Thromboprophylaxis continued for up to 1 month postoperatively.

> Follow-up appointments until union has been confirmed with X-rays.

⍰ SURGEON'S FAVOURITE QUESTION

What are the two key factors that ensure nailing works properly?

True reduction of the fracture prior to nailing and entry point of initial guide wire to ensure good position of the nail.

LATERAL MALLEOLUS LAG SCREW AND NEUTRALISATION PLATE

Stephanie Eltz

DEFINITION
Open reduction and internal fixation of a lateral malleolar (fibular) fracture using a plate and screw.

✓ INDICATIONS
- Unstable fractures.
- Displacement of fracture following non-operative management.
- Open ankle fractures.

✗ CONTRAINDICATIONS
Relative
- Peripheral vascular disease.
- High-risk patient with poor bone quality.

Absolute
- Patients suitable for non-operative management (e.g., undisplaced stable ankle fracture).

ANATOMY

Gross anatomy
- The ankle, or the talocrural joint, is the articulation between fibula, tibia, and talus. The inferior and superior tibiofibular syndesmosis hold the tibia and fibula together and form part of the soft tissue stabiliser of the joint.
- The medial and posterior malleoli (of the tibia) and the lateral malleolus (the base of the fibula) are all palpable on clinical examination.
- Ligaments of the ankle joint:
  - Four different groups of ligaments stabilise the ankle joint: lateral ligaments, medial ligaments, syndesmosis and subtalar ligaments.
  - The lateral group of ligaments comprise the anterior talofibular ligament, calcaneofibular ligament, lateral talocalcaneal ligament, and posterior talofibular ligament.
  - The medial group of ligaments consists of the two parts of the deltoid ligament (superficial and deep).
  - The syndesmosis is the membranous band distally between the fibula and tibia. It is made up of three ligaments: anteroinferior tibiofibular ligament, posteroinferior tibiofibular ligament, and interosseous tibiofibular ligament.

- The lateral malleolus:
  - The lateral malleolus is formed by the distal fibula and provides attachment for the posterior and anterior talofibular ligaments and the lateral ligament complex.
  - Passing anterior to the lateral malleolus are the tendons of extensor digitorum longus and peroneus tertius.
  - Passing posterior to the lateral malleolus are the tendons of peroneus brevis and longus and, more posteriorly, the sural nerve, which descends along the posterolateral aspect of the leg to innervate the overlying cutaneous surface.

Neurovasculature
- The superficial peroneal nerve is at risk during the surgical approach to the fibula, as it leaves the lateral muscle compartment 10–12 cm above the tip of the distal fibula to run superficial to the anterior compartment, where it provides motor innervation to the peroneus longus and brevis.

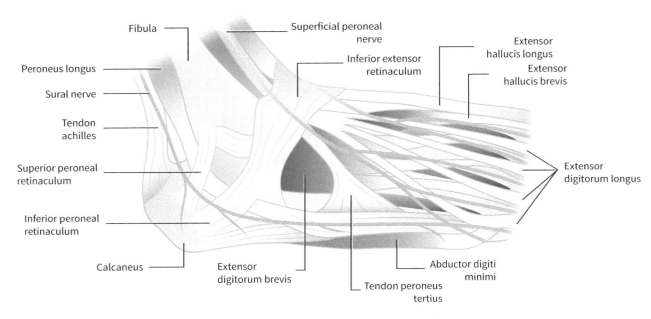

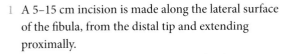

Figure 10.23 Anatomy of the lateral malleolus and surrounding nerves

STEP-BY-STEP OPERATION

Anaesthesia: general or regional.

Position: supine position, with a tourniquet; a sandbag is under the ipsilateral buttock.

Considerations: The procedure is guided by a portable image intensifier (II).

1 A 5–15 cm incision is made along the lateral surface of the fibula, from the distal tip and extending proximally.

2 The subcutaneous fat is divided and the deep fascia incised. Special attention is paid to avoid the superficial peroneal nerve, which is at risk if the incision reaches within 10 cm of the proximal tip of the fibula.

3 The fracture site is exposed and cleared of haematoma and soft tissue.

4 Using pointed reduction clamps, the fracture is then reduced under direct vision.

5 Using a drill guide, a 3.5 mm hole is drilled perpendicular to the fracture site into the adjacent cortex. A 2.5 mm hole is then drilled into the far cortex.

6 The drill hole is measured, and a 3.5 mm lag screw is inserted, compressing the fracture.

7 A one-third tubular plate is positioned over the fracture site and clamped into place.

8 The most distal hole is drilled first, using a 2.5 mm drill piece into the near cortex only. The depth is measured, and a threaded cancellous screw inserted.

9 The most proximal hole is then drilled with a 2.5 mm drill piece, this time passing through both cortices. The depth is measured and a cortical screw inserted. This process is then repeated for the adjacent hole. Using the II, the position of metal wear is assessed.

10 The wound is then washed, the deep fascia and subcutaneous tissue are closed with absorbable sutures, and the skin is closed with absorbable sutures.

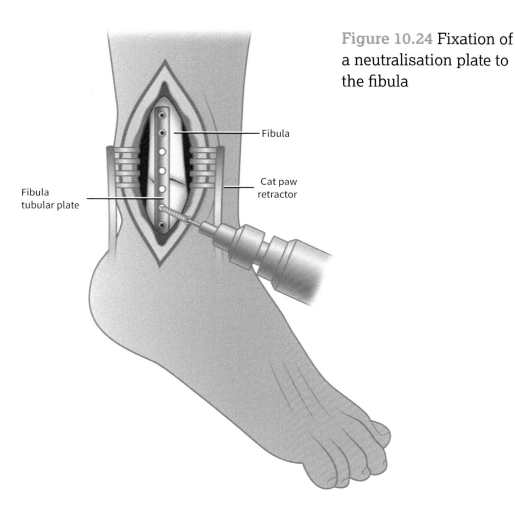

Figure 10.24 Fixation of a neutralisation plate to the fibula

Fibula

Cat paw retractor

Fibula tubular plate

COMPLICATIONS

Early

> Damage to the superficial peroneal nerve or sural nerve, causing sensory loss over dorsal and lateral surfaces of the foot.
> Compartment syndrome (when the pressure within a muscle compartment rises above arterial pressure, resulting in reduced tissue perfusion, ischaemia, and necrosis).

Intermediate and late

> Wound dehiscence and infection.
> Deep Vein Thrombosis (DVT) and Pulmonary Embolism (PE)
> Mal- or non-union of the fracture.
> Metal work prominence/irritation.
> Ankle stiffness.
> Early ankle arthritis.

POSTOPERATIVE CARE

Outpatient

> Non-weight-bearing mobilisation for 6 weeks.
> 2-week fracture clinic review: wound check and change to full lightweight cast.

> 6-week fracture clinic review: X-ray, remove cast, and begin full weight-bearing +/- physiotherapy.

SURGEON'S FAVOURITE QUESTION

How would you assess for a syndesmotic injury?

Stress syndesmosis under II intra-operatively by forced external rotation of the ankle. If syndesmosis opens up, then add syndesmotic screws to stabilise and allow healing of syndesmosis.

LOWER LIMB FASCIOTOMY

John Kennedy

DEFINITION

Decompression of a fascial compartment to relieve vascular tamponade and restore perfusion.

✓ INDICATIONS

> Acute lower limb compartment syndrome, occurring when the pressure within a compartment of the lower limb exceeds arterial pressure resulting in reduced tissue perfusion. Untreated, it has the potential to result in irreversible muscle and nerve damage.

✗ CONTRAINDICATIONS

> Delayed diagnosis of compartment syndrome—there is little benefit obtained in fasciotomies performed more than 12–24 hours after the onset of symptoms, as irreversible tissue damage has usually occurred by this point.

ANATOMY

> The leg has four compartments: anterior (extensor), lateral (peroneal), superficial posterior (flexor), and deep posterior (flexor).

> The compartments are separated by three fascial layers: the interosseous membrane, the transverse intermuscular septum, and the anterior intermuscular septum.

> Superficial posterior compartment:
>   › The superficial posterior compartment is separated from the lateral compartment by the posterior intermuscular septum and from the deep posterior compartment by a fascial layer.
>   › The superficial posterior compartment contains the soleus, gastrocnemius, and plantaris muscles.
>   › There are no major neurovascular structures in this compartment.

> Deep posterior compartment:
>   › The deep posterior compartment is separated from the superficial compartment by the posterior intermuscular septum and from the anterior compartment by the interosseous membrane.
>   › The deep posterior compartment contains the tibialis posterior, flexor hallucis longus, and flexor digitorum longus.

> Importantly, the tibial nerve and the posterior tibial artery descend in the posterior compartment.

> The lateral compartment:
>   › The lateral (peroneal) compartment is bounded by the anterior intermuscular septum (anteriorly), the posterior intermuscular septum (posteriorly), and the fibula (medially).
>   › It is supplied by the superficial peroneal nerve, which arises from the bifurcation of the common peroneal nerve as it winds around the head of the fibula.

> The anterior compartment:
>   › The anterior compartment is bounded medially by the lateral surface of the tibia and laterally by the extensor surface of the fibular and anterior intermuscular septum.
>   › It contains the deep peroneal nerve and the anterior tibial artery as it descends the lower legs before transitioning into the dorsalis pedis artery on the dorsal surface of the foot.

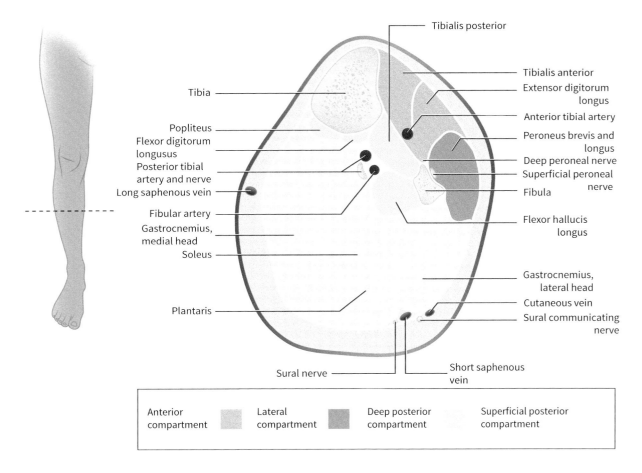

Figure 10.25 **Compartments of the lower limb**

STEP-BY-STEP OPERATION

Anaesthesia: general.

Position: supine, with a sandbag to rotate the leg for approach to the posterolateral aspect of the leg.

No tourniquet.

1 Two 15–18 cm longitudinal incisions are made; the two incisions are separated by an 8 cm bridge of skin.

2 The first incision is over the anterolateral aspect of the leg 2cm anterior to the fibula and runs from the level of the tibial tubercle to 6 cm above the ankle.

3 The superficial peroneal nerve is then identified as it distally penetrates the deep fascia. It is then marked and protected.

4 The fascia overlying the anterior compartment is then incised for the length of the incision decompressing it. The intermuscular septum is incised along its full length, decompressing the lateral compartment.

5 The second incision runs over the anteromedial aspect of the leg 1–2 cm posterior to the medial border of the tibia and runs from the level of the tibial crest to 6 cm above the ankle.

6 The saphenous nerve and vein are identified and protected.

7 The deep fascia anterior to the saphenous vein and overlying the superficial compartment is then incised, decompressing the superficial posterior compartment.

8 The tendon of flexor digitorum longus is identified and the overlying fascia incised. The fascia underlying the belly of soleus is dissected to give access to the deep posterior compartment.

9 The head of soleus is then freed from its origin, decompressing the deep posterior compartment.

10 Ensure vascularisation of muscles. Warm saline swabs can be used to encourage vasodilation. Necrotic tissues can be debrided. Wounds should be left open and covered with non-adhesive dressings.

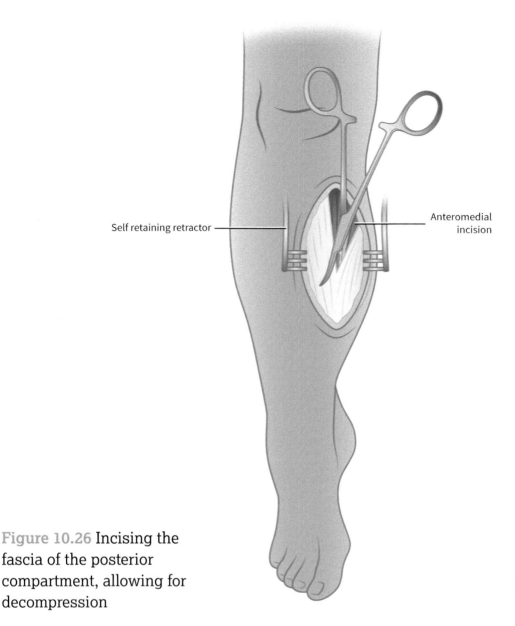

Self retaining retractor

Anteromedial
incision

Figure 10.26 Incising the
fascia of the posterior
compartment, allowing for
decompression

COMPLICATIONS

Early

> Saphenous (loss of sensation in the medial leg) and
  superficial peroneal nerve injury (inability to evert the
  foot and loss of sensation over the dorsum of the foot).

> Exposure of tibia or fibula if incisions are too anterior
  or lateral.

> Rhabdomyolysis—the excessive release of myoglobin
  and electrolytes caused by the rapid breakdown of
  skeletal muscle. These obstruct renal tubules, resulting
  in renal failure.

Intermediate and late

> Wound infection and delayed healing.

> Chronic venous insufficiency.

> Amputation may be required if fasciotomy is
  unsuccessful.

POSTOPERATIVE CARE

Inpatient

› Regular wound checks.

› Second look at 48–72 hours +/- debridement of non-viable tissue.

› Wound closure if possible, otherwise will need soft tissue coverage with skin graft or flap.

› Monitor and treat any renal failure from rhabdomyolysis.

 SURGEON'S FAVOURITE QUESTION

Why are young men especially prone to compartment syndrome?

Greater muscle mass.

DYNAMIC HIP SCREW

Chukwudi Uzoho and Paul Robinson

DEFINITION

Fixation of an extracapsular neck of femur fracture with a plate and a sliding screw to allow dynamisation and predictable fracture healing.

✓ INDICATIONS

› Extracapsular neck of femur fractures.

✗ CONTRAINDICATIONS

› Unstable fracture configurations (e.g., reverse oblique, multifragmentary, or sub-trochanteric).
› Imminent death, although hip hemiarthroplasty is offered as a palliative treatment for pain control.
› Severe hip joint arthritis.

ANATOMY

Gross anatomy

› The proximal femur is composed of the head, neck, and proximal shaft.
› The intertrochanteric ridge runs supero-lateral to infero-medial between the greater and lesser trochanters.
› The neck-shaft angle is 130 +/- 7° in adults, with approximately 10° of anteversion.
› Muscular attachments of the femur
  › The extensor mechanism is composed of the vastus lateralis, vastus intermedius, vastus medialis, and rectus femoris (the quadriceps) inserting into the tibial tuberosity through the sesamoid patella.
  › Obturator internus, the superior and inferior gemelli, the piriformis, and the gluteus medius and minimus muscles all insert into the greater trochanter.
  › Iliopsoas originates from the iliac fossa and lumbar spine and inserts into the lesser trochanter.
  › The tensor fascia lata muscle inserts into the tibia through a tough aponeurosis—the tensor fascia lata—which runs on the lateral aspect of the thigh.

Neurovasculature

› Lying in close proximity with the proximal femur are the sciatic, femoral, and pudendal nerves.
› The sciatic nerve originates from L4–S3 and descends the leg, innervating the hamstring muscles. Within the popliteal fossa, it divides into the common peroneal nerve and the tibial nerve.
› The femoral nerve derives from the rootlets of L2–L4 and within the thigh divides into anterior and posterior branches. The anterior branch supplies the anterior cutaneous surface and sartorius. The posterior branch is responsible for the innervation of the quadriceps muscles.
› The arterial supply to the femoral head is distal to proximal via the medial (predominantly) and lateral circumflex arteries.
› The supply to the femoral head from the artery of the ligamentum teres is insignificant.

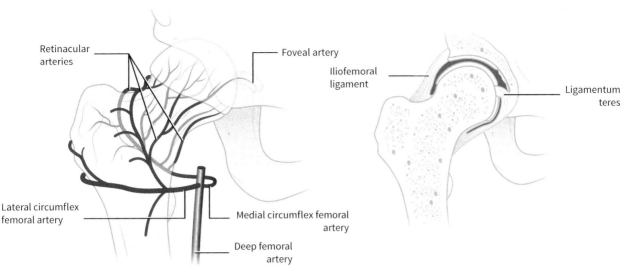

Retinacular arteries

Foveal artery

Iliofemoral ligament

Ligamentum teres

Lateral circumflex femoral artery

Medial circumflex femoral artery

Deep femoral artery

Figure 10.27 Vasculature and ligaments of the hip

STEP-BY-STEP OPERATION

Anaesthesia: general or spinal.
Position: supine on a traction table with the fractured leg in traction and the contralateral hip in stirrup
Considerations: A dynamic hip screw (DHS) is inserted with the aid of a portable image intensifier (II). Antibiotics are administered at induction.

1 Closed manipulative reduction is performed under II control to achieve a satisfactory position.
2 Using the II, an entry point for the hip screw is identified at the level of the lesser trochanter.
3 A longitudinal lateral incision is made to divide the skin.
4 Subcutaneous tissue and the fascia lata are then incised.
5 The vastus lateralis is split to expose the lateral femur.
6 A guide wire is inserted under image guidance into the neck of femur, to the centre of the femoral head.

7 The length of the guide wire is measured, and a hip screw 5 mm shorter than the guide wire length is selected.
8 A reamer is placed over the guide wire to make way for the lag screw, which is inserted under II.
9 A 135° four-hole plate is slid over the lag screw. The most distal hole is drilled, the depth measured, and the cortical screw inserted; this process is then repeated for the remaining three holes.
10 Overlying soft tissues are closed in layers using absorbable sutures.

ORTHOPAEDICS

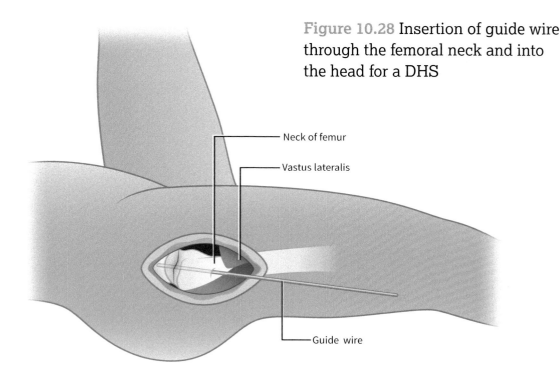

Figure 10.28 Insertion of guide wire through the femoral neck and into the head for a DHS

Neck of femur

Vastus lateralis

Guide wire

COMPLICATIONS

Early

> Peripheral neuropathy (direct versus tractional)—pudendal, sciatic, or femoral nerve damage that can result in paralysis of the supplied muscles and neuralgia or paraesthesia of the supplied cutaneous surfaces.

> Myocardial infarction and stroke at time of surgery due to fat embolism or thrombosis.

Intermediate and late

> Infection.

> Implant failure due to varus collapse.

> Avascular necrosis if fixation is used for undisplaced intracapsular neck of femur fractures (9–18%).

> Deep Vein Thrombosis (DVT) and Pulmonary Embolism (PE)

> Malunion in case of collapse.

> Mortality—average one-year mortality rates are 10–20%.

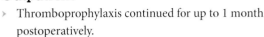
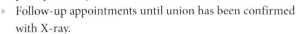

POSTOPERATIVE CARE

Inpatient

> Physiotherapy—most patients should be mobilising and fully weight-bearing from day 1 postoperatively unless there are concerns regarding the strength of the construct.

Outpatient

> Thromboprophylaxis continued for up to 1 month postoperatively.
> Follow-up appointments until union has been confirmed with X-ray.

 SURGEON'S FAVOURITE QUESTION

What makes a DHS dynamic?

The lag screw used to fix the femoral head slides into the barrel of the plate, allowing compression and healing at the fracture site and enabling healing as the patient weight-bears and mobilises after fixation. If this did not happen, the fracture fragments would remain separated and a high rate of non-union would occur.

DYNAMIC HIP SCREW

CEMENTED HIP HEMIARTHROPLASTY

Gareth Rogers

DEFINITION

Replacement of femoral head and neck with a stemmed implant in the treatment of displaced intracapsular fractured neck of femur (NOF).

✓ INDICATIONS

- Displaced intracapsular NOF fractures where viability of head is unlikely.

✗ CONTRAINDICATIONS

Relative

- Imminent death, although hip hemiarthroplasty is offered as a palliative treatment for pain control.
- Extracapsular fractures where fixation is the treatment of choice.
- Young, active patients for whom a total hip replacement is the treatment of choice.

ANATOMY

Gross anatomy

- The hip joint comprises two articulating surfaces: the head of the femur and the acetabulum of the pelvis, which form a stable ball and socket synovial joint.
- The articular surfaces are lined by hyaline cartilage.
- The acetabulum:
  - The acetabulum comprises the acetabular fossa, the location for attachment of the ligamentum teres, and the lunate surface, which surrounds the fossa and articulates with the femur.
  - The lunate surface is crescent shaped and opened at the inferior aspect, forming the acetabular notch, which houses the transverse acetabular ligament.
  - The ligamentum teres connects the acetabular fossa to the head of femur at the fovea.
  - The acetabular labrum deepens the acetabulum, enhancing the stability of the joint.
  - The joint capsule attaches to the pelvis via the margins of the acetabulum, the transverse ligament,

and the margin of the obturator foramen, and to the femur via the intertrochanteric line anteriorly and the intertrochanteric crest posteriorly.

Neurovasculature

- The hip joint is innervated by branches from the femoral, obturator, and superior gluteal nerves, as well as the nerve to the quadratus femoris.
- Vascular supply to the hip joint arises from the obturator artery via the medial and lateral femoral circumflex arteries (the main supply travelling beneath the capsule).
- The femoral head receives minimal blood supply from the artery of the ligamentum teres, which is not clinically significant.
- Additional arteries supplying the hip joint include the superior and inferior gluteal arteries and the first perforating branch of the deep artery of the thigh.

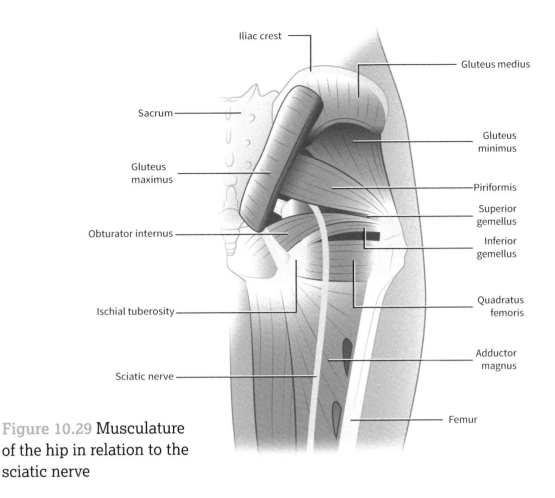

Figure 10.29 Musculature of the hip in relation to the sciatic nerve

Labels: Iliac crest, Sacrum, Gluteus maximus, Obturator internus, Ischial tuberosity, Sciatic nerve, Gluteus medius, Gluteus minimus, Piriformis, Superior gemellus, Inferior gemellus, Quadratus femoris, Adductor magnus, Femur

STEP-BY-STEP OPERATION

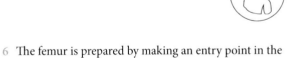

Anaesthesia: general or spinal.

Position: lateral position with the affected leg up.

1 A 10–12 cm longitudinal incision is made centred on the tip of the greater trochanter extending in line with the femur. The subcutaneous tissue is incised.

2 A small incision is made into the tensor fascia lata and the leg is abducted. Using blunt dissection, the fibres of the gluteus maximus are parted.

3 The leg is then rotated externally; the tip of the greater trochanter is identified, and the fibres of gluteus medius are split. The insertion of the gluteus medius into the greater trochanter is freed.

4 Blunt dissection is used to expose the joint capsule, which is then incised. The limb is then externally rotated and the hip dislocated.

5 The neck is osteotomised at the right level, and the femoral head is removed from the acetabulum with a corkscrew and measured for size.

6 The femur is prepared by making an entry point in the postero-lateral aspect of the femoral canal.

7 The femur is reamed sequentially until cortical bone is felt. Rasps are then inserted into the femoral canal to shape it to the prosthesis. A trial reduction is performed to assess stability, positioning, leg length equality, and movement of the hip.

8 The cement restrictor is sized and inserted, and the canal is washed.

9 Cement is then inserted into the femoral canal, and the femoral implant is inserted in the predetermined position. The hip is then manually reduced and stability assessed.

10 The wound is washed. The deep layer of external rotators and joint capsule is closed with non-absorbable sutures, and the superficial subcutaneous tissue is closed with absorbable sutures.

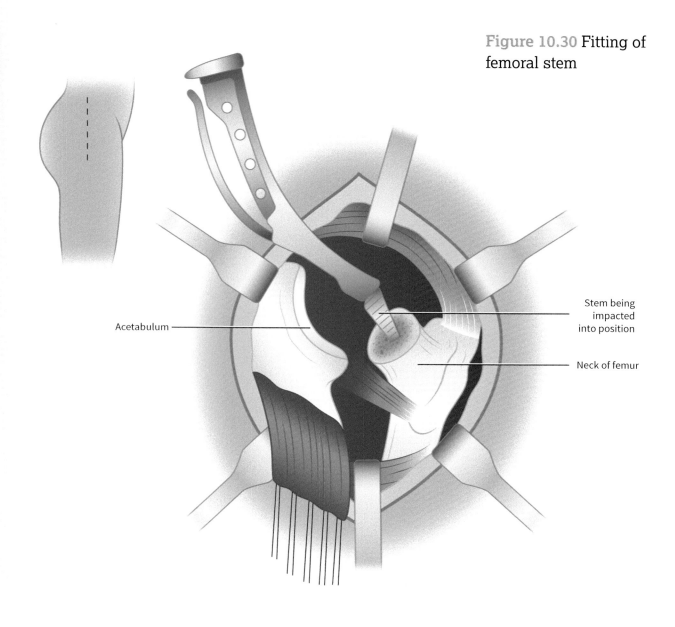

Figure 10.30 Fitting of femoral stem

Acetabulum

Stem being impacted into position

Neck of femur

COMPLICATIONS

Early

> Peripheral neuropathy (direct or tractional) affecting the pudendal, sciatic, or femoral nerves, which can result in paralysis of the supplied muscles and neuralgia or paraesthesia of the innervated cutaneous surfaces.
> Myocardial infarction and stroke at time of surgery due to fat embolus.
> Dislocation.

Intermediate and late

> Infection.
> Deep Vein Thrombosis (DVT) and Pulmonary Embolism (PE).
> Mortality—average one-year mortality rate is 14–36%, highly dependent on comorbidities.

POSTOPERATIVE CARE

Inpatient

‣ Physiotherapy—most patients should be mobilising and fully weight-bearing from day 1 postoperatively.

Outpatient

‣ Thromboprophylaxis for 1 month postoperatively.

‣ Routine follow-up is not usually required.

 SURGEON'S FAVOURITE QUESTION

What sign may result if the abductor muscles are not repaired adequately when closing the wound?

A positive Trendelenburg sign indicates abductor dysfunction.

MEDIAL MALLEOLUS OPEN REDUCTION AND INTERNAL FIXATION

Gareth Rogers

DEFINITION

Fixation of an isolated displaced fracture of the medial malleolus using two partially threaded cancellous screws.

✓ INDICATIONS

> Unstable fractures involving the medial malleolus.
> Displacement following non-operative management.
> Open ankle fractures.

✗ CONTRAINDICATIONS

Absolute

> Fractures suitable for non-operative management, including undisplaced stable ankle fractures.
> Comminuted fracture.

Relative

> Patients with peripheral vascular disease.
> Osteoporotic bone.

ANATOMY

Gross anatomy

> The ankle or the talocrural joint is the articulation between fibula, tibia, and talus. The inferior and superior tibiofibular syndesmosis hold the tibia and fibula together and form part of the soft tissue stabiliser of the joint.
> The medial and posterior malleoli (parts of the tibia) and the lateral malleolus (the base of the fibula) are all palpable on clinical examination.
> Four different groups of ligaments stabilise the ankle joint: lateral ligaments, medial ligaments, syndesmosis and subtalar ligaments.
> > Lateral ligaments comprise the anterior talofibular ligament, calcaneofibular ligament, lateral talocalcaneal ligament, and posterior talofibular ligament.
> > The medial ligaments consist of the two parts of the deltoid ligament (superficial and deep).
> > The syndesmosis is the membranous band distally between the fibula and tibia. It is made up of three ligaments: anteroinferior tibiofibular ligament, posteroinferior tibiofibular ligament, and interosseous tibiofibular ligament.

Neurovasculature

> The tibial nerve and posterior tibial artery lie posterior to the medial malleolus.
> The anterior tibial artery (which continues in the foot as the dorsalis pedis artery) and the deep peroneal nerve pass anterior to the ankle joint.

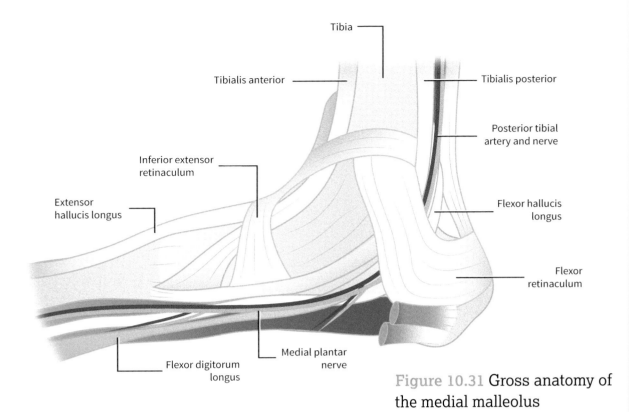

Tibia

Tibialis anterior

Tibialis posterior

Posterior tibial artery and nerve

Inferior extensor retinaculum

Extensor hallucis longus

Flexor hallucis longus

Flexor retinaculum

Flexor digitorum longus

Medial plantar nerve

Figure 10.31 Gross anatomy of the medial malleolus

STEP-BY-STEP OPERATION

Anaesthesia: general or spinal.

Position: supine, with a tourniquet.

Considerations: A portable image intensifier (II) is used to check position throughout the procedure.

1 A 4–6 cm longitudinal curved incision, starting 2 cm distal to the anterior tip of the medial malleolus, is made.

2 The skin flaps are then carefully elevated to protect the great saphenous vein and the saphenous nerve, which lie anterior to the medial malleolus.

3 The periosteum is incised to expose the fracture site.

4 The fracture fragments are retracted. The site is debrided of any soft tissue and any haematoma and is irrigated.

5 Using pointed reduction clamps and under direct vision, the fracture is then reduced.

6 The fracture is then temporarily fixated with a 1.6 mm K-wire.

7 A stab incision through the deltoid ligament is made, and a 2.5 mm hole for the anterior lag screw is drilled parallel to the K-wire and perpendicular to the fracture. The position of the metal work is then assessed using the II.

8 The depth of the anterior hole is measured, and the malleolar fragment is tapped with a 4 mm cortical tap.

9 An appropriately sized 4 mm partially threaded cancellous screw is inserted, compressing the fracture. The K-wire is then removed and replaced with a second partially threaded cancellous screw.

10 The wound is then washed and the skin closed with absorbable sutures

Figure 10.32 Insertion of cancellous screw to compress a medial malleolus fracture

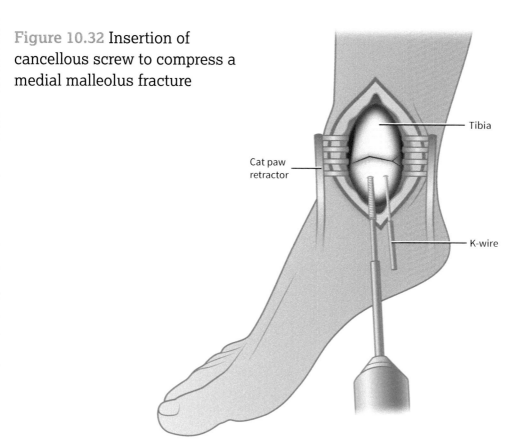

COMPLICATIONS

Early

> Damage to the saphenous nerve, potentially resulting in sensory loss over the dorsum of the foot.

> Compartment syndrome (when the pressure within a muscle compartment rises above arterial pressure, resulting in reduced tissue perfusion, ischaemia, and necrosis).

Intermediate and late

> Wound dehiscence and infection.

> Deep Vein Thrombosis (DVT) and Pulmonary Embolism (PE)

> Mal- or non-union of the fracture.

> Metal work prominence/irritation.

> Ankle stiffness.

> Early ankle arthritis.

POSTOPERATIVE CARE

Outpatient

- Non-weight-bearing mobilisation for 6 weeks.
- 2-week fracture clinic review: wound check and change to full lightweight cast.
- 6-week fracture clinic review: X-ray, remove cast, and begin full weight-bearing +/- physiotherapy.

SURGEON'S FAVOURITE QUESTION

What is meant by talar shift?

Opening/widening of the gap between the talus and the calcaneus in the ankle.

DISTAL RADIUS VOLAR LOCKING PLATE

Rebecca Telfer

DEFINITION

Open reduction and internal fixation of unstable or displaced distal radius fracture using a volar locking plate with screws.

✓ INDICATIONS

› Unstable displaced fracture of the radius.
› Intra-articular fracture.
› Fracture with associated nerve or vessel damage.
› Delayed presentation.
› Failed conservative management.
› Mal- or non-union of fracture.

✗ CONTRAINDICATIONS

Absolute

› Very distal fractures where purchase into distal fragments for plate attachment is not achievable.

Relative

› Severe soft tissue injury is a relative contraindication, as these patients may first require wound debridement and external fixation.

ANATOMY

Gross anatomy

› The wrist joint:
  › The wrist joint is a synovial joint composed of the articulation between the radius and an articular disc formed by the adjacent surfaces of the distal ulnar, scaphoid, lunate, and triquetrum bones.
  › The complex arrangement of articulations allow for a range of movements: abduction, adduction, flexion, and extension.
  › The wrist joint capsule is supported by the palmar radiocarpal, palmar ulnocarpal, and dorsal radiocarpal ligaments. There is additional ligament support from the radial and ulnar collateral ligaments.
› Muscles at the wrist joint:
  › Flexor carpi radialis (FCR) originates from the medial epicondyle of the humerus and inserts into the palmar aponeurosis. It is innervated by the median nerve, and it flexes and abducts the wrist.
  › Flexor pollicis longus (FPL) originates from the anterior surface of the radius and the adjacent

portion of the interosseous membrane and inserts into the base of the distal phalanx of the thumb. It is innervated by the median nerve and is responsible for flexion of the thumb. It runs in close proximity to FCR.
  › Pronator quadratus originates from the ulna and inserts on the radius. Innervated by the median nerve, it enables pronation of the forearm.

Neurovasculature

› The median nerve descends the forearm on the deep surface of the flexor digitorum superficialis and passes onto the palmar surface of the hand through the carpal tunnel.
› The radial artery leaves the forearm by passing around the lateral surface of the wrist and onto the posterolateral aspect of the hand.
› The ulnar nerve and ulnar artery leave the forearm and enter the palmar surface of the hand by passing over the flexor retinaculum of the wrist.

Figure 10.33 Ligament components of the wrist joint capsule

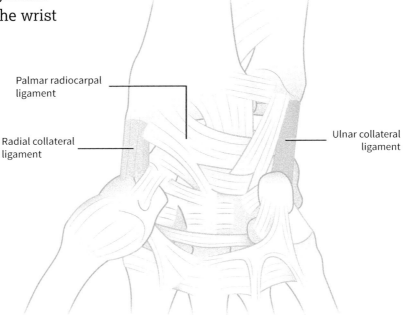

Palmar radiocarpal ligament

Radial collateral ligament

Ulnar collateral ligament

STEP-BY-STEP OPERATION

Anaesthesia: general and/or local nerve blocks to the ulnar, radial, and median nerves.

Position: supine, with a tourniquet on the affected arm and using an arm board.

Considerations: Prophylactic antibiotics are administered at induction. The procedure is guided by a portable image intensifier (II).

1. A longitudinal volar incision is made in the plane between FCR and the radial artery.
2. The radial artery is retracted radially and the median nerve and FCR in the ulnar direction.
3. Pronator quadratus is dissected to expose the fracture.
4. To reduce the fracture, longitudinal traction and flexion of the distal segment are applied. Reduction is under direct vision.
5. A wire is used to temporarily fixate the fracture, and position is checked with the II.
6. An appropriately sized volar locking plate is placed across the fracture and is temporarily held in place by drilling a K-wire through the plate's most distal screw hole. The position is then checked with the II.
7. The plate is fixed with locking and non-locking screws and the final position assessed.
8. The positioning K-wire is removed.
9. Finally, the wound is irrigated and closed in two layers with absorbable sutures.

Figure 10.34 Fixation of distal radius fracture with a volar locking plate

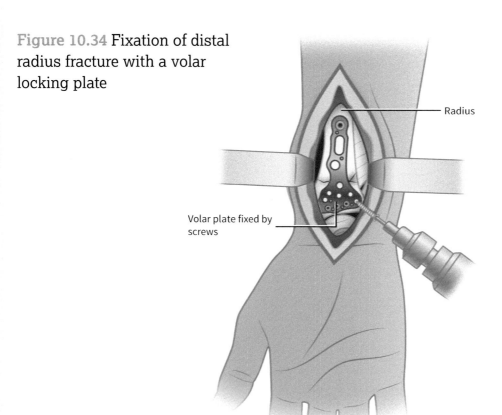

Radius

Volar plate fixed by screws

COMPLICATIONS

Early

> Radial artery injury, which in the absence of an ulnar artery has the potential to result in vascular insufficiency of the hand. The presence of an ulnar artery can be confirmed with the Allen's test.

Immediate and late

> Infection.
> Median nerve injury resulting in carpal tunnel syndrome type symptoms.
> Tendon injury most commonly affecting the tendon of either FPL and extensor pollicis longus; damage to either structure results in weakness and requires repair.
> Mal- or non-union of the fracture.
> Stiffness.
> Complex regional pain syndrome (nociceptive sensitisation causing allodynia and vasomotor dysfunction).

POSTOPERATIVE CARE

Outpatient

> Fracture clinic at 2 weeks for review of wound and simple exercises.

> Repeat X-rays at 6 weeks.

> Fracture clinic at 3 months to check X-rays and to start strengthening exercises.

SURGEON'S FAVOURITE QUESTION

Why is the volar approach preferred over dorsal?

Due to plate irritation of extensor tendons.

TIBIAL NAIL

Gareth Rogers

DEFINITION
Internal fixation of a tibial fracture with an intramedullary nail.

✓ INDICATIONS

▹ All displaced tibial fractures 5 cm from the articular surface.
▹ Minimally displaced tibial fractures with an intact fibula.
▹ Salvage procedure for mal- or non-union of a tibial fracture following failed management.

✗ CONTRAINDICATIONS

▹ Intra-articular fractures extending into the ankle or knee joint.
▹ Existing tibial deformity precluding the use of a straight nail.
▹ An undisplaced fracture that may be managed non-operatively.
▹ Infection.

ANATOMY

▹ The tibia is a major weight-bearing long bone and forms the articular surfaces of both the ankle and knee joints. It is connected to the fibula via the superior and inferior tibiofibular syndesmoses.
▹ The tibia is surrounded by the four muscle compartments of the leg: anterior (extensor), lateral (peroneal), superficial posterior (flexor), and deep posterior (flexor).
  ▸ The superficial posterior compartment is separated from the lateral compartment by the posterior intermuscular septum and from the deep posterior compartment by a fascial layer. The superficial posterior compartment contains the soleus, gastrocnemius, and plantaris muscles. There are no major neurovascular structures in this compartment.
▹ The deep posterior compartment is separated from the anterior compartment by the interosseous membrane. It contains the tibialis posterior, flexor hallicus longus, and flexor digitorum longus, along with the tibial nerve and the posterior tibial artery.
▹ The lateral (peroneal) compartment is bounded anteriorly by the intermuscular septum, posteriorly by the posterior intermuscular septum, and medially by the fibula. It contains the superficial peroneal nerve.
▹ The anterior compartment is bounded medially by the lateral surface of the tibia, laterally by the extensor surface of the fibula, and posteriorly by the anterior intermuscular septum. It contains the anterior tibial artery and the deep peroneal nerve.

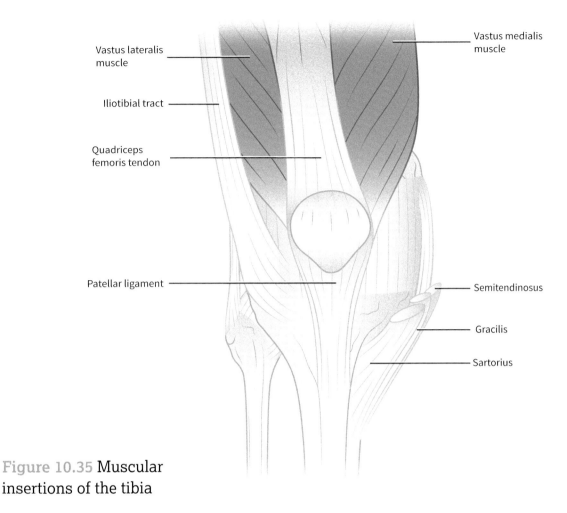

Figure 10.35 **Muscular insertions of the tibia**

Labels: Vastus lateralis muscle · Iliotibial tract · Quadriceps femoris tendon · Patellar ligament · Vastus medialis muscle · Semitendinosus · Gracilis · Sartorius

STEP-BY-STEP OPERATION

Anaesthesia: general.

Position: supine; the fracture is reduced either with the aid of an assistant flexing the knee over a triangular block or by using a tibial traction table with the knee in flexion.

Considerations: Intramedullary nails are inserted with the aid of a portable image intensifier (II). Antibiotics are administered at induction.

1 A vertical incision is made medial to the patellar tendon. The patellar tendon is identified using blunt dissection and retracted laterally to expose the tibial plateau.

2 Using an II, the tibial entry point is made just medial to the lateral tibial spine on AP and entering the canal on lateral view.

3 The guide wire is inserted, and the cannulated entry reamer is then used to open the proximal tibia.

4 The entry guide wire is exchanged for a reaming rod, over which sequential reamers are passed and used to ream the cortex to allow passage of the nail (usually up to 1 mm greater than nail diameter).

5 Using a depth gauge, the guide wire is measured and the appropriate length and diameter nail selected and assembled.

6 The nail is inserted over the guide wire and positioned using an II.

7 The proximal locking jig is used to lock the proximal nail with two to three locking screws.

8 Using the II, the distal nail is locked freehand with two locking screws.

9 Soft tissue is closed in layers, and a pressure dressing is applied.

Figure 10.36 Tibial nail
locking jig

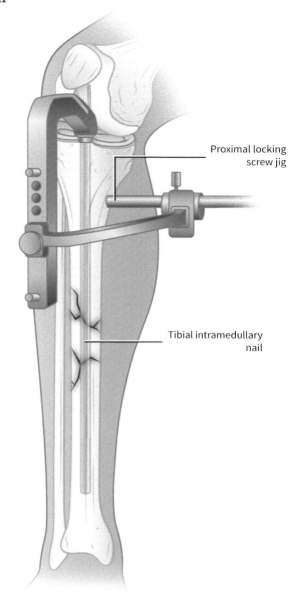

Proximal locking
screw jig

Tibial intramedullary
nail

COMPLICATIONS

Early

> Bleeding.
> Compartment syndrome (when the pressure within
  a muscle compartment rises above arterial pressure,
  resulting in reduced tissue perfusion, ischaemia, and
  necrosis).

Intermediate and late

> Infection, affecting 1% of patient with closed fractures,
  increasing to 6% in open fractures.

> Mal- or non-union.
> Anterior knee pain.
> Deep Vein Thrombosis (DVT) and Pulmonary
  Embolism (PE)
> Stiffness of knee and ankle.
> Metal work prominence or irritation.

POSTOPERATIVE CARE

Inpatient

‣ Thromboprophylaxis.

‣ Weight-bearing as tolerated.

‣ Physiotherapy consisting of a range of motion exercises to the knee and ankle.

Outpatient

‣ Dressing change and suture/staple removal after 14 days by GP nurse.

‣ Outpatient appointment in 4–6 weeks with tibial radiographs.

 SURGEON'S FAVOURITE QUESTION

What would you do if fracture healing is not progressing as expected?

Review patient factors affecting healing—nutrition, smoking, poor circulation, noncompliance, etc. Remove static locking screws and dynamise the nail to aid fracture healing as early as possible. Consider ultrasonic stimulation. Consider bone grafting.

SPLIT-THICKNESS SKIN GRAFT (STSG)

Nigel Mabvuure and Dariush Nikkhah

DEFINITION

The harvesting of the epidermis and variable thickness of dermis from an area of the body and transplanted onto another area of the body. STSGs can be thick (0.45–0.75 mm) or thin (0.2–0.45 mm).

✓ INDICATIONS

> Burns.
> Wounds that cannot be closed by primary intention.

✗ CONTRAINDICATIONS

> Infected wound beds.
> Bones and tendons stripped of periosteum and paratenon (poor blood supply).

ANATOMY

> The skin is formed of two layers:
>   1. Epidermis— superficial and avascular
>   2. Dermis
> The epidermis:
>   › Composed of stratified squamous epithelium and provides a physical barrier to the external environment.
>   › Keratinocytes are the predominant epidermal cell type.
>   › Since the epidermis is devoid of blood vessels, nutrients reach this layer via diffusion from the underlying dermis.

> The dermis:
>   › The dermis is a complex layer containing structural components such as collagen, blood vessels, hair follicles, sweat glands, and cells, including fibroblasts and other immune cells.
>   › The dermis is responsible for nourishing the epidermis, as harbouring epithelial cells are able to replenish the epidermis should the need arise (e.g., in the lining of hair follicles).
> Larger blood vessels and nerves, fat, and connective tissue compose the subcutaneous tissue layer.

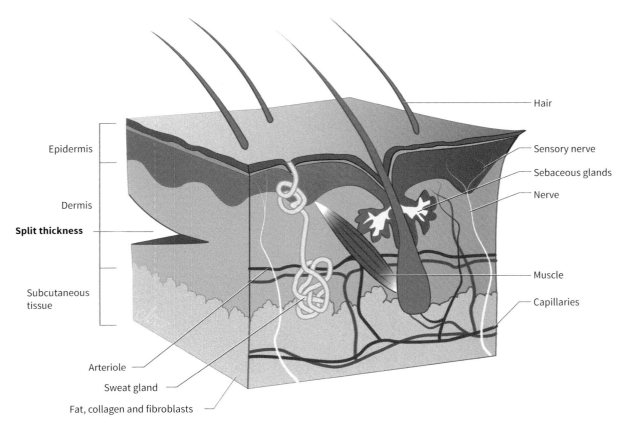

Figure 11.1 Layers and components of the skin and underlying subcutaneous tissue

STEP-BY-STEP OPERATION

Anaesthesia: general, regional, or local, dependant on whether skin grafting is being performed as a sole procedure or as part of a more complex operation.

Position: dependant on the harvest and recipient sites.

1 Both the donor site and the harvest instrument are lubricated using Aquagel, paraffin, or normal saline.

2 The graft can be harvested using an electric or air-powered dermatome or a Watson or Humby knife (non-electric) with an assistant flattening the donor site by providing proximal and distal traction.

   A *Using an electric or air-powered dermatome:*
   - The device is set to the required thickness.
   - Power is switched on before the dermatome contacts the skin.
   - The dermatome is pressed firmly on the skin at 45° and advanced slowly in one smooth passage.
   - Power is only switched off when the dermatome is completely off the skin.

   B *Using a Watson or Humby knife*
   - The sharp edge of the knife is held to the skin with the knife at 45°.
   - Small oscillating movements are made to advance the knife forward.

3 The graft is prepared by trimming it to size or by meshing (a process of placing slits in the graft to allow it to expand to cover larger areas (e.g., burn wounds. This can be performed manually or through a meshing machine).

4 The recipient site is prepared by rasping it with a scalpel or curette until it bleeds.

5 After bleeding is controlled, the skin graft is placed onto the wound bed with the dermal (shiny) side abutting the wound bed and secured with absorbable sutures.

6 The recipient site is closed, and sponge is secured with staples above the new graft to prevent graft shear.

7 The donor site is closed, and an alginate dressing (Kaltostat) is applied directly to the wound and bandaged in place. It is often soaked in local anaesthetic to reduce postoperative pain, but adhesive retention tape (e.g., Mefix) may also be used.

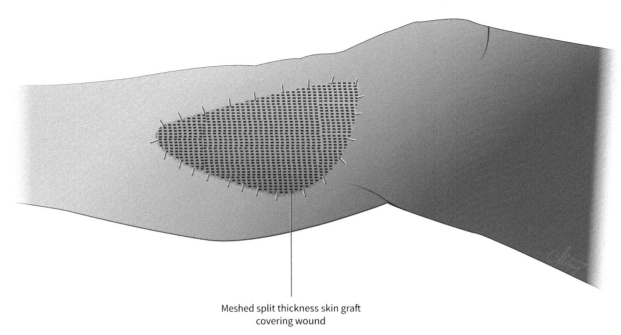

Meshed split thickness skin graft
covering wound

Figure 11.2 Meshed split thickness graft secured with staples

COMPLICATIONS

Early
> Bleeding and/or haematoma formation.

Intermediate and late
> Skin graft failure.
> Infection at either the donor or the recipient site.

> Altered sensation at the recipient site.
> Aberrant scarring at both donor and recipient sites.
> Poor cosmetic outcome due to pigment/texture mismatch and wound contraction (greater than with full thickness graft)

POSTOPERATIVE CARE

Recipient site
> Apply wet dressings twice daily until the graft has taken (approximately 2 weeks).
> Graft take and complications can be assessed in the wound dressing clinic after 7 days.
> A well-healing graft assumes the colour of the surrounding skin and is well-adherent to the wound bed.

Donor site
> Remove dressing after 2 weeks to allow undisturbed re-epithelialisation.

SURGEON'S FAVOURITE QUESTION

Define and describe the process of 'graft take'.

Graft take is the process by which the graft adheres to the recipient site. Following transplantation, a fibrin network 'glues' the graft to the wound bed. The graft is initially nourished via imbibition, the process by which severed vessels within the graft dilate and draw nutrient-rich serous fluid into the graft. Inosculation (anastomosis of graft and wound bed vessels of similar diameter) occurs after 24–72 hours, providing a more secure nutrient source.

FULL-THICKNESS SKIN GRAFT (FTSG)

Nigel Mabvuure and Dariush Nikkhah

DEFINITION

The harvesting of epidermis and dermis from one body area and transplantation onto another body part.

✓ INDICATIONS

- Small defects in cosmetically and functionally sensitive areas such as the face and hands.
- Where local flaps or primary closure are not feasible or contraindicated.

✗ CONTRAINDICATIONS

- Infected wound beds.
- Systemic disease resulting in unreliable vascularisation of the recipient bed.
- Bones and tendons stripped of periosteum and paratenon, respectively, should be avoided, as they have poor blood supply that will lead to failure of the graft to take.

ANATOMY

- The skin is formed of two layers:
  1. Epidermis—superficial and avascular.
  2. Dermis.
- The epidermis:
  - Composed of stratified squamous epithelium and provides a physical barrier to the external environment.
  - Keratinocytes are the predominant epidermal cell type.
  - Since the epidermis is devoid of blood vessels, nutrients reach this layer via diffusion from the underlying dermis.

- The dermis:
  - The dermis is a complex layer containing structural components such as collagen, blood vessels, hair follicles, sweat glands, and cells, including fibroblasts and other immune cells.
  - The dermis is responsible for nourishing the epidermis, as harbouring epithelial cells are able to replenish the epidermis should the need arise (e.g., in the lining of hair follicles).
- Larger blood vessels and nerves, fat, and connective tissue compose the subcutaneous tissue layer.

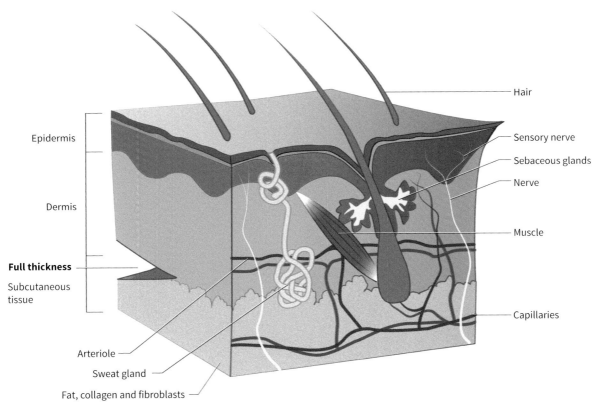

Epidermis

Dermis

Full thickness

Subcutaneous tissue

Arteriole

Sweat gland

Fat, collagen and fibroblasts

Hair

Sensory nerve

Sebaceous glands

Nerve

Muscle

Capillaries

Figure 11.3 Layers and components of the skin and underlying subcutaneous tissue

STEP-BY-STEP OPERATION

Anaesthesia: general, regional, or local, dependant on whether skin grafting is being performed as a sole procedure or as part of a more complex operation (regional or general).

Position: dependant on the harvest and recipient site.

Considerations: Common areas for FTSG harvest include pre- and post-auricular skin, supraclavicular skin, groin skin, or the inner arm or forearm.

1 The graft is harvested by scoring the outline of an ellipse of appropriately sized skin with a scalpel.

2 The skin is then lifted from the corner with forceps and is separated under tension from the underlying subcutaneous fat using a scalpel.

3 The graft is prepared under tension by wrapping it around the surgeon's finger. Fat is then carefully removed using scissors.

4 Fenestrations are made to reduce the accumulation of exudates between the graft and the wound bed (FTSGs should not be finely meshed like split-thickness grafts).

5 The recipient site is prepared by rasping it with a scalpel or curette until it bleeds (making graft take and survival more likely).

6 After bleeding is controlled, the skin graft is placed onto the wound bed with the dermal (shiny) side abutting the wound bed.

7 The graft is then secured with absorbable sutures.

8 The recipient site is closed with sponge dressings being sutured above the new graft (these act as a 'bolster dressing' to prevent graft shear).

9 The donor site is closed with absorbable subcuticular sutures.

PLASTICS

Figure 11.4 Lift and excision of a full thickness skin graft under tension

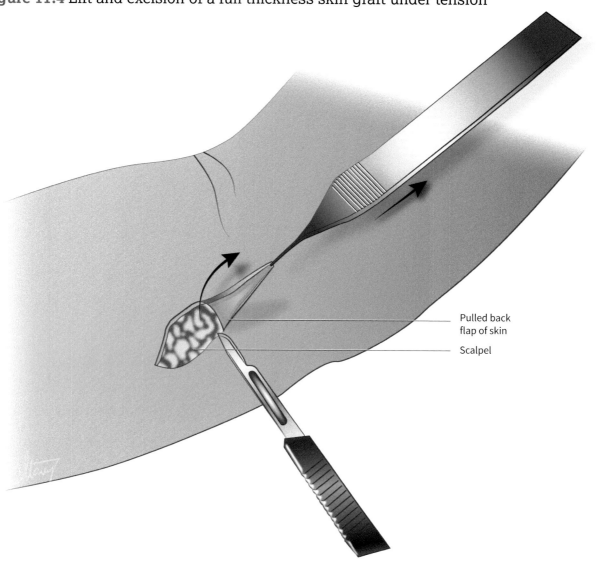

Pulled back
flap of skin

Scalpel

COMPLICATIONS

Early
> Bleeding and/or haematoma formation.

Intermediate and late
> Skin graft failure (greater risk than STSGs), since nutrients have a longer distance to diffuse.

> Infection at either the donor or the recipient site.
> Altered sensation at the recipient site.
> Aberrant scarring at both donor and recipient sites.
> Poor cosmetic outcome due to colour pigment/texture mismatch and wound contraction.

POSTOPERATIVE CARE

Inpatient

> Recipient site:
>> Care should be taken to ensure no pressure of shearing forces are applied to the recipient site.
>> The recipient site should remain elevated and immobilised.
>> The initial dressing should not be removed for the first 3–7 days unless signs of complications including pain, odour, or discharge occur.

Outpatient

> Recipient site:
>> Graft take and complications can be assessed in the wound-dressing clinic within 7 days.
> Donor site:
>> Remove dressing (if applied) in the same dressing clinic.

SURGEON'S FAVOURITE QUESTION

What is the reconstructive ladder?

This describes wound management in increasing complexity.

1. 'Secondary intention': leaving the wound to heal from the bottom up.
2. 'Primary intention': Approximating the wound edges.
3. Skin grafts.
4. Local tissue transfer such as local flaps, covering defects anatomically close to their origin.
5. Free flaps—flaps reattached from their original blood supply to vessels at the defect site.

DEEP INFERIOR EPIGASTRIC PERFORATOR (DIEP) FREE-FLAP FOR BREAST RECONSTRUCTION

Georgios Pafitanis

DEFINITION

An elective procedure to rebuild the breast mound following mastectomy, either as immediate or delayed reconstruction. Tissue that includes fat and skin with a vascular pedicle (a 'free-flap') is taken from the lower abdomen and transferred to the breast.

✓ INDICATIONS

> Breast cancer reconstruction following mastectomy or wide local excision.
> Congenital syndromes of the breast (e.g., breast agenesis or Poland syndrome).

✗ CONTRAINDICATIONS

Relative

> Previous abdominal liposuction.
> Active heavy smokers or those on nicotine replacement therapy (nicotine-induced vasoconstriction will compromise flap survival).

> Abdominal scars near the abdominal donor site.
> Radiotherapy to chest within previous 6 months.
> Thrombophilic conditions.
> Very obese patients.

Absolute

> Inadequate abdominal donor site (e.g., previous abdominal surgery with scar through the lower abdomen).
> Thin patients with insufficient skin and fat.

ANATOMY

> The deep inferior epigastric artery (DIEA) and vein (DIEV) are branches of the external iliac vessels and run from lateral to medial, deep to or within the rectus abdominis muscle. The DIEA supplies the lower abdominal muscles, fat, and skin.
> The Decp inferior epigastric (DIE) vessels either branch before entering the muscle or within it and then perforate through the muscle into the subcutaneous fat. These perforating vessels, 'perforators' of the DIE, range from 0.3 to 1.0 mm and form the vascular pedicle of the free-flap.

> The superficial inferior epigastric artery (SIEA) and vein (SIEV) originate from the external iliac vessels and contribute to the superficial vascular supply of the lower abdominal muscles, fat, and skin.
> Due to the bilateral vascular supply, two DIEP free-flaps can be raised from each side of the lower abdomen (this is done for bilateral breast reconstruction).
> The intercostal nerves T11 and T12 provide sensory innervation to the skin of the lower abdomen.

Figure 11.5 The deep inferior epigastric arteries and veins

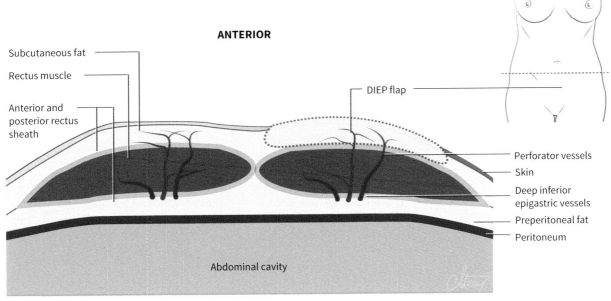

ANTERIOR

Subcutaneous fat

Rectus muscle

Anterior and posterior rectus sheath

DIEP flap

Perforator vessels

Skin

Deep inferior epigastric vessels

Preperitoneal fat

Peritoneum

Abdominal cavity

POSTERIOR

STEP-BY-STEP OPERATION

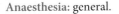

Anaesthesia: general.

Position: supine with both arms outstretched on arm boards.

Considerations: This operation involves two operative fields and can therefore involve two surgical teams working simultaneously. Preoperatively, a Doppler ultrasound is used to locate the DIE perforator supplying the lower abdominal fat and skin. CT angiogram can also be used preoperatively to locate the DIE perforators.

1. An elliptical incision is made across the lower abdomen, preserving the umbilicus.
2. The free-flap is raised by dissecting out the DIE perforator vessel (low-energy diathermy is used to prevent vessel damage).
3. A longitudinal incision is made through the anterior rectus sheath onto the muscle and the muscle fibres are split, allowing the DIE vessels to be traced through the muscle to their origin (this ensures a long vascular pedicle for the flap).
4. Smaller vessels branching off the DIE perforator are carefully ligated with metal clips.
5. The recipient vessels in the chest are simultaneously identified and dissected (either the internal mammary vessels of the anterior chest wall or the thoracodorsal vessels of the axilla). This may include the resection of a rib or costal cartilages.

(To minimise ischaemic time, the free-flap pedicle is ligated only when the recipient vessels are ready).

6. The free-flap vessels are anastomosed to the donor site vessels (artery to artery, vein to vein) under microscopic vision.
7. Vacuum-assisted drains are inserted in the abdomen and the chest wounds.
8. The free-flap is sutured into position, ensuring no tension or pressure on the anastomosed vessels (the skin of the free-flap must be accessible and visible for essential 'flap observations' postoperatively).
9. Closure of the abdominal wound is done in layers, and the umbilicus is repositioned.
10. Once the abdominal wound is dressed, a corset is applied to offer support and prevent seroma/haematoma formation.

PLASTICS

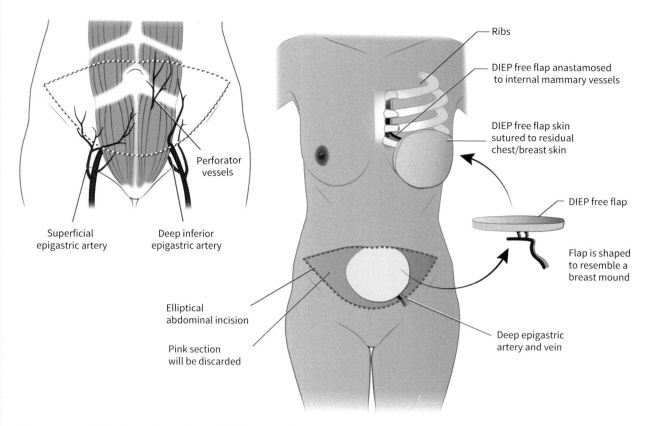

Figure 11.6 Relocation of a DIEP from the recipient to donor site

COMPLICATIONS

Early

> Abdominal donor site:
>> Seroma or haematoma.
> Free-flap related:
>> Flap failure—total or partial flap necrosis from vascular compromise due to:
>>> Extrinsic compression (e.g., haematoma, tight dressing, or overly tight closure).
>>> Venous thrombus.
>>> Arterial thrombus or spasm.
>>> Anastomotic failure.

Intermediate and late

> Abdominal donor site:
>> Abdominal hernia or abdominal muscle weakness.
>> Wound infection (<5%).
> Free-flap-related:
>> Fat necrosis causing a lumpy appearance of the breast (<5%).
>> Wound infection (<5%).
>> Seroma or haematoma (<10%).
>> Asymmetry and alteration of body image.

POSTOPERATIVE CARE

Inpatient

> Hourly 'flap observations' postoperatively, including blood pressure, urine output, and flap checks to assess for warmth, congestion, and turgor, all signs of vascular compromise of the flap.
> Surgical drains removed at surgeon's discretion, commonly when output <30ml/24hrs after mobilisation.

Outpatient

> Review by the Breast Clinical Nurse Specialist within a week of discharge to assess wound healing and monitor for seroma formation.
> Consultant-led outpatient clinic in 4–6 weeks.

SURGEON'S FAVOURITE QUESTION

What are clinical consequences of using a transverse rectus abdominis muscle (TRAM) flap instead of a DIEP flap?

The TRAM uses a portion of the rectus abdominis muscle, not just fat and skin, and therefore has a higher risk of abdominal wall weakness and herniation.

LOCAL FLAP RECONSTRUCTION OF SOFT TISSUE DEFECTS

Evgenia Theodorakopoulou

DEFINITION

A local flap (an area of tissue with its own blood supply) that is moved to treat adjacent soft tissue defects.

✓ INDICATIONS

> Provide robust coverage in areas of tissue loss that cannot be closed directly.
> Provide an alternative to skin grafts in:
>   1. Areas of exposed bone, tendon, or cartilage.
>   2. Areas where grafts may fail due to shear forces.
>   3. Areas where grafts may become traumatised/ulcerated.
>   4. Areas where contraction must be avoided (e.g., over a joint and the hand dorsum).

✗ CONTRAINDICATIONS

Relative
> Smoking.
> Peripheral arterial disease.

Absolute
> Active infection (delay coverage until this is resolved).
> Injured, poor-quality tissue around the defect and/or donor site.
> When raising a flap could compromise function (e.g., in the hand).

ANATOMY

Core characteristics of a flap:

1. Tissue composition:
   a. Cutaneous—skin only.
   b. Fasciocutaneous—fascia and skin.
   c. Musculocutaneous—muscle and skin.
   d. Muscle—muscle only.
   e. Osteocutaneous—bone, soft tissue, and skin.
2. Vascularity:
   > Random flaps—these are not based on a specific vessel. Their blood supply has a random pattern, derived from the subdermal plexus.
   > Axial flaps—these receive their blood supply from a specific known vessel (pedicle). This enables a larger area to be detached. These flaps tend to exhibit better survival, as they are more optimally perfused than random flaps.
3. Geometrical design/movement:
   > Advancement flap—the flap is advanced directly forward with no rotation or lateral movement (e.g., simple, bi-pedicled, or V-Y advancement flaps).

> Rotational flap—these flaps are rounded in shape and are rotated about a pivot point. Their circumference should be 5–8 x the width of the defect. The secondary defect can then be closed directly.
> Transpositional flap—these flaps tend to be quadrilateral and are moved laterally about a pivot point. The flap becomes shorter as it is rotated. The resultant defect often needs wound coverage with a graft or a secondary local flap (e.g., rhomboid flap). Transpositional flaps are the most frequently utilised flap.
> Interpolation flap—this flap is lifted off the donor site to cover a defect that is close but not adjacent, while maintaining its vascular pedicle. The flap often must be moved under or over an intervening soft tissue bridge.

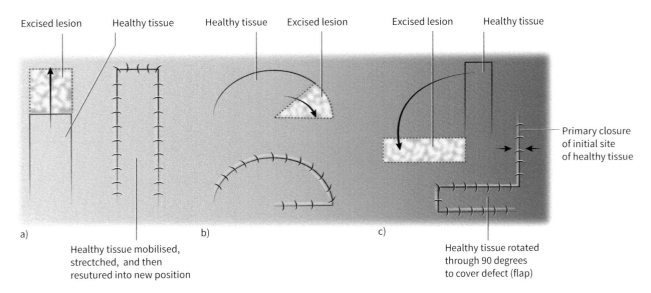

Figure 11.7 Geometric designs of a flap. A) Advancement flap. B) Rotational flap. C) Transpositional flap

STEP-BY-STEP OPERATION

Anaesthesia: general or regional.

Position: dependant on the harvest and recipient sites.

Considerations: In a V-Y advancement flap (as described below), the initial V-shaped incision is eventually converted into a Y-shaped scar (described here in relation to fingertip loss/coverage).

1 A triangular incision (the height of the triangle tends to be 1.5–2 x the base) is made from the edges of the wound (including skin and subcutaneous tissue). This becomes the 'flap' that will be moved to cover the defect. The triangle may need to have a curvilinear rather than a straight shape so that the incisions follow the natural skin creases ('Horn Flap').

2 The tissues surrounding the flap and laterally are undermined.

3 The apex and base of the flap are slightly undermined to further increase mobility and prevent tethering (care is taken to preserve a small amount of subcutaneous tissue and to not overly undermine the underlying subdermal plexus).

4 Any excess recipient subcutaneous tissue is removed to ensure that the original defect is the same thickness as the flap.

5 A skin hook is used to advance the flap base into position and to check there is no excessive tension.

6 The first securing suture is placed in the middle of the triangle base (or 'leading edge').

7 The remainder of the flap is then sutured into position.

8 The linear defect extending from the apex is then sutured directly.

9 The wound is dressed, ensuring there is adequate compression to prevent haematoma formation, but not so much as to compromise blood supply.

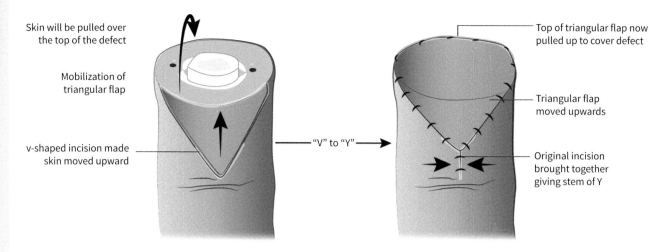

Figure 11.8 V-Y advancement flap to cover finger tip loss

COMPLICATIONS

Early

> Haematoma and/or seroma formation.
> 'Dog-ears'—small triangular soft tissue bulges at the edge of a scar, which can be unsightly.

Intermediate and late

> Compromised flap perfusion or flap necrosis due to:
  1. Tense closure.

2. Insufficient length-to-width ratio.
3. Flap raised outside of its pedicle's vascular territory.
4. Excessive external pressure from dressings or a developing haematoma.

> Wound breakdown.
> Infection.

POSTOPERATIVE CARE

Inpatient

> Large local flaps may require formal monitoring postoperatively for signs of vascular compromise and/or haematoma formation.

Outpatient

> Wound check at 7–10 days in clinic to assess healing and to rule out infection.

 SURGEON'S FAVOURITE QUESTION

Explain the difference between local, regional, and distant flaps.

Local: flap is adjacent to the defect. Regional: flap is composed of tissue from the same body region as the defect. Distant: the flap originates in a different area than the defect and can be pedicled or free.

DIGITAL TENDON REPAIR

Evgenia Theodorakopoulou

DEFINITION

Surgical repair of the digital flexor or extensor tendon(s) to restore function following tendon trauma.

✓ INDICATIONS

Complete and partial tendon injuries (>30%), including:

▸ Laceration—traumatic or iatrogenic.

▸ Avulsion—usually a closed injury.

▸ Rupture secondary to:
  1. Trauma—unrepaired partial laceration.
  2. Failed repair.
  3. Inflammatory disease (e.g., rheumatoid arthritis).

✗ CONTRAINDICATIONS

▸ Repair should be delayed until wound and soft tissues are optimised in:
  › Gross wound contamination or active infection.
  › Human-bite injuries.
  › Lack of soft tissue coverage.

ANATOMY

▸ Tendons attach muscle to bone.

▸ Tendons are composed of dense, uniform connective tissue composed mainly of Type I collagen, elastin, and mucopolysaccharides.

▸ Flexor tendons:
  › Originate from:
    □ Flexor digitorum profundus (FDP) and flexor digitorum superficialis (FDS) muscles, which flex the fingers.
    □ Flexor pollicis longus (FPL) muscle, which flexes the thumb.
  › Tendons are enclosed within a protective flexor sheath that offers nourishment and enables smooth gliding.
  › Each FDS tendon starts superficial to the FDP, then divides on either side of it (over the proximal interphalangeal joint). These two slips then re-join proximally, deep to the FDP.
  › FDS tendons insert into the middle phalanx and cause flexion across the proximal interphalangeal joints (PIPJ).
  › FDP tendons insert into the distal phalanx and cause flexion across the distal interphalangeal joints (DIPJ).

› Eight thickened areas known as pulleys (five annular and three cruciform) overlie the tendons and provide stability, preventing bow-stringing and increasing functional efficiency.

▸ Extensor tendons:
  › Extrinsic extension of the digits originates in the forearm and is influenced by the extensor digitorum communis (EDC), extensor indicis (EI), extensor digiti minimi (EDM), extensor pollicis longus (EPL), and extensor pollicis brevis (EPB).
  › Intrinsic extension of the digits originate in the hand via the seven interossei and four lumbrical muscles.
  › The extensor tendon divides into three, forming one central slip and two lateral bands.
  › The central slip inserts at the base of the middle phalanx and causes extension across the PIPJ.
  › The lateral slips combine with the lateral bands of the intrinsics, reuniting distally. Together they form the terminal extensor, which inserts into the distal phalangeal base and causes extension across the DIPJ.

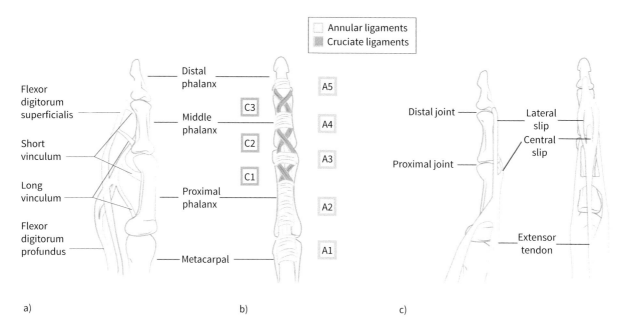

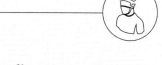

Figure 11.9 Flexor and extensor tendons of the hand

STEP-BY-STEP OPERATION

Anaesthesia: general, regional, or local (distal extensor injuries only).
Position: arm outstretched on an arm board.

1 Extend the wound to allow both divided ends to be visualised and accessed (avoid longitudinal incisions across finger creases, as this may cause scar contractures and affect mobility).
2 The wound is irrigated and debrided.
3 The neurovascular bundle is located to assess for associated injury.
4 Both ends of the tendon are identified, assessed, and retrieved.
5 For the core repair, the 'Modified Kessler' with a two- or four-strand repair is employed using a 3/0 or

4/0 non-absorbable monofilament suture. During the repair, the tendon ends are temporarily secured by pinning them in place with a hypodermic needle (in the Modified Kessler technique, the strength of the repair is proportional to the number of strands).
6 The epitendinous repair is then performed by placing a continuous running suture to the outer circumference of the tendon using a 5/0 or 6/0 suture (overly tight suturing can compromise the tendon's blood supply).
7 The wound is closed to ensure coverage of the repair.
8 The hand is placed in a splint.

Figure 11.10 Core and epitendinous stages of tendon repair

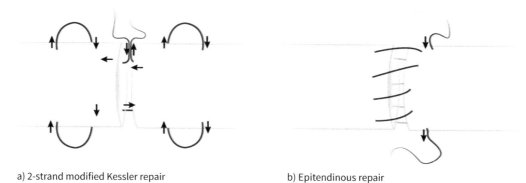

a) 2-strand modified Kessler repair   b) Epitendinous repair

COMPLICATIONS

Early

> Iatrogenic damage to the neurovascular bundle.
> Rupture of tendon repair (5%).

Intermediate and late

> Postoperative infection and/or wound breakdown.
> Poor mobility due to scarring, contractures, adhesions, poor repair, prolonged immobilisation, and non-compliance with therapy.

> Joint deformities—e.g., swan-neck, boutonniere (in extensor complications).
> Complex regional pain syndrome (CRPS)—a rare condition that can occur even after minor hand injuries.

POSTOPERATIVE CARE

Inpatient

> Commonly performed as a day-case procedure.

Outpatient

> Wound check at 7–10 days to assess for healing and infection.

> Hand therapy and rehabilitation by specialist hand physiotherapists—a vital component of successful tendon repair.
> Generally, early active mobilisation is advocated, though a short period of immobilisation may initially be required—duration of splinting is variable depending on type of injury.

SURGEON'S FAVOURITE QUESTION

When is a tendon repair at its weakest?

At around 10–12 days postoperatively, with most ruptures occurring at day 10.

NAIL BED INJURY REPAIR

Katrina Mason

DEFINITION

Repair of a traumatic laceration involving the nail bed with the aim of ensuring continued nail growth and prevention of nail deformity.

✓ INDICATIONS

- Repair of a nail bed laceration is done to ensure the best cosmetic outcome with regards to future nail growth in the following situations:
  - Crush injuries to nail bed.
  - Simple nail bed laceration.
  - Stellate lacerations of nail bed.
  - Avulsion of nail plate from nail fold.
  - Subungual haematoma >50% of visible nail.

✗ CONTRAINDICATIONS

- Grossly contaminated or devitalised wound with complex underlying phalangeal fracture. These injuries may be more suitable for digital terminalisation and/or nail avulsion matrixectomy (removal of nail and germinal matrix to prevent nail regrowth).

ANATOMY

- The nail plate is composed of hard, keratinised squamous cells attached to the nail bed inferiorly.
- The nail fold is where the nail plate proximally attaches to the underlying tissues and consists of the dorsal roof superiorly and the ventral floor inferiorly. The ventral floor is the site of the germinal matrix. The germinal matrix is responsible for the majority of nail production.
- The sterile matrix is the distal portion of the nail bed and is tightly adherent to both the overlying nail plate and the underlying periosteum. Along with the dorsal roof, it is a secondary site of nail production.
- The nail plate is loosely attached to the germinal matrix but is densely attached to the sterile matrix.
- The eponychium (cuticle) is the distal portion of the nail fold.
- The paronychium is the soft tissue along the lateral borders of the nail plate.
- Nails grow at roughly 3–4 mm per month (0.1 mm/day).

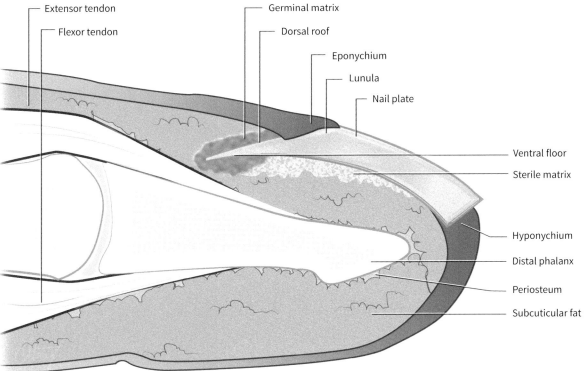

Figure 11.11 Anatomy of the nail bed

Labels (clockwise from top left): Extensor tendon, Flexor tendon, Germinal matrix, Dorsal roof, Eponychium, Lunula, Nail plate, Ventral floor, Sterile matrix, Hyponychium, Distal phalanx, Periosteum, Subcuticular fat

STEP-BY-STEP OPERATION

Anaesthesia: general with digital ring block (paediatrics), digital ring block only (adults). NB: local anaesthetic should not contain adrenaline due to the risk of avascular necrosis.

Position: arm and hand outstretched on an arm board.

Considerations: Apply a tourniquet to the digit to ensure a bloodless field for optimal visualisation of structures. Following hand trauma, these injuries may require additional surgical management, such as k-wire fixation.

1 The nail plate is removed with a Kutz or Freer elevator and fine tenotomy scissors.

2 The nail bed is irrigated with saline.

3 Any grossly contaminated and non-viable tissue is excised.

4 Any associated finger pad laceration and/or distal phalanx injury is first repaired to minimise flailing of the distal segment.

5 Using fine absorbable sutures, the nail margin is then repaired to ensure anatomical alignment.

6 The nail bed is then sutured from the distal segment to proximal tissue.

7 The tourniquet is released and, using bipolar diathermy, haemostasis is achieved.

8 The removed nail plate acts as a dressing (often glued down over the nail bed repair). If the nail plate has been lost, Xeroform® gauze or a silastic plate can be used.

9 A non-adherent dressing such as Mepitel®, then gauze, tape, and a protective digital splint, are applied. Children require extensive bandaging of the hand ('boxing glove bandaging') to prevent picking or further injury.

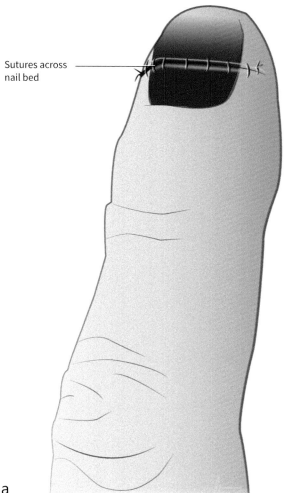

Sutures across
nail bed

Figure 11.12 Suturing of a
nail bed laceration

COMPLICATIONS

Early
> Bleeding.
> Pain and discomfort.

Intermediate and late
> Infection.
> Absence of nail growth secondary to damage to the
germinal matrix.

> Abnormal nail growth secondary to damage to
the sterile matrix—ridged nail, hook nail, and nail
spikes.
> Hypersensitivity—this can be transient or persistent.
> Complex regional pain syndrome—a rare condition
that can occur even after minor hand injuries.

POSTOPERATIVE CARE

Inpatient

▸ Commonly performed as a day-case procedure.

▸ Antibiotics in the case of contaminated wounds.

Outpatient

▸ Dressing clinic in 7 days for removal of dressings and wound assessment.

▸ Protective splinting for 2 weeks.

▸ Outpatient follow-up in 6 weeks.

▸ Note: It takes approximately 100 days to grow a complete nail and see the final result of the nail bed repair.

SURGEON'S FAVOURITE QUESTION

What are the causes of a hook nail?

These are often caused by trauma to the nail bed—for example, in distal phalangeal bone loss resulting in poor support of the sterile matrix, causing a curved growth of the nail.

12 | PAEDIATRICS

MARY PATRICE EASTWOOD

RAMSTEDT PYLOROMYOTOMY

Ivana Capin

Ivana Capin

PAEDIATRICS

DEFINITION

A procedure to relieve outlet obstruction of the stomach caused by hypertrophy of the circular muscle of the pylorus.

✓ INDICATIONS

> Hypertrophic pyloric stenosis.

✗ CONTRAINDICATIONS

> Uncorrected metabolic abnormalities.

ANATOMY

Gross anatomy

> The stomach comprises of five parts:
>> 1 Cardia.
>> 2 Fundus.
>> 3 Body.
>> 4 Antrum.
>> 5 Pylorus.
> The stomach has two sphincters:
>> 1 Inferior oesophageal—this is a physiological sphincter created by the acute angle between the cardia and the oesophagus (angle of His).
>> 2 Pyloric—an anatomical sphincter between the stomach and the duodenum made of a thick layer of circular smooth muscle. It is located at the level of the transpyloric plane (L1), 1 cm right of the midline.

Neurovasculature

> The parasympathetic nerve supply to the stomach is via the vagus nerve.
> The sympathetic innervation of the stomach is derived from segments T6–T9 via the coeliac plexus.

> The blood supply to the stomach is via the coeliac trunk, which branches from the abdominal aorta at T12.
> The left gastric artery (LGA), a direct branch of the coeliac trunk, supplies the superior lesser curvature of the stomach, whereas the right gastric artery (RGA), a branch of the common hepatic artery, supplies the inferior portion.
> The right gastro-epiploic artery (RGE) arises from the gastroduodenal artery and runs along the greater curvature from the distal aspect of the stomach.
> At the hilum of the spleen, the splenic artery divides into the short gastric arteries, which supply the fundus, and the left gastro-epiploic artery, which supplies the proximal greater curvature.
> The venous drainage of the stomach follows the arterial supply. An important vein to note in Ramstedt's pyloromyotomy is the pre-pyloric vein of Mayo, which runs anteriorly over the pylorus and drains into the right gastric vein.

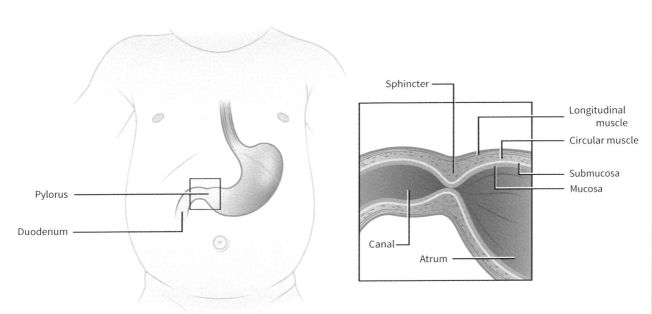

Figure 12.1 Pyloric stenosis

STEP-BY-STEP OPERATION

Anaesthesia: general.

Position: supine.

Considerations: Pre-operatively, the patient should be fluid resuscitated, and any electrolyte abnormalities should be corrected.

1 A 3 cm incision is made in the supraumbilical region over the palpable pylorus.

2 The layers of abdominal wall are dissected, and the peritoneum is breeched.

3 Traction is applied inferiorly to the transverse colon, and laterally to the antrum of the stomach, to deliver the pylorus into the wound (the thickened pylorus is easily identified from the adjacent pink duodenum by its whitish appearance and the vein of Mayo that demarcates the boundary between the two).

4 The pylorus is held between the thumb and forefinger.

5 A longitudinal incision is made on the anterior surface from the non-hypertrophied stomach antrum and extended distally, but not beyond the vein of Mayo.

6 The thickened muscle is then split along the length of the incision until the mucosa bulges upwards and the two halves of the pyloromyotomy move freely.

7 An air leak test, submerging the pylorus in saline and insufflating the stomach with air, is performed to identify any mucosal perforation.

8 The abdomen is closed in layers.

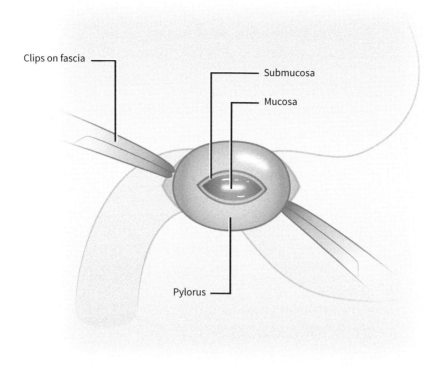

Clips on fascia

Submucosa

Mucosa

Pylorus

Figure 12.2 Split fibres of the thickened pylorus

COMPLICATIONS

Early
› Mucosal perforation (1–2%).

Intermediate and late
› Wound infection.
› Inadequate pyloromyotomy (4%).

POSTOPERATIVE CARE

Inpatient
› Feeding can be commenced 4 hours postoperatively and progressively built up.

Outpatient
› No routine clinic follow-up is required.

SURGEON'S FAVOURITE QUESTIONS

In cases of mucosal perforation, how does one proceed?

The perforation can be closed with an absorbable suture and an omental patch attached. Alternatively, the myotomy can be closed and then a second pyloromyotomy performed following a 90° rotation of the pylorus.

OESOPHAGEAL ATRESIA/TRACHEOESOPHAGEAL FISTULA LIGATION WITH REPAIR

Ivana Capin

DEFINITION
A surgical procedure to correct and restore continuity of the oesophagus.

✓ INDICATIONS

- Presence of oesophageal atresia (OA) with or without tracheoesophageal fistula (TOF).

✗ CONTRAINDICATIONS

- Abdominal X-ray showing no air below the diaphragm signifies the absence of a distal TOF. In these cases, a gastrostomy is formed for feeding, and the primary repair is delayed.

ANATOMY

Embryology

- Between the third and fourth gestational week, the foregut gives rise to a ventral diverticulum, which becomes the respiratory primordium.
- The trachea is derived from a laryngotracheal tube.
- Separation of the developing trachea and oesophagus (foregut) is tightly regulated within the developing embryo.
- OA occurs when the oesophagus is not completely formed and ends in a pouch, failing to connect with the stomach.

Gross anatomy

- The trachea connects the pharynx and larynx to the lungs.
- The trachea comprises C-shaped cartilage with an inferior wall of muscle.
- The upper third of the oesophagus is composed of striated muscle that transitions to smooth muscle in the lower two-thirds.

Neurovasculature

- The trachea derives parasympathetic innervation from branches of the vagus nerve and the recurrent laryngeal nerve, and sympathetic innervation from the sympathetic trunk via the posterior and anterior pulmonary plexus.
- The oesophagus is parasympathetically innervated by the vagus nerve and sympathetically innervated by the thoracic spinal nerves.
- The trachea is perfused by branches of the subclavian, internal mammary, and brachiocephalic arteries.
- The upper third of the oesophagus is supplied by the inferior thyroid arteries.
- The middle third of the oesophagus is supplied by the oesophageal branches of the thoracic aorta.
- The lower third of the oesophagus is supplied by the left gastric artery.

Pathology

- Gross classification is used to describe OA:
  - Type A—OA with no TOF (8%).
  - Type B—OA with TOF between the trachea and the upper portion of the oesophagus (1%).
  - Type C—OA with TOF between the trachea and the lower portion of the oesophagus (86%).
  - Type D—OA with TOF between the trachea and both the upper and lower portions of the oesophagus (1%).
  - Type E—TOF with no atresia of the oesophagus ("H-type") (4%).

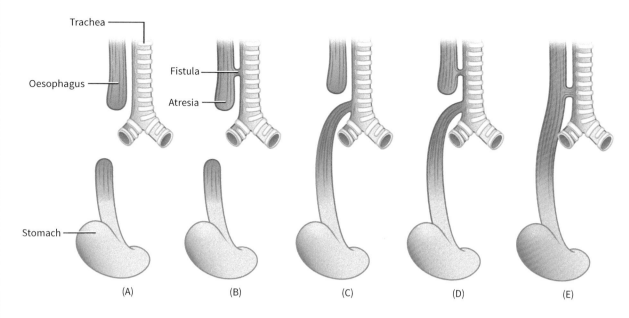

Trachea

Fistula

Oesophagus

Atresia

Stomach

(A)   (B)   (C)   (D)   (E)

Figure 12.3 Classification of oesophageal atresia (OA)

STEP-BY-STEP OPERATION

Anaesthesia: general.

Position: The patient is positioned on the left side with the right arm extended over the head.

1 A thoracotomy incision is made 1 cm below the right scapula extending from the mid-axillary line posteriorly. The muscle layers are split, and entry is made into the pleural cavity at the fourth to fifth intercostal space.

2 The right lung is gently retracted to visualize the oesophagus and trachea.

3 The azygos vein running across the trachea is identified and ligated.

4 The TOF is carefully dissected with care taken to avoid the vagus nerve.

5 A loop is placed around the fistula and the lungs insufflated before separation to ensure the loop is not around a major airway.

6 Sutures are placed across the oesophageal fistula close to the trachea, and the fistula is then divided distal to these sutures and the tracheal defect over-sewn.

7 The distal end of the fistula is checked for patency and occasionally divided again a few centimetres distal from the first dissection to create a wider end for anastomosis.

8 The distal oesophagus (previously the fistula) is mobilized superiorly to meet the proximal oesophagus.

9 An end-to-end anastomosis is performed with care taken to include both mucosal and muscle layers.

10 A small nasogastric (NG) tube, also known as a trans-anastomotic tube (TAT), is placed to enable early NG feeding postoperatively. A chest drain is only necessary in cases of a difficult dissection. The chest wall is closed in layers.

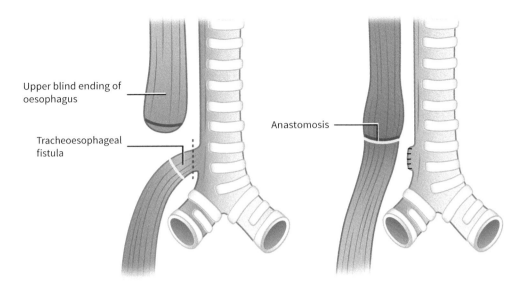

Figure 12.4 Sites of fistula ligation and oseophageal anastomosis

COMPLICATIONS

Early
> Anastomotic leak (15–20%).

Intermediate and late
> Anastomotic stricture (30–40%).
> Recurrent TOF (5–14%).

POSTOPERATIVE CARE

Inpatient
> The patient is transferred to neonatal intensive care postoperatively.
> TAT feeds may commence on the second or third postoperative day, and oral feeding may be introduced gradually.

> Occasionally, an oesophageal contrast study may be performed to ensure no leak at the anastomotic site.

Outpatient
> Omeprazole is prescribed for 1 year to minimize oesophageal reflux.

 SURGEON'S FAVOURITE QUESTIONS

What other abnormalities should be ruled out preoperatively in OA neonates?

OA is associated with VACTERL syndrome (20%), encompassing vertebral, anal atresia, cardiovascular, tracheoesophageal, renal, and limb defects. It is particularly important to rule out a cardiac defect (20-50%), the most common being ventricular septal defect, as these are associated with a higher mortality rate.

LAPAROTOMY FOR NECROTISING ENTEROCOLITIS (NEC)

Stephen Ali

DEFINITION

Closure of isolated intestinal perforations and the resection of necrotic bowel and/or formation of a stoma.

✓ INDICATIONS

> Intestinal perforation.
> Failure of NEC to respond to medical management.
> Abdominal mass with signs of intestinal obstruction or sepsis.

✗ CONTRAINDICATIONS

> Total intestinal gangrene—treatment withdrawal should be considered.

ANATOMY

Embryology

> The embryological development of the gut is derived from a primitive endodermal tube that is divided into three parts:
>> 1 Foregut—oesophagus to upper duodenum (d2) (supplied by the coeliac axis).
>> 2 Midgut—lower duodenum (d3) to proximal two-thirds of the transverse colon (supplied by the superior mesenteric artery).
>> 3 Hindgut—distal one-third of transverse colon to ectodermal part of the anal canal (supplied by the inferior mesenteric artery.

Gross anatomy

> The small bowel starts at the duodenal jejunal (DJ) flexure (ligament of Treitz) and travels obliquely and downwards towards the right sacroiliac joint within the free edge of a mesentery attached to the posterior abdominal wall.
> The first two-fifths of the small intestine is termed the jejunum and the remainder the ileum; the distinction between the two is histological.

> The colon comprises the caecum, ascending colon, transverse colon, descending colon, and sigmoid colon.
> The ascending colon extends upwards from the caecum to the under surface of the liver at the hepatic flexure and turns left to become the transverse colon.
> The transverse colon is covered completely by peritoneum.
> The transverse colon runs from the hepatic flexure to the left colic flexure (splenic flexure), where it becomes the descending colon.
> The descending colon passes from the splenic flexure to the sigmoid colon.
> The mesenteries of the ascending and descending colon blend with the posterior abdominal wall (retro-peritoneal), except for the sigmoid colon, which retains a mesentery.
> The pelvic brim marks the beginning of the sigmoid colon, which extends to the recto-sigmoid junction.
> Any part of the bowel may be affected by necrotising enterocolitis (NEC), but the most frequent sites (respectively) are the terminal ileum, right hemi-colon, left hemi-colon, and sigmoid colon.

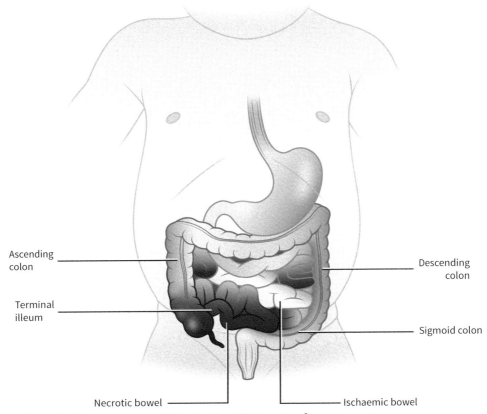

Ascending colon

Terminal illeum

Descending colon

Sigmoid colon

Necrotic bowel

Ischaemic bowel

Figure 12.5 Necrotising enterocolitis in the GI tract of a neonate

STEP-BY-STEP OPERATION

Anaesthesia: general.

Position: supine.

Considerations: An exploratory laparotomy is conducted with the aim of controlling sepsis and removing areas of frankly necrotic bowel whilst preserving bowel length.

1 A transverse supraumbilical incision is made (in pre-term neonates, extra care should be taken not to damage the liver, which is extremely fragile; in these patients, a left-sided incision should be considered to avoid the liver).

2 Intraoperative options depend upon the amount of disease found:

a Isolated simple perforations –"focal NEC" (frequently occur in the terminal ileum) are closed with sutures placed transversely to prevent narrowing of the bowel lumen.

b Isolated necrotic or perforated segments (2 to 3 cm) with no involvement of the remaining bowel—are treated with resection and primary anastomosis. The intestine is cut at an angle of 30° to 45° to increase the anastomotic circumference. Non-viable bowel is discarded, with healthy bowel ends sewn together. Anastomotic ends should bleed briskly when cut, indicating bowel viability.

c Multiple perforations and necrotic segments—can be treated with a combination of over-sewing, resection with primary anastomosis, or 'clip and drop' in the case of an unstable neonate. 'Clip and drop' involves resecting and removing segments of necrotic bowel and closing the end independently using a LIGACLIP (metal clip) rather than performing a primary anastomosis. The most proximal piece of bowel can be formed into an enterostomy.

d Pan-intestinal NEC—usually results in the formation of a proximal jejunotomy. Again, 'clip and drop' is an option.

3 A defunctioning loop ileostomy or terminal stoma with distal mucosal fistula is formed.

4 Closure:
  a Abdominal wound closure is performed in two fascial layers using a running absorbable suture.
  b If the fascia is friable or difficult to identify, single-layer closure including both fascial layers and the rectus muscle is performed.

  c In case of massive inflammation or difficulties in closing the abdominal cavity, a temporary patch should be considered to avoid the risk of compartment syndrome. In the latter, a second-look operation may be performed at 24 hrs to check viability.

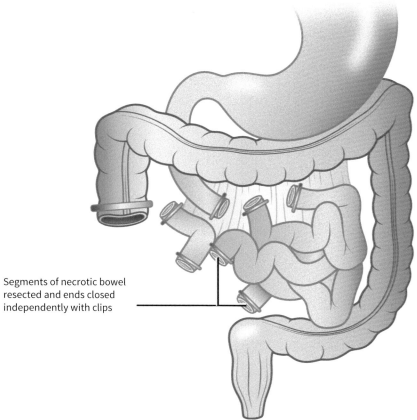

Segments of necrotic bowel resected and ends closed independently with clips

Figure 12.6 Sites of clip and drop in NEC

COMPLICATIONS

Early
> Mortality is dependent on disease severity and gestational age at birth (overall around 30%).

Intermediate and late
> Neurodevelopmental delay (50%).
> Stricture formation (30–40%).
> Short gut syndrome (up to 23%).
> Vitamin B12 deficiency if ileal resection is required.

POSTOPERATIVE CARE

Inpatient

- ▸ Postoperatively the patient is managed in the Neonatal Intensive Care Unit (NICU).
- ▸ Parental nutrition is commenced for feeding with complete bowel rest and intravenous antibiotics for at least 1 week.
- ▸ Future management depends on the surgical technique performed. Bowel continuity will need to be restored in the case of a 'clip and drop' when the neonate is stable and no longer septic.
- ▸ Total parental nutrition is established in cases where there may be a delay in enteral feeding (>5 days). When bowel continuity is restored, a trophic feed can be started and gradually built up as tolerated.

- ▸ Re-anastomosis of a stoma is around the eight to twelfth postoperative week. A contrast enema is performed before re-anastomosis to detect intestinal strictures that usually occur within the large bowel.

Outpatient

- ▸ Children are followed up in the outpatient clinic and subsequently on a yearly basis to monitor for growth and late complications.
- ▸ In case of terminal ileum resection, long-term follow-up is needed to rule out possible vitamin B12 deficiency.

 SURGEON'S FAVOURITE QUESTION

What are the radiographic findings in necrotising enterocolitis?

Pneumatosis intestinalis is the pathognomonic X-ray finding. This signifies the presence of gas-producing organisms in the bowel wall. Other signs include a dilated bowel loop or a fixed loop 'signet sign', portal venous gas, and, importantly, pneumoperitoneum.

LADD'S PROCEDURE

Christina Cheng

DEFINITION

Division of Ladd's bands, widening of the small intestine mesentery, and return of the bowel to a non-rotated state. Ladd's bands are fibrous stalks of peritoneum that attach the right lower quadrant retroperitoneum to the caecum.

✓ INDICATIONS

> Intestinal malrotation.
> Midgut volvulus—a surgical emergency.

✗ CONTRAINDICATIONS

> None

ANATOMY

Embryology

> The embryological development of the gut is derived from a primitive endodermal tube that is divided into three parts:
>   1 Foregut—oesophagus to upper duodenum (d2) (supplied by the coeliac axis).
>   2 Midgut—lower duodenum (d3) to proximal two-thirds of the transverse colon (supplied by the superior mesenteric artery).
>   3 Hindgut—distal one-third of transverse colon to ectodermal part of the anal canal (supplied by the inferior mesenteric artery).
> The midgut herniates through the umbilical ring in the fourth week of embryological development and returns to the abdominal cavity between the 10th and 12th weeks when space is adequate.
> The caecocolic loop returns last to the left lower quadrant and subsequently rotates counterclockwise 270° anterior to the superior mesenteric artery, finally positioning itself in the right lower quadrant.
> The duodenojejunal loop fixes in the left upper quadrant after rotating counterclockwise 270° to sit posterior and to the left of the superior mesenteric artery.

> At the 12th gestational week, fascial connections form, fixing these structures in place.
> The ligament of Treitz, a muscular structure, connects the diaphragm (at the right crus) to the small intestine at the junction of the duodenum and jejunum.
> The caecum becomes fixed as the posterior parietal peritoneum fuses.

Pathology

> Non-rotation—the duodenojejunal and caecocolic segments don't rotate; therefore, the small bowel predominantly lies on the right and the large bowel on the left of the abdomen.
> Malrotation—rotation halts at 180°, resulting in the caecum lying in the right upper quadrant and the duodenojejunal flexure to the right of the midline. The base of the mesenteric vessels is narrow and prone to volvulus. Ladd's bands are peritoneal bands that extend across the duodenum and attach the abnormally sited caecum to the right paracolic gutter, liver, and gallbladder.

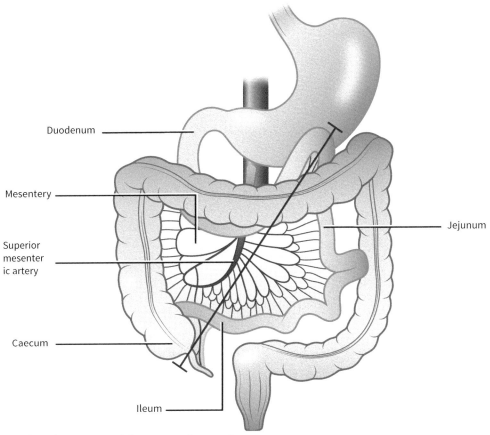

Duodenum

Mesentery

Superior
mesenter
ic artery

Caecum

Ileum

Jejunum

Figure 12.7 The GI tract with normal rotation

STEP-BY-STEP OPERATION

Anaesthesia: general.

Position: supine

1. A transverse upper abdominal incision is made.
2. The small bowel is delivered from the abdominal cavity, and the midgut volvulus is untwisted in a counterclockwise direction (this is opposite to the direction of volvulus, which usually occurs clockwise).
3. To increase perfusion, manual massage of the mesenteric vessels is performed to assist with the breakdown of the blood clot (tissue plasminogen activator (tPA) is considered postoperatively in the most severe cases).
4. 10 minutes following reperfusion, the bowel is assessed for ischaemic or necrotic areas, and a resection with stoma formation is performed where necessary.

5. The duodenum is mobilised from the abdominal wall by dividing the Ladd's bands.
6. Adhesions at the base of the mesentery are divided, and the mesentery is subsequently widened to increase mobility of the bowel.
7. The ligament of Treitz is divided and the duodenum straightened out.
8. An appendicectomy is performed to avoid diagnostic errors in the patient's future life.
9. The small bowel is repositioned with the duodenum placed on the right of midline and the caecum placed in the left upper quadrant in a non-rotated position.
10. The wound is closed in layers.

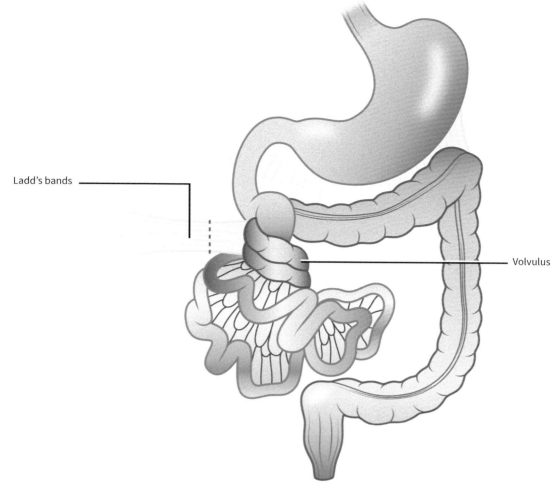

Figure 12.8 Ladd's bands with a malrotational-volvulus

COMPLICATIONS

Early

> Intestinal infarction (<6%).

Intermediate and late

> Adhesive small bowel obstruction (8–10%), which seems to be avoided with the laparoscopic approach.
> Recurrent volvulus (<2%).

> Short bowel syndrome—occurs when there is insufficient length of functional small intestine, resulting in insufficient absorptive capacity. Most patients require total parenteral nutrition. Small bowel transplantations can be performed, but long-term results in children are still unsatisfactory.

POSTOPERATIVE CARE

Inpatient

> Monitor fluid status and electrolytes.
> Total parenteral nutrition until full oral feeds tolerated.

Outpatient

> Regular long-term follow-up is not necessary.

SURGEON'S FAVOURITE QUESTION

What is the finding in the investigation of choice in a patient with suspected malrotation (bilious vomiting)?

Any infant presenting with bilious i.e. green vomiting should have an urgent upper gastro-intestinal contrast study. The duodenojejunal flexure will be to the right of the midline below the pylorus in cases of malrotation. In cases of midgut volvulus, there may be a 'corkscrew' or 'beaked' appearance of the duodenum, suggesting incomplete duodenal obstruction.

HEPATOPORTOENTEROSTOMY (KASAI PORTOENTEROSTOMY)

Jane Lim

DEFINITION
Removal of obstructed biliary tree and restoration of bile flow by anastomosing the jejunum to the patent hepatic ducts.

✓ INDICATIONS

> Infants diagnosed with biliary atresia in the first 120 days of life (best outcomes within 60 days after birth).

✗ CONTRAINDICATIONS

> If the patient presents after 120 days postnatally, a liver transplant should be considered instead.

ANATOMY

Gross anatomy

> The liver is found in the right hypochondrium and has four anatomical lobes:
>   1 Left.
>   2 Right.
>   3 Caudate.
>   4 Quadrate.
> The liver can also be divided into two functional lobes (left and right), with each lobe having its own hepatic portal vein and hepatic artery.
> Anatomically, the divide between the left and right functional lobes is from the fundus of the gallbladder to the inferior vena cava (IVC).
> The gallbladder sits in a fossa on the underside of the right lobe of the liver, near the quadrate lobe.
> The gallbladder is divided into fundus, body, and neck, which follow into a narrow infundibulum and the cystic duct.
> Bile produced in the liver drains through the left and right hepatic ducts into the common hepatic duct. The cystic duct joins the common hepatic duct to form the common bile duct.
> The common bile duct is joined by the pancreatic duct to form the ampulla of Vater, which drains into the second part of the duodenum through the sphincter of Oddi.
> In biliary atresia, the extrahepatic ducts are obliterated, and this is classified by the level of obstruction:

> Type 1 (5%)—common bile duct.
> Type 2 (3%)—common hepatic duct.
> Type 3 (>90%)—porta hepatitis with no visible bile containing lumen.

Neurovasculature

> The gallbladder and liver are both innervated by the coeliac plexus (sympathetic) and the vagus nerve (parasympathetic). The right phrenic nerve innervates the peritoneum of the gallbladder and liver, providing sensory information.
> Blood drains from the liver via the right, left, and intermediate (middle) hepatic veins into the IVC.
> The hepatic portal vein is formed from the superior mesenteric vein and the splenic vein. It carries nutrients absorbed from the intestines. The hepatic artery proper originates from the coeliac trunk. Both these vessels form the portal triad with the bile duct and enter the liver at the porta hepatis.
> The superficial and deep branches of the cystic artery supply the gallbladder. They originate from the right hepatic artery. Multiple cystic veins drain the neck and cystic duct. These enter the liver directly or drain through the hepatic portal vein to the liver.
> The veins from the fundus and the body drain directly into the hepatic sinusoids.

Figure 12.9 The biliary tree

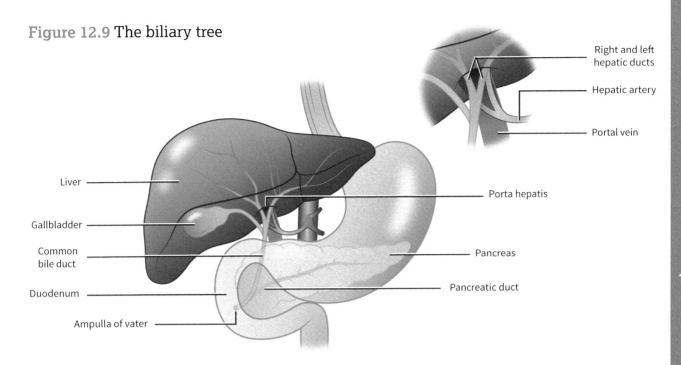

Right and left hepatic ducts

Hepatic artery

Portal vein

Liver

Gallbladder

Common bile duct

Duodenum

Ampulla of vater

Porta hepatis

Pancreas

Pancreatic duct

STEP-BY-STEP OPERATION

Anaesthesia: general.

Position: supine.

Considerations: A urinary catheter and a nasogastric (NG) tube are inserted. Prophylactic antibiotics are administered at induction.

1 A short subcostal incision is made in the hepatic area to facilitate an operative cholangiogram. A small catheter is secured in the gallbladder and contrast instilled to delineate the biliary tree (biliary atresia is confirmed when the cholangiogram shows no passage of radiographic contrast media into the liver).

2 After confirming biliary atresia, the initial incision is extended to a full subcostal incision.

3 The falciform and coronary ligaments of the liver are divided to allow the liver to be brought out of the body and rotated so regions of fibrotic biliary tree can be dissected under direct vision whilst avoiding the vascular structures.

4 The fibrous bile duct is dissected, starting from the junction of the cystic duct.

5 The gallbladder is mobilised and removed.

6 Dissection then proceeds upwards until the porta hepatis is reached with excision of any biliary remnants (care should be taken to ligate the small communicating branches of the portal vein if necessary).

7 Next, the jejunal Roux-en-Y loop is constructed, the jejunum is divided, and the distal end is brought up behind the transverse colon and anastomosed directly to the region of the porta hepatis, encompassing the bile ducts. The vascular structures at the porta hepatis must not be incorporated within this anastomosis.

8 The proximal end of the divided jejunum is anastomosed (end on side) to the roux-en-Y-loop of the jejunum.

9 The liver is replaced into the abdominal cavity; a drain may be placed.

10 The subcostal incision is closed in layers with absorbable sutures.

PAEDIATRICS

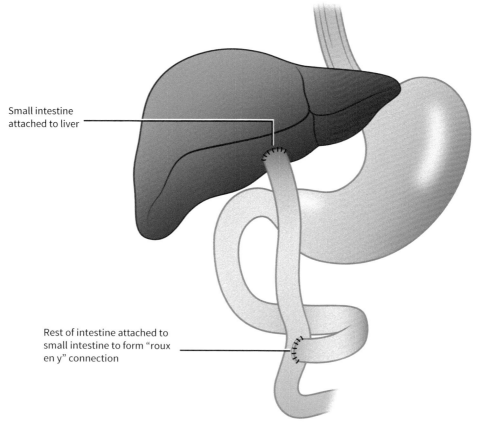

Small intestine attached to liver

Rest of intestine attached to small intestine to form "roux en y" connection

Figure 12.10 Anastomosis between the porta hepatis and the jejunum

COMPLICATIONS

Early
> Failure to resolve/restore biliary drainage (10–20%).

Intermediate and late
> Cholangitis (40–50%).
> Portal hypertension and oesophageal varices.

POSTOPERATIVE CARE

Inpatient
> Monitoring of liver function.
> IV antibiotics are given to reduce the early risk of postoperative cholangitis. Oral antibiotic prophylaxis continues for 3 to 6 months.

Outpatient
> Long-term oral ursodeoxycholic acid is given for its choleretic effect and to relieve symptoms of cholestasis, such as pruritus.
> Fat-soluble vitamin (A, D, E, and K) supplements should be continued until normal bilirubin has been achieved.
> Many of these patients will ultimately require a liver transplant at some point in their lives.

SURGEON'S FAVOURITE QUESTION

What is the most important initial investigation in a baby with prolonged jaundiced?

Split bilirubin, looking at the conjugated fraction of bilirubin.

ORCHIDOPEXY

Jane Lim

DEFINITION

Repositioning of the testis into the scrotum.

✓ INDICATIONS

- Testicular torsion with a viable testicle (bilateral fixation is required).
- To reduce the risk of infertility and malignancy in:
  - Congenital cryptorchidism—when the testicle has not descended into the scrotum by 6 months of age. Orchidopexy should be performed before the patient turns 1 year old.
  - Acquired cryptorchidism—orchidopexy is performed within 6 months of testicular ascent.

✗ CONTRAINDICATIONS

- If the testis is impalpable, a two staged procedure may be required.

ANATOMY

Embryology

- The gonadal structures form in the urogenital ridge on the posterior abdominal wall at around seven weeks *in utero*.
- The gonads descend from the abdominal cavity through the inguinal canal into the scrotum, guided by a fibrous structure called the gubernaculum.

Gross anatomy

- The muscle and fascial layers of the anterior abdominal wall give rise to the layers of the spermatic cord.
- The spermatic cord contains the vas deferens, testicular and deferential arteries, a venous network known as the pampiniform plexus, testicular nerves, lymphatic vessels, and the tunica vaginalis.
- The layers of the scrotum, from skin to testes, are the skin, dartos fascia and muscle, external spermatic fascia (external oblique muscle), cremasteric muscle and fascia (internal oblique muscle), internal spermatic fascia (transversalis fascia), and parietal layer of the tunica vaginalis.

Neurovasculature

- The testis and the spermatic cord are innervated by sympathetic fibres from the thoracic spinal cord segments T1–12.
- The scrotum is mainly innervated by the posterior scrotal nerves (branches of the perineal nerve, arising from the pudendal nerve).
- The spermatic cord and testis derive their blood supply mainly from the testicular artery, which arises from the abdominal aorta. There is also collateral blood supply from the deferential artery and the cremasteric artery (internal and external iliac artery).
- The scrotum gets its blood supply from the anterior and posterior scrotal arteries.
- Venous drainage of the testis and spermatic cord is via the pampiniform plexus into the testicular vein. The left testicular vein drains into the renal vein and the right testicular vein into the inferior vena cava.
- Blood is drained from the scrotum into the pudendal veins.
- The lymphatic vessels of the testis and spermatic cord drain into the para-aortic lymph nodes, while that of the scrotum drains into the superficial inguinal lymph nodes.

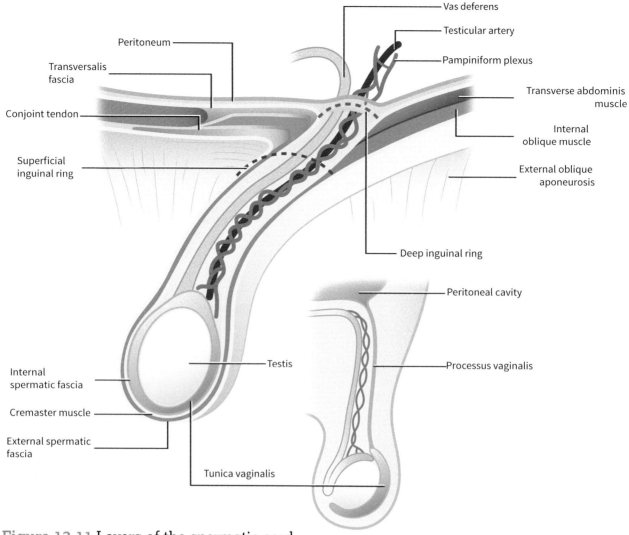

Figure 12.11 Layers of the spermatic cord

STEP-BY-STEP OPERATION

Anaesthesia: general with a caudal block.
Position: supine.

1 A transverse skin incision is made along the Langer's lines over the mid inguinal point.

2 The incision is deepened through the subcutaneous tissue to Scarpa's fascia. The superior inferior epigastric vein is identified and protected.

3 The external oblique aponeurosis is cleared, the reflection of the inguinal ligament and the external inguinal ring is identified, and an incision is made in the external oblique muscle and extended towards the external inguinal ring. The ilioinguinal nerve is protected.

4 The spermatic cord superior to the testis is mobilised and delivered out of the wound. The gubernaculum is then detached.

5 The spermatic cord is stripped of remaining cremasteric fibres.

6 To gain maximal length, the patent processus vaginalis or hernial sac is separated from the cord structures; care is taken to avoid injury to the vas deferens and vessels.

7 The hernial sac is divided and dissected from the cord structures to the level of the internal ring. It is twisted to the point of the internal ring, then transfixed and ligated.

8 A finger is passed from the incision into the scrotum, and a second horizontal incision is made over the fingertip in the ipsilateral scrotal skin. A subdartos pouch is developed just under the scrotal skin.

9 A pair of fine artery forceps are passed through the scrotal incision and guided into the inguinal incision as the fingertip is retracted.

10 The testis is brought through the opening of the fascia, ensuring the spermatic cord does not twist in the process. The testis is placed in the pouch and is fixed to the scrotum.

11 The scrotal skin is closed with absorbable sutures. The incisions, namely the external oblique aponeurosis to the external ring, Scarpa's fascia, and the skin incision, are closed in layers.

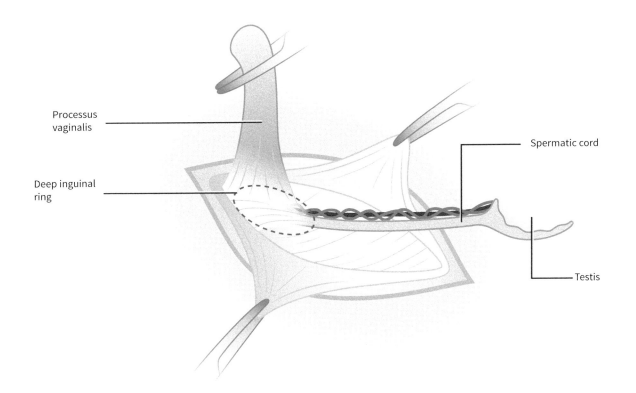

Figure 12.12 Separation of the processus vaginalis from the spermatic cord

COMPLICATIONS

Early
▸ Scrotal haematoma.
▸ Injury to vas deferens (1–2%).

Intermediate and late
▸ Wound infection.

▸ Testicular atrophy (<5%).
▸ Retraction of testis is dependent on testicular position—i.e., external ring, inguinal canal, or intra-abdominal (8–16%).

POSTOPERATIVE CARE

Inpatient

› Commonly performed as a day-case procedure.

Outpatient

› Vigorous or strenuous activities and straddle-type toys (e.g., bicycle) should be avoided for 2 weeks postoperatively.

› Clinic follow-up at 6 months to check for testicular atrophy or retraction.

⦿ SURGEON'S FAVOURITE QUESTION

If the testis cannot reach the scrotum, what other techniques can be employed to gain extra length?

The retroperitoneal plane above the internal ring can be developed by pulling the peritoneal membrane anteriorly using a retractor. If the vas deferens is a limiting factor, the inferior epigastric vessels can be divided to gain up to 1 cm in length.

13 OBSTETRICS AND GYNAECOLOGY

JENNIFER ROBERTSON, KATRINA MASON

HYSTERECTOMY

Jenny Robertson

DEFINITION

Removal of the uterus either laparoscopically, via a laparotomy ("open"), or transvaginally. A hysterectomy can be:

> Total—removal of the uterus and the cervix.

> Subtotal—removal of the uterus but the cervix is preserved.

> Radical—removal of the cervix, upper third of the vagina, and the parametrium, including lymph nodes.

✓ INDICATIONS

General

> Malignancy.
> Dysfunctional uterine bleeding.
> Endometriosis.
> Fibroids.
> Pelvic organ prolapse.
> Pelvic infection or pain.
> Final life-saving option in massive post-partum haemorrhage.

✗ CONTRAINDICATIONS

Relative

> Large uterus—an open abdominal approach may be preferred.
> A vaginal approach may be preferred in patients with multiple previous abdominal operations.

Absolute

> Advanced uterine/cervical/ovarian malignancy.

ANATOMY

Gross anatomy

> The uterus lies within the pelvis and is divided into:
> › Fundus—most commonly orientated anteriorly.
> › Cornua.
> › Corpus.
> › Cervix.
> The uterus is held within the broad ligament, which is continuous between the sides of the pelvis in the form of two leaves (anterior and posterior).
> The ovaries arise from the posterior surface of the broad ligament and are attached to the cornua of the uterus by the ovarian ligaments, and to the side pelvic walls by the infundibulo-pelvic ligament (IP)/suspensory ligament. The suspensory ligament contains the ovarian blood vessels and nerves.
> The round ligaments travel anteriorly from the cornua to the inguinal canals.
> The uterosacral ligaments travel from the cervix to the second part of the sacrum.
> The cardinal ligaments travel from the cervix and upper vagina to the root of the internal iliac vessels and contain the nerves, arteries, and veins that travel from the pelvic sidewall to the genital tract.
> The uterus is connected through the cervix to the vagina, which lies immediately posterior to the urethra and bladder and anterior to the anal canal and rectum.

Neurovasculature

> Parasympathetic fibres of the uterus are derived from the pelvic splanchnic nerves (S2, 3, 4). Sympathetic fibres arise from the uterovaginal plexus, a division of the inferior hypogastric plexus. Afferent sensory fibres ascend through the inferior hypogastric plexus and enter the spinal cord at T10, 11 ,12, and L1. Epidural analgesia therefore provides sensory block to these fibres.
> The main blood supply to the uterus is via the uterine arteries, which travel medially in the base of the broad ligament before ascending along the lateral aspect of the uterus and anastomosing with the ovarian arteries.

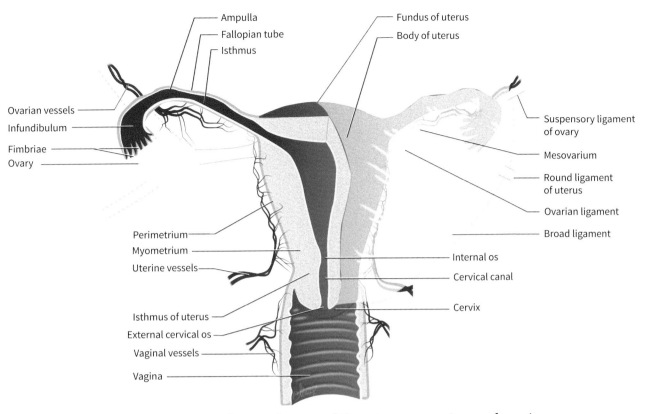

Figure 13.1 Gross anatomy and vasculature of the uterus, ovaries and vagina

STEP-BY-STEP OPERATION

Anaesthesia: general or regional (epidural or spinal).

Position: Trendelenburg for open and laparoscopic (described here) or lithotomy for transvaginal.

1 The cervix is dilated, and a uterine manipulator is inserted into the uterus.

2 Three to four laparoscopic trocars are positioned, and pneumoperitoneum is achieved via the Hasson technique:
   a Umbilical x1.
   b Supra-pubic (optional) x1.
   c Medial to the anterior superior iliac spines x2.

3 The uterus is mobilised to expose the round ligaments, which are then cut using bipolar diathermy.

4 Scissors are used to dissect the broad ligament's anterior leaf from the posterior leaf.

5 In ovarian conservation, the fallopian tube and utero-ovarian ligament are cut. However, in cases of salpingo-oophorectomy (removal of the fallopian tubes and ovaries), the infundibulopelvic ligament is cut.

6 The ureters are displaced laterally and posteriorly (where they are less susceptible to accidental iatrogenic injury). The vesico-peritoneum is cut and elevated from the anterior uterine segment, and then the posterior leaf of the broad ligament is opened up to the uterosacral ligaments.

7 The vaginal mucosa is then cut near to the cervix and through the anterior section. Dissection is made caudally until the peritoneal cavity can be entered through the previous opening made in the vesico-peritoneum. The posterior vaginal mucosa is then incised just above the uterosacral ligaments to free the vagina.

8 The uterine arteries are clamped and ligated, and the uterus (+/- ovaries and fallopian tubes) is removed through the vagina.

9 Drains are inserted into the pelvis and exiting through the abdomen, the edges of the vaginal cuff are sutured and the vagina is returned to the pelvis. The uterosacral ligaments are plicated to ensure suspension of the vaginal cuff and to prevent prolapse.

10 The abdomen is deflated, and port sites are closed with sutures.

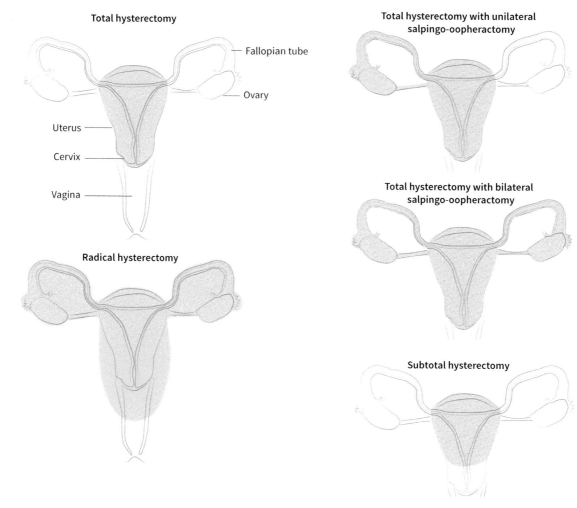

Figure 13.2 Subtypes of hysterectomy

COMPLICATIONS

Early

> Bleeding.
> Injury—ureter, bladder, and bowel.
> Ileus.
> Urinary retention.

Intermediate and late

> Infection—wound, vagina, urinary tract, intra-abdominal.
> Vaginal cuff dehiscence.
> Abdominal adhesions—may cause bowel obstruction.
> Vaginal prolapse.

POSTOPERATIVE CARE

Inpatient

> Patients can be discharged once mobile, passing urine after catheter removal, and drains have been removed.

> Most patients are discharged home within 48 hours following surgery as long as no complications occur.

Outpatient

> Consultant outpatient appointment 2 weeks postoperatively.

> Patients are advised to avoid heavy lifting.

> Vaginal intercourse is discouraged for 6 weeks post-surgery to facilitate healing and prevent infection.

💬 SURGEON'S FAVOURITE QUESTION

When would you choose open versus laparoscopic versus transvaginal hysterectomy?

Open hysterectomy:

> Multiple previous abdominal operations.

> Large uterus.

> Extensive disease.

Laparoscopic hysterectomy:

> Uterine size smaller than the equivalent of a 12-week pregnancy.

> Anatomical barriers to transvaginal—narrow subpubic arch or a long and narrow vagina.

> Obesity—easier to visualise the pelvis.

Transvaginal hysterectomy:

> Obesity—enhanced recovery compared to abdominal wound.

> General anaesthesia contraindicated, as can be performed under regional (spinal) anaesthesia.

> Vaginal prolapse.

TENSION-FREE VAGINAL TAPE (TVT)

Jenny Robertson

DEFINITION

The placement of a sling/tape beneath the urethra to provide support to the neck of the urethra in order to treat stress urinary incontinence (SUI).

✓ INDICATIONS

SUI, the involuntary leakage of urine when pressure is applied to the bladder (e.g., on sneezing or coughing, effort, or exertion) that affects quality of life and is unresponsive to conservative measures.

✗ CONTRAINDICATIONS

> Pure urge incontinence with no element of SUI present (can be worsened by TVT).

> Previous hernia surgery in the groin (when using the retro-pubic approach).
> Vulval, vaginal, or cervical malignancy.
> Previous radiotherapy to the vulval, vaginal, or cervical tissue.
> Current pregnancy (plans for future pregnancy is a relative contraindication)

ANATOMY

> The urethra and bladder lie posterior to the pubic symphysis and the space of Retzius (extraperitoneal space between the pubic symphysis and bladder) and anterior to the vagina.
> The female urethra is approximately 4 cm long and is embedded in the anterior vaginal wall immediately posterior to the pubic rami.
> The internal urethral sphincter (IUS) lies at the inferior end of the bladder and the proximal end of the urethra. It contains smooth muscle fibres in a horseshoe arrangement and is continuous with the detrusor muscle of the bladder. The IUS is controlled involuntarily though the autonomic nervous system.
> The external urethral sphincter (EUS) surrounds the urethra, is made up of striated muscle, and is under voluntary control. It includes three parts: the annular

sphincter around the urethra (urethral sphincter), a part encircling both the vagina and the urethra (urethrovaginal sphincter), and a muscle attaching to the ischial rami and passing anterior to the urethra (compressor urethral muscle). It is innervated by the pudendal nerve (S2, 3, 4).
> At the bladder neck, the urethra is surrounded by multiple elastic fibres that also help to maintain urethral closure.
> The urethra passes through the levator ani muscles, which insert into the perineal body.
> The action of this group of muscles is to elevate the urethrovesical junction and to create an angle between the fixed lower portion and the flexible upper portion of the urethra. This also helps maintain urinary continence.

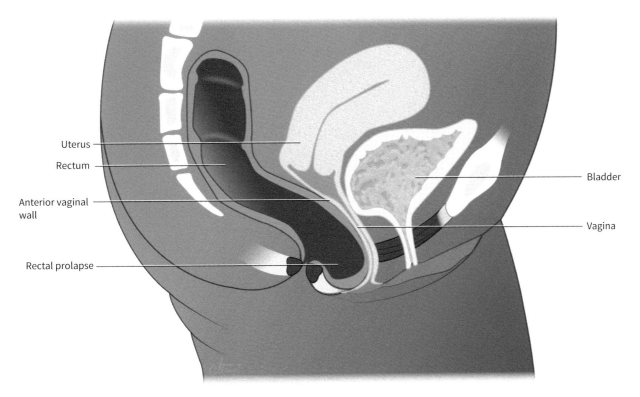

Uterus

Rectum

Anterior vaginal wall

Rectal prolapse

Bladder

Vagina

Figure 13.3 Cross sectional anatomy of the female pelvis

STEP-BY-STEP OPERATION

Anaesthesia: general, regional (epidural or spinal), or local.
Position: lithotomy.

1 The bladder is examined cystoscopically to ensure that there is no pathology within the bladder or within its walls, and a Foley catheter is then inserted into the bladder via the urethra.

2 Two exit sites are marked 2 cm immediately above and lateral to the pubic symphysis and at the level of the urethra. Local anaesthetic is injected submucosally.

3 At the two implant exit sites, a local anaesthetic solution mixed with adrenaline or plain saline is used to hydrodissect the bladder walls and the urethra off the surrounding tissue and organs. It is applied:
  i Just above the pubic tubercle on both sides of the midline.
  ii To the anterior vaginal wall.

4 A sagittal incision is made at the urethral meatus, and dissection is performed paraurethrally towards the endopelvic fascia to dissect the urethra free of the anterior vaginal wall.

5 The bladder is drained, and a rigid catheter guide is inserted into the Foley catheter. The handle is pivoted to the left of the surgeon to expose the left endopelvic fascia.

6 The trochar is padded through the right paraurethral dissection. The right endopelvic fascia is punctured, and the trochar is then advanced through the space of Retzius and the anterior abdominal wall towards the right exit site. At the surface, the skin is incised to allow the needle to emerge.

7 The Foley catheter is removed, and a cystoscopy is performed to ensure bladder integrity. The Foley catheter is reinserted, along with the rigid catheter guide.

8 The procedure is repeated on the contralateral side, ensuring the sling/ tape does not twist during insertion. The tape now forms a 'U' shape around the urethra. A further check via cystoscopy is performed.

9 The tape should be tension free. This is tested by filling the bladder with 250 ml of saline and applying pressure to the anterior abdominal wall. The sling/tape is pulled upwards gently on both sides until only a few drops leak out when pressure is applied.

10 The abdominal ends of the tape are cut, and the wounds are sutured. The vaginal wall is inspected, and the vaginal incision is sutured. If there has been significant bleeding, a vaginal gauze pack may be left in situ for 24 hours.

407

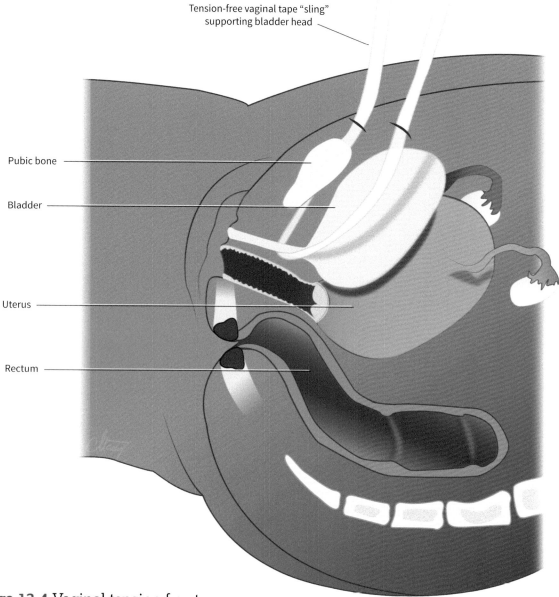

Tension-free vaginal tape "sling" supporting bladder head

Pubic bone

Bladder

Uterus

Rectum

Figure 13.4 Vaginal tension free tape

COMPLICATIONS

Early
> Bleeding.
> Urinary retention.
> Bladder perforation.

Intermediate and late
> Infection.
> De novo or worsening urge incontinence.
> Voiding dysfunction.

POSTOPERATIVE CARE

Inpatient

‣ To have a trial without catheterisation (TWOC) and, if passing urine, can be discharged home.

Outpatient

‣ Outpatient appointment in 3 months to evaluate success of operation and check for wound healing and complications.

 SURGEON'S FAVOURITE QUESTION

What causes stress urinary incontinence?

Stress urinary incontinence results from weakening of the pelvic floor muscles or displacement of the bladder neck. This can be caused by pregnancy (even if birth is by caesarean section), vaginal delivery (operative and spontaneous), and menopause (lack of oestrogen atrophies the pelvic floor muscles). In all cases, there is damage to the pelvic floor and ligament support of the bladder neck and urethra, thus resulting in leakage when pressure is applied.

HYSTEROSCOPY

Jenny Robertson and Katrina Mason

DEFINITION

The diagnostic insertion of a camera (hysteroscope) through the cervix into the uterus. Can be combined with several therapeutic procedures (see below).

✓ INDICATIONS

- Diagnosis and management of abnormal uterine bleeding (AUB):
  - Endometrial biopsy for diagnosis of malignancy.
  - Polypectomy for uterine polyps.
  - Myomectomy for uterine fibroids.
  - Endometrial ablation therapy.
- To rule out, diagnose, and treat causes of subfertility:
  - Division of intrauterine adhesions.
  - Division of uterine septum.
  - Polypectomy.

- Removal of intrauterine devices (IUD) if conservative attempts (e.g., ultrasound-guided removal) have failed.
- Removal of retained products of conception.
- Tubal sterilisation.

✗ CONTRAINDICATIONS

- Active cervical or uterine infection.
- Known cervical or uterine cancer.
- Viable intrauterine pregnancy.

ANATOMY

Gross anatomy

- The uterus lies within the pelvis and is divided into:
  - Fundus—most commonly orientated anteriorly.
  - Cornua.
  - Corpus.
  - Cervix.
- The uterus is held within the broad ligament, which is continuous between the uterus and the sides of the pelvis in the form of two leaves (anterior and posterior).
- The ovaries arise from the posterior surface of this ligament and are attached to the cornua of the uterus by the ovarian ligaments and to the side pelvic walls by the infundibulo-pelvic ligament (IP)/suspensory ligament. The suspensory ligament contains the ovarian blood vessels and nerves.
- The round ligaments travel anteriorly from the cornua to the inguinal canals.
- The uterosacral ligaments travel from the cervix to the second part of the sacrum.
- The cardinal ligaments travel from the cervix and upper vagina to the root of the internal iliac vessels and contain the nerves, arteries, and veins that travel from the pelvic sidewall to the genital tract.

- The uterus is connected through the cervix to the vagina, which lies immediately posterior to the urethra and bladder and anterior to the anal canal and rectum.

Neurovasculature

- The parasympathetic and sympathetic nerves supplying the vagina are derived from the uterovaginal nerve plexus. The pudendal nerve (S2, 3, 4) has both motor and sensory functions; branches of the pudendal nerve supply sensation to the labia, clitoris, and anal canal as well as innervating the muscles of the pelvic floor, the external anal sphincter, and the external urethral sphincter.
- The main blood supply to the uterus is via the uterine arteries, which travel medially in the base of the broad ligament before ascending along the lateral aspect of the uterus and anastomosing with the ovarian arteries.

Histology

- The endometrium has varying thickness throughout:
  - Anterior and posterior walls 15–25 mm (anterior wall often slightly thicker).
  - Fundus 15–22 mm.
  - Isthmus 8–12 mm.
  - Corpus 4–7 mm.

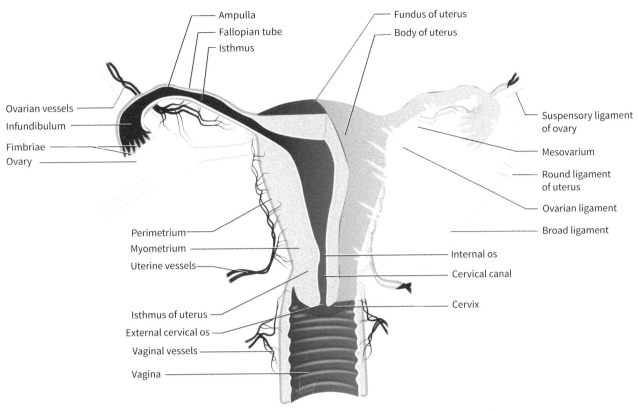

Figure 13.5 Gross anatomy and vasculature of the uterus, ovaries and vagina

STEP-BY-STEP OPERATION

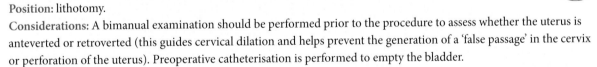

Anaesthesia: general, regional (epidural or spinal), or local.

Position: lithotomy.

Considerations: A bimanual examination should be performed prior to the procedure to assess whether the uterus is anteverted or retroverted (this guides cervical dilation and helps prevent the generation of a 'false passage' in the cervix or perforation of the uterus). Preoperative catheterisation is performed to empty the bladder.

1. A speculum is inserted, and the cervix is visualised.
2. Under direct visualisation, the cervix is grasped with a tenaculum at the 12 o'clock position.
3. The cervical canal is then progressively dilated with straight Hegar dilators to allow the hysteroscope to pass. Dilation depends on the choice of hysteroscope (e.g., 4 mm for a small diagnostic mini-hysteroscope, or 8+ mm for a therapeutic procedure using a resectoscope).
4. The hysteroscope is inserted, and dilation fluid (usually isotonic sodium chloride, but a hypotonic, non-electrolyte non-conductive media such as glycine is used if electrocautery is to be performed) is flushed into the uterus, causing distension and allowing visualisation of the structures. A careful record of the amount of dilation fluid used must be recorded to ensure against excessive fluid absorption.
5. Diagnostic or therapeutic procedures are then performed accordingly.
6. Pre-, intra-, and postoperative photographs are recorded.
7. The instruments and hysteroscope are carefully removed under direct vision.
8. If there has been significant bleeding, a vaginal gauze pack may be left in situ for 24 hours.

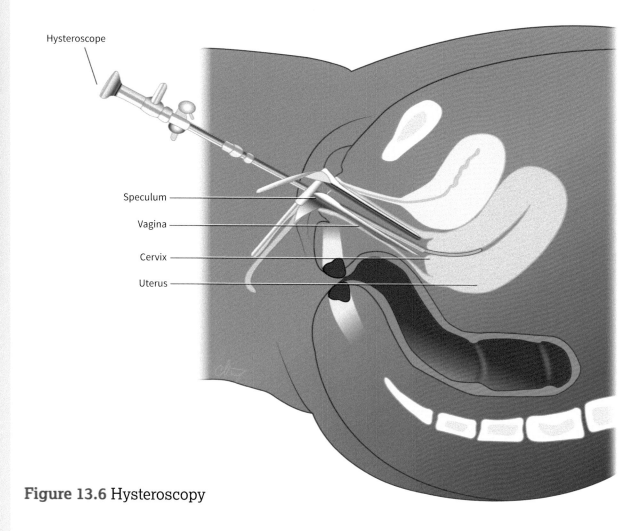

Hysteroscope

Speculum

Vagina

Cervix

Uterus

Figure 13.6 Hysteroscopy

COMPLICATIONS

Early

> Uterine trauma—perforation (increased risk if peri-pregnancy).
> Cervical trauma.
> Urinary tract or bowel injury.
> If excessive hypotonic infiltration media is absorbed, this can lead to hyponatraemia, hypervolemia, hypotension, pulmonary oedema, cerebral oedema, and cardiovascular collapse.
> Bleeding.
> Air embolus.

Intermediate and late

> Infection.
> Uterine adhesions (Asherman's syndrome), leading to an increased subsequent risk of ectopic pregnancy, miscarriage, or abnormal placentation.

POSTOPERATIVE CARE

Inpatient

> This is usually a day-case procedure; patients can be discharged home once recovered from the general anaesthetic (if used).

Outpatient

> Outpatient follow-up at 2–6 weeks, depending on indications of procedure and operative findings.

 SURGEON'S FAVOURITE QUESTION

What key symptoms should prompt a patient to seek medical review following hysteroscopy?

Heavy or prolonged bleeding, severe abdominal pain, fever, or foul-smelling vaginal discharge.

CAESAREAN SECTION

Jenny Robertson and Katrina Mason

DEFINITION

› Delivery of the foetus through an incision in the lower abdomen and uterus.

✓ INDICATIONS

› Caesarean sections can be performed for either maternal or foetal indications and may be planned elective or emergency procedures.

Elective

› category 4 section (performed at a time to suit the woman and maternity services):
  › Malpresentation (e.g., breech).
  › Multiple pregnancy.
  › Abnormality of placenta (placenta previa, vasa previa, placenta accreta).
  › Previous caesarean section.
  › Maternal infection (HSV, HIV).
  › Foetal bleeding tendency (haemophilia).
  › Macrosomia (large baby unlikely to be safely delivered vaginally).
  › Mechanical obstruction to vaginal birth (e.g., large fibroid).
  › Maternal choice.

Emergency

› Category 3 section—needing early delivery but no maternal or foetal compromise (e.g., failure to progress during labour).
› Category 2 section—maternal or foetal compromise that is not immediately life-threatening.
› Category 1 section (aim for delivery within 30 minutes)—immediate threat to life of woman or foetus (e.g., umbilical cord prolapse, eclampsia, foetal bradycardia).

✗ CONTRAINDICATIONS

› Gestation under 39 weeks—a relative contraindication (as the foetal lungs may not be mature), but caesarean sections are commonly performed earlier than this in emergencies.

ANATOMY

Gross anatomy

› Layers of the abdominal wall:
  › Skin.
  › Subcutaneous tissue.
  › Rectus abdominus muscles—contained within the rectus sheath.
  › Parietal peritoneum.
› The uterus is usually located within the pelvis immediately posterior to the bladder and anterior to the rectum.
› The full-term gravid uterus extends up to the xiphisternum and is the most anterior organ in the abdomen.
› Layers of the uterine wall:
  › Peritoneum—outermost.
  › Myometrium—consists of three layers of smooth muscle.
  › Endometrium—the inner lining of the uterus into which the placenta implants.
› The cervix, which communicates with the upper vagina, is composed of dense collagenous tissue that retains the foetus in utero.

Neurovasculature

› Parasympathetic fibres of the uterus are derived from the pelvic splanchnic nerves (S2, 3, 4). Sympathetic fibres arise from the uterovaginal plexus, a division of the inferior hypogastric plexus. Afferent sensory fibres ascend through the inferior hypogastric plexus and enter the spinal cord at T10, 11, 12, and L1. Epidural analgesia therefore provides sensory block to these fibres.
› The main blood supply to the uterus is via the uterine arteries, which travel medially in the base of the broad ligament before ascending along the lateral aspect of the uterus and anastomosing with the ovarian arteries.

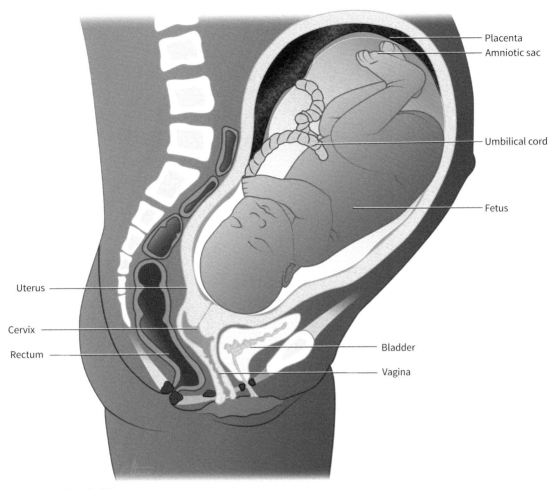

Placenta
Amniotic sac
Umbilical cord
Fetus
Uterus
Cervix
Rectum
Bladder
Vagina

Figure 13.7 The full term gravid uterus

STEP-BY-STEP OPERATION

Anaesthesia: regional or general.

Position: supine with left tilt to reduce aorto-caval compression.

Considerations: Prior to surgery, a urinary catheter is inserted to drain the bladder.

1 A 10–15-cm-long transverse 'Pfannenstiel' or 'Joel-Cohen' incision is made 2–3 cm above the pubic symphysis, and subcutaneous fat is dissected using sharp or blunt dissection with bipolar diathermy for haemostasis.

2 The rectus sheath is incised bilaterally for the full length of the incision. The sheath is then separated from the underlying rectus muscles by sharp and blunt dissection.

3 The rectus muscles are then separated in the midline, exposing the peritoneum.

4 Once intra-abdominal, the loose peritoneum over the lower segment is opened and the bladder is pushed down and protected with a Doyen's retractor.

5 Using a scalpel, a small transverse incision is made along the lower uterine segment of the uterus until the uterine cavity is entered or membranes are seen.

6 The baby should be delivered with minimal delay by applying firm fundal pressure (only if cephalic lie). Once delivered, the cord is clamped in two places and divided. The baby can then be passed to the midwife or paediatric team.

7 Syntocinon is then administered to enhance uterine contractions and expulsion of the placenta (unless contraindicated) while gentle traction is applied to the cord.

8 Once the placenta is delivered, the uterus should be explored and cleaned to ensure that there is no

retained placental tissue. The fallopian tubes and ovaries are inspected for any undiagnosed pathology, and the bladder is carefully inspected for any damage. The para-colic gutters are cleared of clots.

9 Clamps are placed at the angles of the uterine incision, then the uterus is closed in two layers of running

and/or interlocking dissolving sutures, ensuring haemostasis.

10 The rectus sheath is closed with a running suture, then the skin is closed with subcutaneous non-absorbable sutures or staples.

Figure 13.8 Exposure and incision of the uterus during a Caesarean Section

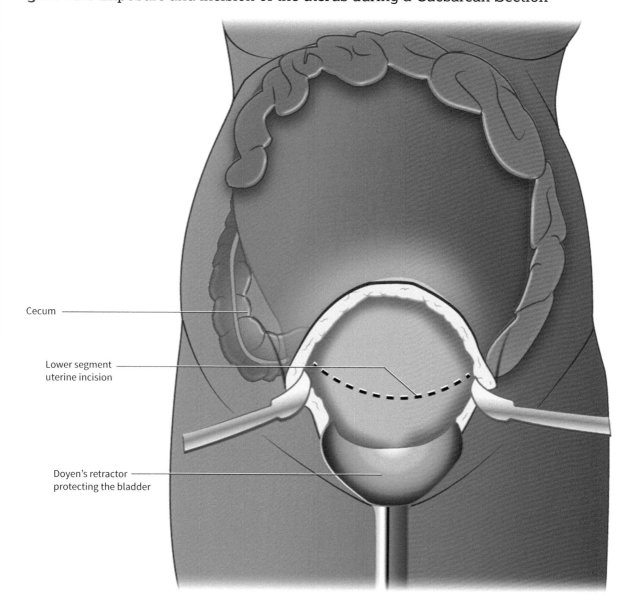

Cecum

Lower segment uterine incision

Doyen's retractor protecting the bladder

COMPLICATIONS

Early

> Haemorrhage.
> Uterine atony.
> Injury to local structures—bladder, ureter, and gastrointestinal tract (<1%).
> Ileus.
> Venous thromboembolism (1%).
> Foetal injury—cut to skin.

Intermediate and late

> Infection—endometritis, septic pelvic thrombophlebitis, and wound infection (2–20%—increased if chorioamnionitis at time of section).
> Abnormal placentation in future pregnancies—placenta previa and placenta accrete.
> Scar complications—ectopic pregnancy, incisional endometriosis, numbness, pain, and uterine rupture in subsequent pregnancy (<1%).
> Abdominal adhesions.

POSTOPERATIVE CARE

Inpatient

> Catheter removed once mobile.
> Home when pain is well controlled and vaginal bleeding is minimal.
> Patients are commonly discharged 2–4 days postoperatively.

Outpatient

> The community midwife should assess the wound at 1 week—the non-absorbable suture can be removed at this visit.
> Breastfeeding should be established and checked on by the community midwife.
> Women should be reviewed at 6 weeks by their primary care physician.

SURGEON'S FAVOURITE QUESTION

Why is the uterine incision made transversely wherever possible?

A transverse incision in the lower segment of the uterus heals better than a vertical incision, ruptures less frequently, and is less dangerous to make, as the placenta is less likely to be damaged because it is normally positioned antero-superiorly.

ANTERIOR VAGINAL WALL REPAIR

Jenny Robertson and Katrina Mason

DEFINITION
The surgical repair of anterior vaginal wall prolapse.

✓ INDICATIONS

➤ Symptomatic anterior vaginal wall prolapse of the bladder (cystocele) that has failed conservative treatments such as vaginal pessary and pelvic floor exercises.

✗ CONTRAINDICATIONS

Relative

➤ Women planning future pregnancies and vaginal deliveries.

➤ Obliterative procedures, such as removing or closing in a portion of the vaginal canal, can be preferred in repair for women who cannot tolerate a more extensive surgery or are not planning future vaginal intercourse.

Absolute

➤ Asymptomatic cystocele.
➤ Vaginal carcinoma.

ANATOMY

Gross anatomy

➤ The bladder lies in the pelvis immediately anterior to the vagina.
➤ The female urethra is approximately 4 cm long and is embedded in the anterior vaginal wall. The smooth muscle layers of the urethral wall intermingle with those of the vagina and are continuous with those of the bladder above.
➤ Where the urethra meets the neck of the bladder, the urethra is surrounded by the urethral sphincters, which maintain urethral closure.
➤ The urethra passes through the pelvic diaphragm, which consists of the levator ani and coccygeus muscles (attached to the inner surface of the minor pelvis).
➤ The levator ani muscles elevate the urethrovesical junction, creating an angle between the fixed lower portion and the flexible upper portion of the urethra. This helps maintain urinary continence.
➤ Supporting the vagina:
  › Superiorly—cardinal-uterosacral ligaments.
  › Anteriorly—perineal membrane.
  › Posteriorly—the perineal body posteriorly.
  › Laterally—pelvic fascia.

Neurovascular

➤ The parasympathetic and sympathetic nerves supplying the vagina are derived from the uterovaginal nerve plexus. The pudendal nerve (S2, 3, 4) has both motor and sensory functions; branches of the pudendal nerve supply sensation to the labia, clitoris, and anal canal as well innervating the muscles of the pelvic floor, the external anal sphincter, and the external urethral sphincter.
➤ Branches of the uterine artery supply the upper vagina, the vaginal artery supplies the middle portion, and the internal pudendal artery supplies the lower portion of the vagina and vulva. All are branches of the internal iliac artery.
➤ The venous drainage of the vagina is via a plexus of veins that drain into the internal iliac veins.
➤ Lymphatic drainage is via the iliac and superficial inguinal lymph nodes.

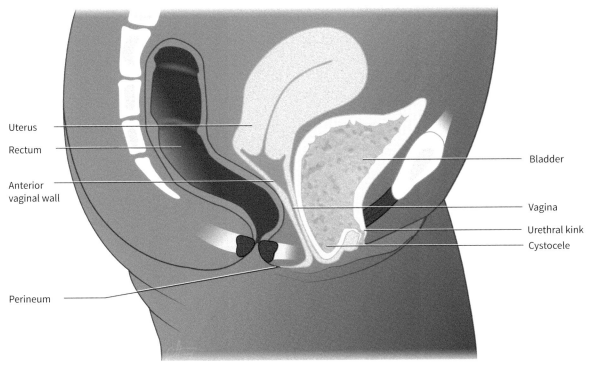

Figure 13.9 Cross sectional anatomy of the female pelvis with a cystocele

STEP-BY-STEP OPERATION

Anaesthesia: general, regional or local.

Position: dorsal lithotomy.

Considerations: Prior to surgery, a urinary catheter is inserted to drain the bladder.

1 The anterior vaginal wall and cystocele are retracted.

2 The anterior vaginal wall is then infiltrated with a mixture of local anaesthetic solution with adrenaline or simply with normal saline to help hydrodissect the bladder wall off the vaginal wall.

3 A longitudinal incision is made from just proximal to the bladder neck.

4 Using scissors, the anterior vaginal wall is then incised up to within 2 cm of the urethral meatus.

5 The edges of the vaginal mucosa are held on lateral traction. Using a mixture of blunt and sharp dissection, the bladder and urethra are moved off from the vaginal mucosa, and the pubo-cervical fascia is defined.

6 Excess vaginal mucosa is trimmed with care.

7 The left and right pubo-cervical fascia are sutured together in the midline 2 cm below the urethral meatus using an absorbable suture. This suture should continue until the entire cystocele has been reduced.

8 A second layer may need to be performed if the cystocele is unduly large and difficult to reduce with the first layer.

9 A urethral Foley catheter is inserted into the bladder for 24–28 hours.

10 A vaginal pack is placed in the vagina.

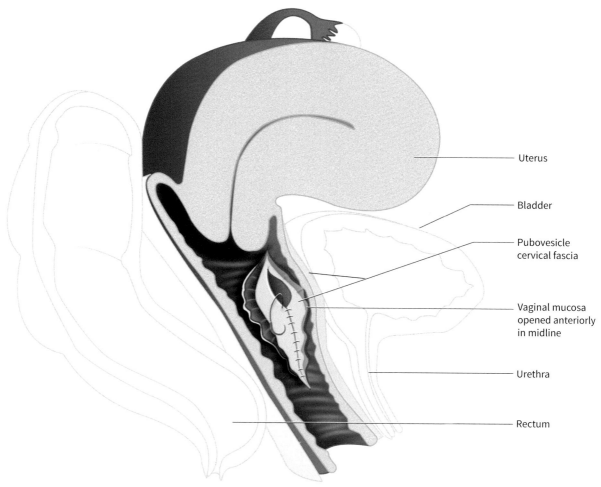

Uterus

Bladder

Pubovesicle cervical fascia

Vaginal mucosa opened anteriorly in midline

Urethra

Rectum

Figure 13.10 Suturing of the pubovesicle cervical fascia in an anterior vaginal wall repair

COMPLICATIONS

Early

- Bleeding.
- Damage to bladder, bowel, ureters, or urethra.
- Urinary retention.

Intermediate and late

- Infection—urinary tract, vagina, and pelvis.
- Urinary urgency, frequency, incontinence, or inability to completely empty bladder.
- Wound infection or dehiscence.
- Dyspareunia (painful sexual intercourse).
- Cystocele recurrence (30%).
- Urogenital fistula.

POSTOPERATIVE CARE

Inpatient

> The vaginal pack and catheter are usually removed the following day; patients should be observed for retention.

> Oestrogen pessaries or creams may be prescribed to aid mucosal healing.

Outpatient

> Follow up at 6 weeks to 3 months postoperatively; women are advised to prevent putting undue stress on the pelvic floor.

💬? SURGEON'S FAVOURITE QUESTION

How would you assess possible damage to the bladder or ureters postoperatively?

Cystourethroscopy would be performed, as this would show if the ureters are failing to perform peristalsis or eject urine from the orifices. If damage is still queried, then fluoroscopy on the table, with a radio-opaque solution, would be recommended to look at the entire renal tree. If damage to the bladder is suspected, then the bladder is filled with a methylene blue-coloured solution, and the vagina is observed. If blue is seen emanating into the vagina, then a bladder injury should be suspected.

LARGE LOOP EXCISION OF THE TRANSFORMATION ZONE (LLETZ)

Jenny Robertson and Katrina Mason

DEFINITION

Electrosurgical excision of the transformation zone of the cervix for diagnosis and treatment of cervical pathology.

✓ INDICATIONS

> Evidence (abnormal biopsy results) or suspicion (history, risk factors, and colposcopy) of high-grade dysplasia, carcinoma in situ, or glandular abnormality.
> Lesion extending into the endocervical canal.

✗ CONTRAINDICATIONS

> Pregnancy—a relative contraindication.
> Suspected adenocarcinoma of the cervix—'cold-knife' excision is preferred, as it has lower recurrence rates.

ANATOMY

Gross anatomy

> The cervix is the lower part of the uterus and is ~ 2.5 cm long and cylindrical in shape.
> The central cervical canal connects the uterine cavity (via the internal os) with the vagina (via the external os).
> The bladder is anterior to the upper cervix.

Neurovasculature

> Somatic sensation of the cervix is from the pelvic splanchnic nerves (S2–3).
> The arterial supply to the cervix is via the descending uterine artery, a branch of the internal iliac artery.
> Venous blood from the cervix drains into the uterine venous plexus.
> The anterior and lateral cervix drains into the para-aortic lymph nodes, while the posterior cervix drains into the obturator and presacral lymph nodes.

Histology

> The outer surface of the cervix is lined with exocervical mucosa, and the central canal of the cervix is lined with endocervical mucosa. Underlying both layers of mucosa is a layer of collagen and one of smooth muscle.
> The transformation zone of the cervix is the squamocolumnar junction of the cervix, where the squamous epithelium of the exocervix meets the columnar epithelium of the endocervical canal.
> In premenopausal women, the transformation zone extends from the canal over the lip of the everted cervix—these cells are most at risk of cancerous transformation.

Figure 13.11 Histology and location of the transformation zone of the cervix

External os

Cervical cleft opening

Columnar cells
Basal cells
Squamous cells

Squamous epithelium
Original squamocolumnar junction
Transformation zone
Active squamocolumnar junction
Columnar epithelium

STEP-BY-STEP OPERATION

Anaesthesia: local ± sedation.
Position: dorsal lithotomy.

1 An insulated speculum with a smoke evacuation tube is introduced into the vagina to visualise the cervix.

2 The transformation zone of the cervix is infiltrated with a mixture of a vasoconstrictor and local anaesthetic (e.g., epinephrine 1:100,000 and 1% lidocaine).

3 Acetic acid or Lugol's solution (iodine and potassium iodide in water) is applied to the cervix to allow visualisation of the lesion (the lesion turns white because of the high density of nuclei in cancerous and pre-cancerous cells if acetic acid is used, or yellow if Lugol's solution is used).

4 The loop electrode is passed around and under the transformation zone with the aim of excising all the transformation zone and suspicious lesions in one pass (the loop excisions should be to a depth of at least 5–8mm; if the lesion extends deeper than this, additional tissue may be excised with a smaller rectangular loop).

5 Additional passes may be required if the lesion or the cervix is particularly large (ideally, however, the tissue should be excised in a single quick pass, reducing thermal damage to healthy tissues).

6 The excised specimen is sent for histology.

Figure 13.12 Wide loop excision of the transformation zone of the cervix

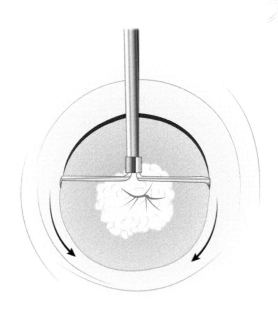
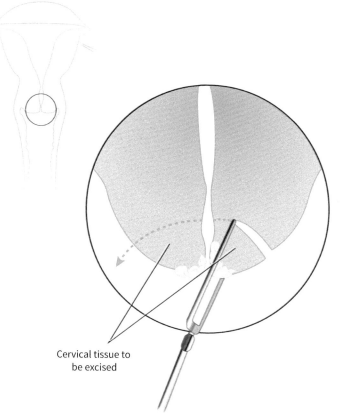

Wire loop cutting through
tissue encompassing cervical lesion

Cervical tissue to
be excised

COMPLICATIONS

Early

> Bleeding—usually easily controlled with electrocautery or Monsel's solution.

Intermediate and late

> Infection.

> Cervical stenosis.
> Cervical insufficiency—a condition in which the cervix begins to widen and dilate before a pregnancy reaches full term, predisposing to miscarriage or preterm birth.
> Recurrence of cervical dysplasia or carcinoma in situ.

POSTOPERATIVE CARE

Inpatient

> Normally a day-case procedure with minimal bleeding.
> Patients are discharged home once mobile and if no complications.

Outpatient

> Patients should avoid intercourse, bathing or swimming, and use of tampons for 2–4 weeks.

> Patients should have repeat cervical cytology at 6 months and 12 months post-procedure and be tested for Human Papillomavirus (HPV) at 12 months.
> Need for repeat colposcopy if there is a suspicion of recurrence or the biopsy result suggests the margins are not clear of abnormal changes.
> If the above tests are negative, routine screening every 12 months for the next 20 years is recommended.

SURGEON'S FAVOURITE QUESTION

What is the most common time frame for recurrence of cervical cancer?

Most recurrence occur within the first five years. A single HPV test at one year is, however, very sensitive and identifies most recurrences.

POSTERIOR VAGINAL WALL REPAIR

Jenny Robertson and Katrina Mason

DEFINITION
The surgical repair of posterior vaginal wall prolapse.

✓ INDICATIONS

- Symptomatic posterior vaginal wall prolapse of the rectum (rectocele) causing:
  - Feeling of a lump in the vagina.
  - Difficulty emptying rectum.
  - Vaginal pain +/- painful sexual intercourse.

✗ CONTRAINDICATIONS

Relative
- Women planning future pregnancies and vaginal deliveries.

Absolute
- Asymptomatic rectocele.
- Vaginal carcinoma.

ANATOMY

Gross anatomy
- The perineum is the skin located between the vaginal orifice and the anus.
- The transverse perinei and bulbocavernosus muscles intermesh at the outlet of the pelvis to form the perineal body located between the lower third of the posterior vaginal wall and the anal canal.
- The upper two-thirds of the vagina is anterior to the rectum and the pouch of Douglas (the extension of the peritoneal cavity between the rectum and posterior wall of the uterus).
- The pelvic floor spans the area beneath the pelvis. It is made up of the levator ani muscles, which pass horizontally on either side of the urethra, vagina, and rectum, and the coccygeus, which passes behind them from the ischial spine to the sacrum and coccyx.

Neurovascular
- The parasympathetic and sympathetic nerves supplying the vagina are derived from the uterovaginal nerve plexus. The pudendal nerve (S2, 3, 4) has both motor and sensory functions; branches of the pudendal nerve supply sensation to the labia, clitoris, and anal canal as well innervating the muscles of the pelvic floor, the external anal sphincter, and the external urethral sphincter.
- Branches of the uterine artery supply the upper vagina, the vaginal artery supplies the middle portion, and the internal pudendal artery supplies the lower portion of the vagina and vulva. All are branches of the internal iliac artery.
- The venous drainage of the vagina is via a plexus of veins that drain into the internal iliac veins.
- Lymphatic drainage is via the iliac and superficial inguinal lymph nodes.

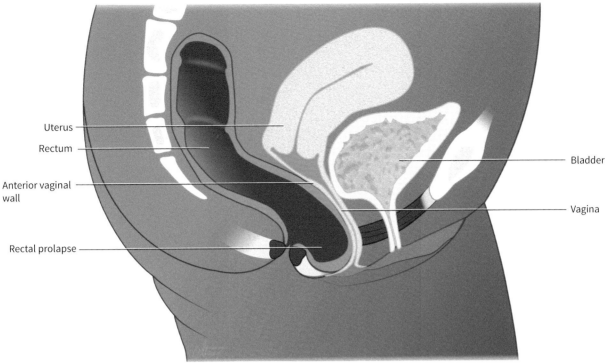

Uterus

Rectum

Anterior vaginal wall

Rectal prolapse

Bladder

Vagina

Figure 13.13 Cross sectional anatomy of the female pelvis with a posterior wall prolapse

STEP-BY-STEP OPERATION

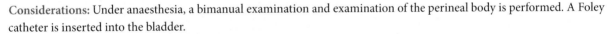

Anaesthesia: general or regional (spinal or epidural).

Position: lithotomy.

Considerations: Under anaesthesia, a bimanual examination and examination of the perineal body is performed. A Foley catheter is inserted into the bladder.

1 The posterior vaginal wall defect is exposed using vaginal wall retractors.

2 The posterior vaginal wall is then infiltrated with a mixture of local anaesthetic solution with adrenaline or simply with normal saline in order to hydrodissect the rectum off the vaginal wall.

3 The posterior vaginal mucosa is clamped at the mucocutaneous junction of the vaginal opening and at the maximum apex point of the rectocele (this may reach up to the vaginal vault).

4 A longitudinal incision is made on the posterior vaginal wall between the two clamps, and the posterior vaginal mucosa is then dissected away from the rectovaginal fascia (the dissection should continue to a point slightly above the defect and transversely as far as the sidewalls).

5 If perineoplasty, repair of the perineum is to be incorporated, a triangular section of skin overlying the perineal body is removed to expose the

aponeurosis of the superficial transverse muscle of the perineum and the bulbocavernosus muscle.

6 The exposure of the rectovaginal fascia and perineal body allows for visualisation of any defects. The edges are grasped and brought into position in the midline. Absorbable sutures are used to bring the left and right sides of the fascial defects together.

7 Depending on the location of the defect, the rectovaginal fascia may be attached to the remaining portion of the uterosacral ligaments at the top of the vagina or to the superficial transverse perinei muscle at the base.

8 Following repair of the rectovaginal fascia, the vaginal mucosa is closed over, and the perineal body should be reconstructed using two to three long-acting absorbable sutures (the sutures should be placed into the separated ends of the perineal muscle group on the left and the right and brought together in the midline).

9 The vaginal mucosa should be carefully aligned and be trimmed with caution. A suture at the top of the vaginal wall can be tied to that at the level of the hymen to pull the vagina posteriorly and into a more anatomical position. The remainder of the vagina is then sutured.

10 A vaginal exam should be performed to exclude narrowing of the orifice, and a rectal exam to ensure no sutures are palpable in the rectum. A vaginal pack is inserted at the end of the operation.

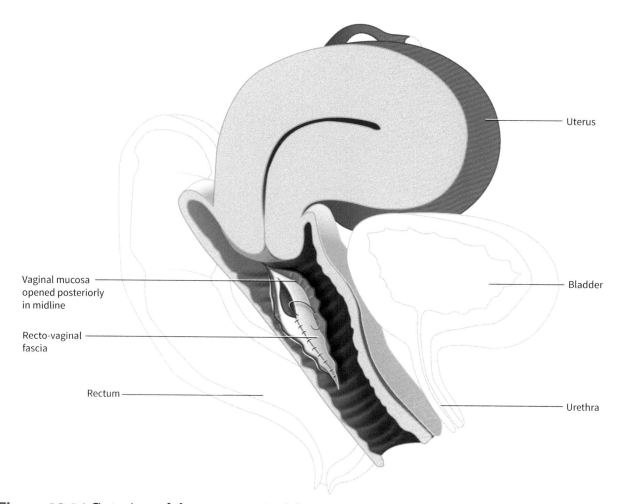

Figure 13.14 Suturing of the recto-vaginal fascia in a posterior vaginal wall repair

COMPLICATIONS

Early

> Bleeding.
> Damage to local structures—rectum and small bowel.
> Urinary retention.

Intermediate and late

> Infection—bladder, vagina, or pelvis.
> Dyspareunia (painful sexual intercourse).
> Bowel and defecatory dysfunction (e.g., faecal impaction or faecal incontinence).
> Rectovaginal or rectoperineal fistula.

POSTOPERATIVE CARE

Inpatient

> The vaginal pack and urinary catheter are usually removed the day after surgery.

Outpatient

> Follow-up at 6 weeks to 3 months after the operation; women are advised to prevent putting undue stress on the pelvic floor.

☁ SURGEON'S FAVOURITE QUESTION

What alternative surgical procedures are available for posterior vaginal wall prolapse?

In those in whom the vaginal vault is also affected, a vaginal procedure to hitch the posterior vaginal wall onto the sacro-spinous ligament (known as the sacro-spinous fixation) may be used to improve the support of the entire wall. In those in whom a prior vaginal procedure has failed, a laparoscopic/open sacro-colpopexy may be used to support the posterior vaginal wall and the vaginal vault by utilising native tissue reconstruction or applying a non-absorbable mesh and securing it onto the sacral promontory. If offering non-absorbable mesh, consent must include risks/benefits, including the permanence of the mesh, the alternatives, and mesh complications which may not be resolved if the mesh is removed.

ANGIOPLASTY +/- STENTING

Brendan S Kelly

Brendan S Kelly

INTERVENTIONAL RADIOLOGY

DEFINITION

The introduction of a balloon, with or without a stent, into a blood vessel to widen or open a pathological narrowing.

✓ INDICATIONS

- Atherosclerosis of the coronary arteries.
- Carotid artery disease (causing significant stenosis or neurological sequelae).
- Peripheral artery disease (refractory to medical treatment, causing life-limiting claudication, rest pain, or ischaemic ulceration).
- Renovascular hypertension secondary to atherosclerosis of the renal artery or fibromuscular dysplasia (in selected cases).

✗ CONTRAINDICATIONS

Relative

- Kidney dysfunction—care must be taken in patients with poor renal function if iodinated contrast is being used (it is used in most cases).
- Allergy to iodinated contrast media (depending on severity of prior reaction).
- Inability of the patient to lie flat and still.
- Uncorrected bleeding disorder or anticoagulation/antiplatelet therapy.
- Long segment of multifocal stenoses.
- Eccentric, calcified stenosis.
- Stents may not be used in patients where dual antiplatelet therapy is contraindicated.

ANATOMY

- In the vascular tree, there are:
  - Arteries.
  - Arterioles.
  - Capillaries.
  - Venules.
  - Veins.
- Arteries and veins have three layers—the tunica intima, the media, and the adventitia.
- The tunica intima is 1 layer thick and is made up of squamous epithelium and internal elastic lamina forming connective tissue.
- The media is thicker in arteries than in veins and contains smooth muscle that can contract to change the diameter of the vessel. It also contains the external elastic lamina.
- The adventitia is thicker in veins and consists purely of connective tissue. In larger vessels, this layer contains the vasa vasorum (the vessels supplying the vessel wall).
- Capillaries are one cell layer of endothelium thick.

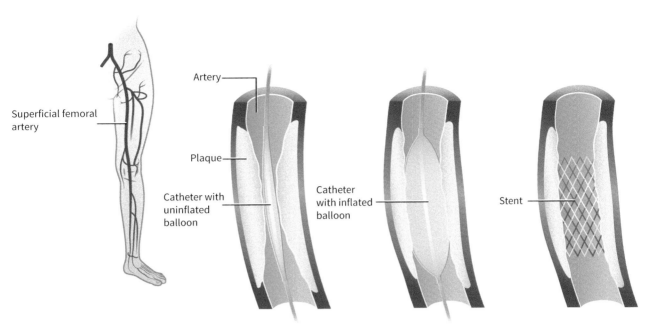

Figure 14.1 Balloon angioplasty and stenting of an atherosclerotic narrowing of the superficial femoral artery

STEP-BY-STEP OPERATION

Anaesthesia: general or local with IV sedation.
Position: supine.

1 Using ultrasound guidance, the desired vessel is cannulated (this is often the right common femoral artery).
2 Via a short introducer sheath (usually 4, 5, or 6 French), a guide wire is inserted and, under fluoroscopic guidance, is passed along the vessel beyond the stenosis, using a catheter for direction and support.
3 The catheter is then threaded over the guide wire and through the stenosis (the Seldinger technique).
4 The catheter can be used to measure the pre- and post-stenosis pressure and calculate the pressure gradient.
5 Using angiography or pre-procedure imaging, the diameter of the normal vessel is measured, and an appropriately sized balloon is selected.
6 After removing the catheter, the angioplasty balloon is passed through the sheath over the wire so that it bridges the stenosis.

7 The angioplasty balloon is inflated with a mixture of contrast and saline (for anything from a few seconds to a few minutes).
8 The angioplasty balloon is deflated, and the post-stenosis pressure gradient can be measured (in the arterial system a gradient of less than 20 mmHg is acceptable).
9 Depending on the pressure gradient and/or angiographic appearance, a stent may be deployed to achieve vessel patency.
10 Angiography is then used to confirm the success of the procedure. The guide wire and introducer sheath are removed and haemostasis at the sheath insertion site achieved with either compression or an arterial closure device.

INTERVENTIONAL RADIOLOGY

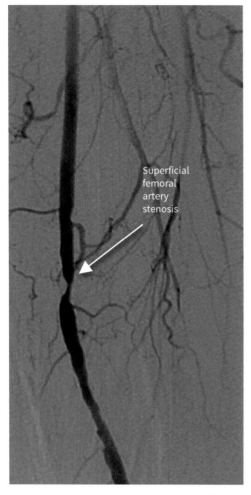

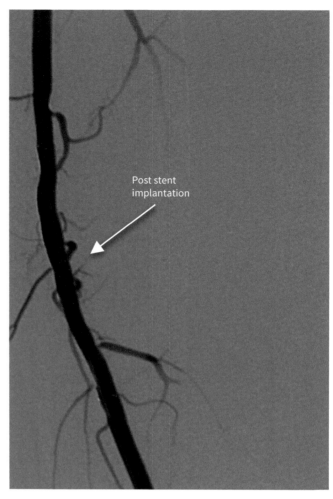

Figure 14.2 Pre-stenting and post-stenting angiography of the superficial femoral artery

COMPLICATIONS

Early

> Allergic reaction to iodine-based contrast.
> Bleeding/haematoma at the vascular sheath insertion site.
> Dissection/rupture of the target vessel.
> Embolisation of atheroma or thrombus into distal vessels.

Intermediate and late

> Recurrence of the stenosis.
> Pseudoaneurysm.
> Stent thrombosis.
> In-stent stenosis.
> Stent fracture.

POSTOPERATIVE CARE

Inpatient

▹ Usually a day-case procedure, with patients discharged home on the same day provided there are no complications. Mobilisation is encouraged.

Outpatient

▹ Patients are usually given a long-term single antiplatelet agent such as aspirin (75 to 100 mg/day) or clopidogrel (75 mg/day).

▹ Follow-up, if required, is either via the interventional radiologist or the vascular surgeon 4–6 weeks after discharge.

▹ Patients are advised to seek urgent medical attention if ischaemic symptoms reoccur (pain, pallor).

SURGEON'S FAVOURITE QUESTION

How do you differentiate veins from arteries on ultrasound?

1. By anatomical knowledge (e.g., Nerve-Artery-Vein in the femoral sheath).

2. Pulse: Arteries are more pulsatile than veins.

3. Compressibility: Veins are more readily compressible compared to arteries (the most important feature).

4. Colour Mode Doppler: While flow towards the transducer is red and away is blue by convention, this distinction is relative to the position of the probe. The flow waveform can also help distinguish arteries from veins.

TRANSJUGULAR INTRAHEPATIC PORTOSYSTEMIC SHUNT (TIPSS)

Brendan S Kelly

DEFINITION

Creation of a tract between the portal vein and the hepatic vein to shunt blood away from the portal venous system, thereby reducing portal pressure.

✓ INDICATIONS

- Indications are the sequelae of decompensated liver disease:
  - Uncontrolled variceal haemorrhage (usually from oesophageal varices).
  - Refractory ascites.
  - Hepatic pleural effusion (hydrothorax).
- TIPSS may also be beneficial in Budd-Chiari syndrome and hepatorenal syndrome.

✗ CONTRAINDICATIONS

Relative contraindications

- Uncorrected bleeding disorder or anticoagulation/ antiplatelet therapy.
- Obstructing neoplasm.

Absolute contraindications

- Severe liver failure (those with a model for end-stage liver disease, MELD score >40 and have a 71% 3-month mortality after TIPSS).
- Severe encephalopathy.
- Polycystic liver disease.
- Severe right-sided heart failure.

ANATOMY

- The internal jugular vein (IJV):
  - The IJV forms at the jugular foramen and drains the inferior petrosal sinus, the sigmoid sinus, and the veins of the face.
  - The IJV lies superficially in the neck and descends within the carotid sheath. Within the sheath, it sits lateral to the carotid artery; the vagus nerve sits posteriorly between the two vessels.
  - This superficial position makes the IJV amenable to cannulation. However, its close proximity to the vagus nerve and carotid artery mean that these structures are at risk of iatrogenic damage during TIPSS.
- The liver:
  - The liver has a dual vascular supply: the hepatic artery (25%) and the portal vein (75%). Together, these vessels supply the liver with approximately 1.5 L of blood per minute.
  - The common hepatic artery is a branch of the coeliac trunk. It gives off the gastroduodenal and right gastric branches and then becomes the proper hepatic artery. At the hilum of the liver, the proper hepatic artery gives off the cystic branch and then further divides into the right and left hepatic arteries.
  - The portal vein, formed from the superior mesenteric and splenic veins, carries nutrients absorbed from the intestines for 'first pass' metabolism. At the hilum of the liver, the portal vein divides into right and left branches.
  - Blood drains from the liver via the right, left, and intermediate (middle) hepatic veins directly into the IVC.
  - The portal triad consists of the hepatic portal vein, the hepatic artery proper, and the common bile duct. The portal triad enters the liver at the porta hepatis and is bounded by a fibrous capsule called Glisson's capsule.

Figure 14.3 Intrahepatic Portosystemic Shunt - Post-procedure imaging

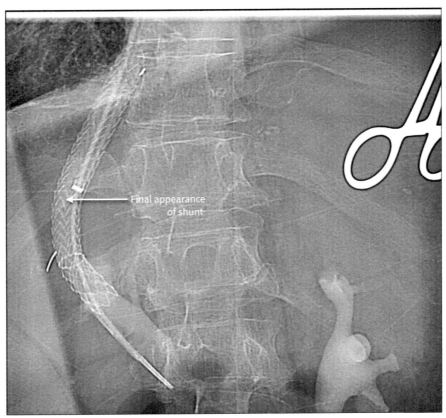

STEP-BY-STEP OPERATION

Anaesthesia: general.

Position: supine.

1. Ultrasound guidance is used to cannulate the right IJV.
2. A long sheath is inserted into the right atrium, and the right atrial pressure is measured.
3. Under fluoroscopic guidance, a guide wire is advanced into the inferior vena cava and then into the right hepatic vein. A stiff catheter is then inserted over the guide wire into the right hepatic vein.
4. A needle is advanced through the stiff sheath and is passed from the right hepatic vein towards the right portal vein (ultrasound can be used for guidance).
5. Once the right portal vein has been punctured, access is secured by advancing a wire. The sheath can then be pushed forward over the wire into the right portal vein. The pressure in the main portal vein is measured using a catheter through the sheath.

6. In cases of variceal bleeding, the varices can be embolised with coils through a catheter.
7. The tract from the right hepatic vein to the right portal vein is dilated with a balloon, and a covered stent (the TIPSS stent) is inserted through the tract.
8. A portogram is performed to confirm the TIPSS is working. The pressure in the main portal vein and right atrium are remeasured. The portosystemic gradient is calculated and compared with the pre-TIPSS value.
9. The sheath is removed, and haemostasis at the neck is achieved with manual compression.

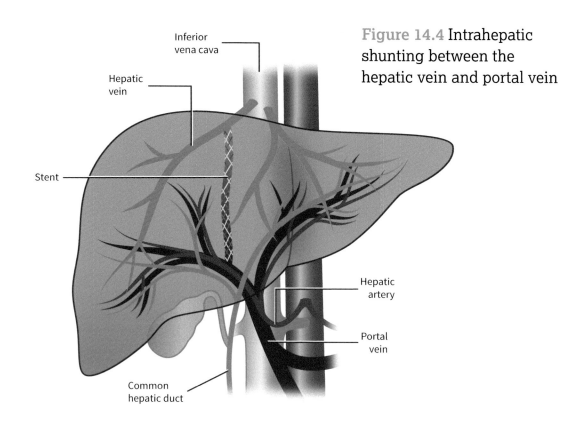

Figure 14.4 Intrahepatic shunting between the hepatic vein and portal vein

COMPLICATIONS

Early
> Bleeding.
> Bile leak causing chemical peritonitis.

Intermediate and late
> Infection.
> Encephalopathy—due to the reduction in first pass metabolism (>15%).
> In-stent stenosis, thrombosis, or occlusion.
> Hepatic ischaemia.
> Mortality (<1%).

POSTOPERATIVE CARE

Inpatient
> In the case of variceal bleeding, the central venous pressure should be kept as low as possible (right atrial pressure is transmitted into the varices through the TIPSS).

Outpatient
> Ultrasound follow-up can be used to ensure the TIPSS remains patent.

⚬ SURGEON'S FAVOURITE QUESTION

What are the signs of decompensated liver failure?

Ascites, encephalopathy and variceal bleeding.

CATHETER-DIRECTED THROMBOLYSIS (CDT)

Brendan S Kelly

DEFINITION

Catheter-directed thrombolysis (CDT) is a technique whereby tissue plasminogen activator (tPA) is injected through a catheter directly into a thrombus.

✓ INDICATIONS

> Acute critical limb ischaemia where symptoms have been present for <14 days and the predicted time to re-establish anterograde flow is short enough to preserve limb viability.
> Acute myocardial infarction (AMI).
> Deep vein thrombosis (DVT).
> Pulmonary embolism (PE).
> Acute ischaemic stroke (AIS).
> CDT versus systemic thrombolysis may be considered in patients at high risk of bleeding and with persistent hemodynamic instability despite systemic thrombolysis. Those at risk of death before systemic thrombolysis can manifest effectiveness.

✗ CONTRAINDICATIONS

Relative minor

> Hepatic failure.
> Bacterial endocarditis.
> Pregnancy.
> Diabetic haemorrhagic retinopathy.

Relative major

> Cardiopulmonary resuscitation within last 10 days.
> Major non-vascular surgery or trauma within last 10 days.
> Severe uncontrolled hypertension: >200 mmHg systolic or >110 mmHg diastolic.
> Intracranial tumour.
> Recent eye surgery.

Absolute

> Established cerebrovascular event (including transient ischaemic attacks within last 2 months).
> Active bleeding diathesis.
> Recent gastrointestinal bleeding (<10 days).
> Neurosurgery (intracranial and spinal) within last 3 months.
> Intracranial trauma within last 3 months.

ANATOMY

> The femoral triangle, also known as Scarpa's triangle, is an anatomical space of the upper thigh. It is of particular importance for CT perfusion (CTP), as vascular access is often obtained through the femoral artery or vein, both of which are located within the triangle.
> The borders of the femoral triangle are:
>> Superiorly—the inguinal ligament running from the pubic tubercle to the anterior superior iliac spine (ASIS).
>> Medially—adductor longus originating at the pubic body to insert into the linea aspera of the femur; contraction results in adduction and flexion at the hip.
>> Laterally—sartorius running from the ASIS to form part of the pes anserinus, which inserts into the medial tibial plateau. Contraction results in abduction, flexion, and lateral rotation at the hip joint and flexion of the knee joint.
>> The floor—pectineus (a quadrangular muscle running from the pectineal line of the pubic tubercle to the pectineal line of the femur) and adductor longus.
>> The roof—fascia lata (a thick fascia that envelops the fascial compartments of the leg; laterally, it thickens to form the iliotibial tract).

> › Contents of the femoral triangle (from lateral to medial, nerve, artery, vein; "NAV-Y-fronts"):
>   › The femoral nerve originates from L2, L3, and L4 and passes into the femoral triangle deep to the inguinal ligament. It descends the thigh in the femoral canal, innervating the anterior compartment of the thigh.
>
> › The external iliac artery becomes the common femoral artery at the inguinal ligament.
> › The common femoral vein drains the popliteal vein and becomes the external iliac vein at the inguinal ligament.
> › Deep inguinal lymph nodes and associated lymphatic vessels.

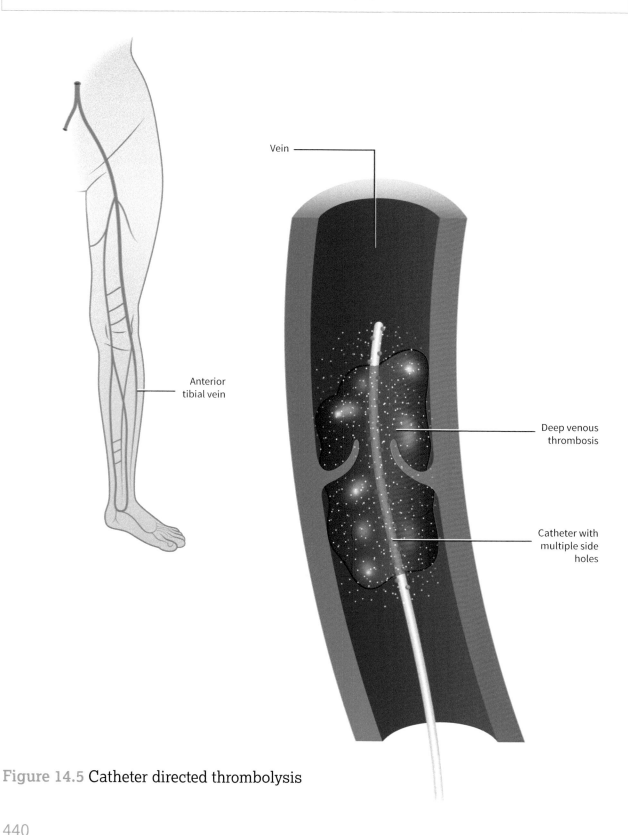

Figure 14.5 Catheter directed thrombolysis

STEP-BY-STEP OPERATION

Anaesthesia: IV sedation.

Position: supine.

Considerations: While this section will focus on CDT for acute lower limb ischaemia, the technique is similar for thrombolysis elsewhere in the arterial and venous system.

1 Using ultrasound guidance, the common femoral artery is cannulated.

2 A diagnostic angiogram is performed by injecting contrast through the catheter.

3 Fluoroscopic imaging is used to ascertain the location of the occlusion (it will appear as a filling defect in the artery).

4 Under fluoroscopic guidance, the occlusion is probed with a soft guide wire. Caution must be used, especially with autologous vessel grafts, as there is a risk of damage to the vessel wall.

5 The occlusion is traversed, and a catheter is pushed beyond the most distal aspect of the occlusion. If this is not possible, thrombolysis can be initiated from the proximal end of the occlusion. The thrombolysis catheter has side holes to allow for the tissue plasminogen activator (tPA) to be dispersed throughout the thrombus.

6 The thrombolytic agent is infused continuously (for a period of time that varies with severity, time of initiation, and patient weight). Alternatively, a series of IV boluses can be used.

7 Post-procedure imaging is used to determine the success of the procedure.

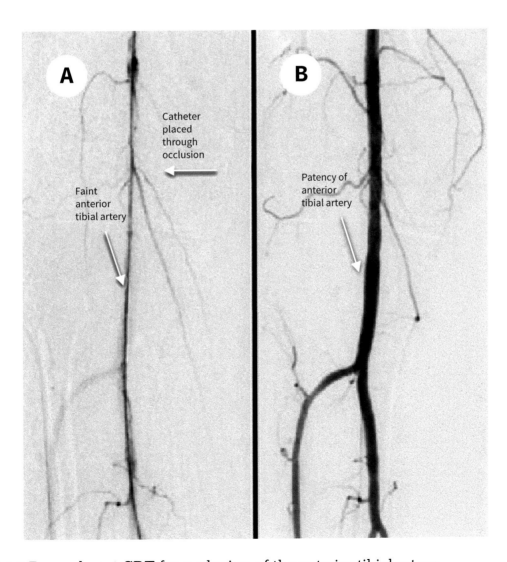

Figure 14.6 Pre and post-CDT for occlusion of the anterior tibial artery

COMPLICATIONS

Early

> Intracranial haemorrhage (up to 3%).
> Major bleeding requiring transfusion or surgery (1–20%).
> Distal embolisation (1–5%).

Intermediate and late

> Compartment syndrome (1–10%).

POSTOPERATIVE CARE

Inpatient

> Patients remain as an inpatient under their appropriate medical team until the cause and complications of their acute critical limb ischaemia, acute myocardial infarction, deep vein thrombosis, pulmonary embolism, or acute ischaemic stroke have been managed.
> On discharge, the patient should be advised to monitor for the return of ischaemic symptoms and for bleeding complications.

Outpatient

> The patent should be followed up by the appropriate medical team according to their presenting thrombotic pathology.

SURGEON'S FAVOURITE QUESTION

What are the 6 P's of acute ischaemia?

Pain, paralysis, paraesthesia, pulselessness, pallor, and perishing cold.

EMBOLISATION

Brendan S Kelly

DEFINITION

Embolisation is an intravascular technique used to occlude blood vessels with the deposition of embolic materials.

✓ INDICATIONS

- Haemorrhage—GI, epistaxis, trauma, post-partum, aneurysms and pseudoaneurysms.
- Vascular anomalies—arteriovenous malformations (AVMs).
- Others—tumours, uterine fibroids, varicoceles and prostatic arteries (for benign prostatic hyperplasia).

✗ CONTRAINDICATIONS

Relative

- Coagulopathy should be corrected prior to embolisation (depending on clinical urgency).
- Pregnancy.
- Wanting future pregnancies (for uterine artery embolisation).
- Contrast agent allergy.

Absolute

- In the context of uterine artery embolisation, concurrent pregnancy is an absolute contraindication unless there is a life-threatening bleed.

ANATOMY

- For the purposes of this chapter, the procedure will focus on embolisation therapy for uterine fibroids.
- The uterus is supplied by branches of the paired ovarian arteries and the uterine arteries.
- Within the broad ligament of the uterus is an extensive anastomosis between the two arterial supplies.
- The ovarian arteries:
  - The ovarian arteries are the main blood supply to the ovaries.
  - The ovarian arteries arise from the abdominal aorta distal to the origin of the renal arteries, they then descend into the pelvis in the uterine suspensory ligament to enter the mesovarium.
- The uterine arteries:
  - The uterine arteries are the major blood supply to the uterus.
  - The paired uterine arteries originate from the internal iliac arteries and travel to the uterus in the cardinal ligament, where they then enter the inferior broad ligament of the uterus.
  - An important anatomical relation to note is that the uterine arteries cross anterior to the ureters (water passes under the bridge).
  - Blood volume through the uterine arteries increase significantly during pregnancy.

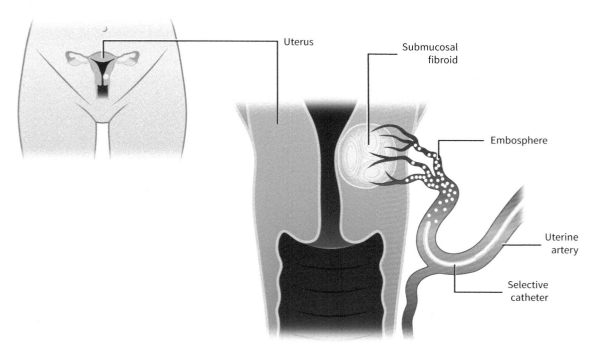

Figure 14.7 Delivery of pro-embolic material via the uterine artery into the blood supply of a submucosal fibroid

STEP-BY-STEP OPERATION

Anaesthesia: local +/- IV sedation (sometimes combined with epidural anaesthesia for postoperative pain relief).

Position: supine.

Considerations: While this section will focus on embolisation for uterine fibroids, the technique is similar for elsewhere in the body.

1 Using ultrasound guidance, the right common femoral artery is punctured and using the Seldinger technique, an introducer sheath is inserted.

2 The guide wire is manoeuvred into the left uterine artery and is followed by the catheter.

3 Uterine supply is confirmed by fluoroscopy and contrast injection, and assessment is made for other vessels that should be excluded from embolisation.

4 Once the catheter has been correctly and safely positioned in the left uterine artery proximal to the uterus, the selected embolisation material is deployed, usually plastic beads or gelatine sponge particles. (Other embolic materials that can be used

in procedures elsewhere in the body include platinum coils, glue, Onyx, lipiodol, and vascular plug devices).

5 This embolisation procedure is then repeated for the right uterine artery.

6 If there is significant fibroid supply from an ovarian artery, embolisation may be considered, depending on the patient's desire to minimise the risk of reduced fertility.

7 The catheter and introducer are then removed and common femoral artery haemostasis achieved with either manual compression or a vascular closure device.

8 A dressing is applied.

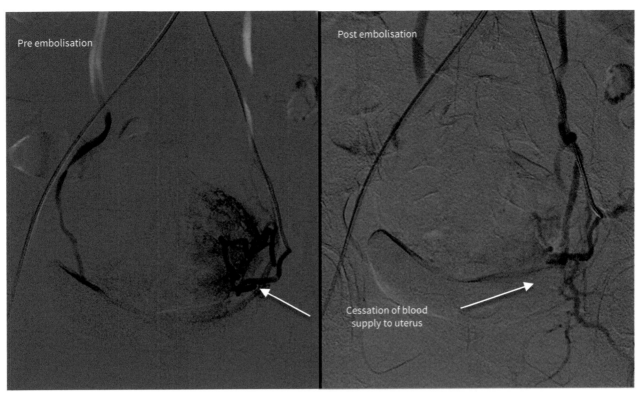

Figure 14.8 Pre and post-embolisation of the uterine blood supply to a fibroid

COMPLICATIONS

Early

> Allergic reaction to iodine-based contrast.
> Bleeding/haematoma at the arterial sheath insertion site.
> Pseudoaneurysm.
> Dissection/rupture of the target vessel.
> Non-target embolisation (embolic material going where not intended).
> Post-embolisation syndrome: a combination of fever, nausea and vomiting, and pain.

Intermediate and late

> Premature menopause.
> Vaginal discharge—usually self-limiting, but if purulent with fever needs assessment +/- antibiotics.
> Amenorrhea.
> Ovarian failure.
> Failure to improve symptoms.

POSTOPERATIVE CARE

Inpatient

> Patients are usually admitted overnight following fibroid embolisation.
> The arterial puncture site and vital signs are monitored.
> There can be significant post-procedural pain, which is often managed with a morphine patient controlled anaesthesia (PCA) pump or epidural if still in place.
> Once the patient's pain is controlled by simple oral analgesia, she can be discharged.

Outpatient

> Shrinkage of fibroids usually continues for 3–6 months, and therefore clinical consultation and repeat imaging can be undertaken after 3–6 months to assess response to therapy.

INTERVENTIONAL RADIOLOGY

 SURGEON'S FAVOURITE QUESTION

What is post-embolisation syndrome?

A syndrome that comprises fever, nausea/vomiting, and other flu-like symptoms. It usually occurs within the first 72 hours, is usually self-limiting, and does not predict infection.

INFERIOR VENA CAVA FILTER

Nick Wroe

DEFINITION

An inferior vena cava (IVC) filter is placed in a patient with lower limb deep vein thrombosis (DVT) to prevent mobilisation of clots causing pulmonary embolism (PE) or stroke if patent foramen ovale (PFO) is present.

✓ INDICATIONS

› Where systemic anticoagulation is contraindicated or has failed.
› Massive PE with residual DVT at risk for further PE.
› Free-floating ilio-femoral or IVC thrombus.
› Severe cardiopulmonary disease with DVT.
› Prophylactic indications include severe trauma (i.e., closed head injury, spinal cord injury, and/or multiple long bone or pelvic fractures).

✗ CONTRAINDICATIONS

Relative

› The presence of an IVC thrombus that carries a risk of iatrogenic PE.
› Sepsis or bacteraemia.

Absolute

› Inaccessible IVC (for example, due to compression by tumour).
› IVC too small or too large to accommodate a filter.

ANATOMY

› Gross anatomy:
  › The deep veins of the leg begin in the calf and unite as the popliteal vein. The popliteal vein becomes the superficial femoral vein and then the common femoral vein in the thigh.
  › The common femoral vein passes under the inguinal ligament, medial to the common femoral artery, and enters the abdomen as the external iliac vein.
  › The external iliac vein travels superiorly, receiving the internal iliac vein (which drains the pelvis) to then form the common iliac vein.
  › The IVC is formed by the confluence of the left and right common iliac veins at L4/5 and acts as the major source of venous drainage from the abdomen and lower limbs.

› The renal veins drain into the IVC at approximately L2. During the deployment of an IVC filter, it is preferable that it be placed below the renal veins.
  › The IVC enters the thorax through the caval opening of the diaphragm at T8 and continues to travel superiorly to the right of the midline and empty into the inferior aspect of the right atrium.
› Pathology:
  › A lower limb DVT is an intraluminal clot formed in the deep veins of the leg.
  › A DVT has the potential to travel through the venous system to enter the right atrium and then continue through to the right ventricle to embolise in a pulmonary artery, resulting in PE. In the presence of a PFO, a PE can cross the heart and travel directly to the brain, causing stroke.

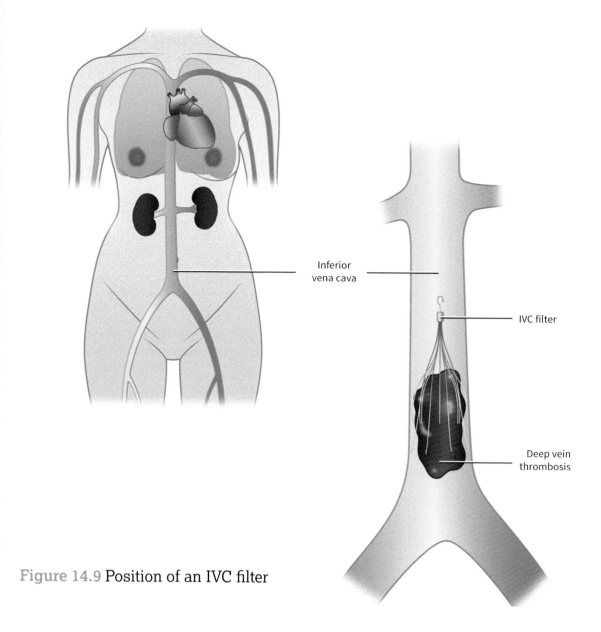

Figure 14.9 Position of an IVC filter

STEP-BY-STEP OPERATION

Anaesthesia: local anaesthetic with IV sedation.

Position: supine.

Considerations: This procedure can be performed using either the jugular (neck) or femoral (groin) approach. Two general types of filter are available: permanent and retrievable.

1 Ultrasound is used to locate the vein; local anaesthetic is infiltrated, and a small incision is made.
2 Using ultrasound guidance, the vein is punctured, and an introducer sheath is inserted into the vein using the Seldinger technique.
3 A wire and catheter are advanced into the IVC.
4 A cavogram is performed by injecting contrast through the catheter, and the patency and size of the IVC are evaluated. The position of the renal veins is also identified.

5 The IVC filter is then inserted through a sheath and deployed in the desired position, usually in the infrarenal IVC.
6 A final venogram is performed to check the filter's position.
7 After confirmation of satisfactory IVC filter position, the sheath is removed. Haemostasis is achieved with manual compression.

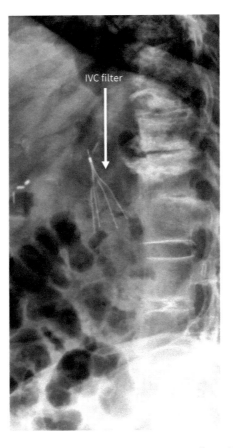

Figure 14.10 Post-procedural imaging for the insertion of an IVC filter

COMPLICATIONS

Early

› Allergy to contrast material.
› Pneumothorax (if jugular approach is used).
› Bruising or bleeding at puncture site.
› PE due to pushing the catheter through a clot.
› Guide wire entrapment within the IVC filter.

Intermediate and late

› Infection of wound or filter.
› Failed procedure (i.e., passage of clots through the filter to the lungs, resulting in a PE).
› IVC obstruction because the filter is clogged with clots. This can result in lower limb oedema.
› Filter migration, erosion, or fracture.
› Chronic thrombosis/recurrent thromboembolism.
› Retrievable filters may scar and become stuck, meaning they must be left in place.

POSTOPERATIVE CARE

Inpatient

› For well patients, ensuring there are no complications, this is usually a day-case procedure.

Outpatient

› Patients who have undergone the femoral approach should avoid heavy lifting and straining activities for 48 hours.
› Retrievable IVC filters should be removed when no longer indicated.

INTERVENTIONAL RADIOLOGY

 SURGEON'S FAVOURITE QUESTION

Explain the mechanism of action of common anticoagulants.

> Warfarin—inhibits vitamin K dependant clotting factors (II, VII, IX, X).
> Heparin—potentiates the action of antithrombin III.
> Abciximab, clopidogrel, aspirin—antiplatelet agents.
> Rivaroxaban—direct factor Xa inhibitor.
> Dabigatran—direct thrombin inhibitor.
> Alteplase—tissue plasminogen activator.

PERCUTANEOUS BILIARY DRAINAGE

Nick Wroe

DEFINITION

Access to and drainage of the biliary system using the Seldinger technique with ultrasound and fluoroscopic guidance.

✓ INDICATIONS

> To relieve biliary obstruction caused by:
>> Gallstones.
>> Head of pancreas tumour.
>> Biliary strictures due to surgery or primary sclerosing cholangitis.
>> Cholangiocarcinoma.

✗ CONTRAINDICATIONS

Relative

> Contrast allergy—depends on severity.
> Uncorrected bleeding disorder or anticoagulation/antiplatelet therapy.
> Multifocal obstruction—multiple points of obstruction may limit the success of the procedure.
> Ascites—paracentesis could be considered.

Absolute:

> No safe access to bile ducts—e.g., overlying bowel.

ANATOMY

> Biliary drainage of the liver:
>> Bile is produced in the liver's bile canaliculi, which come together to form intrahepatic bile ducts within the portal triad.
>> The portal triad consists of an arterial branch of the hepatic artery, a branch of the portal vein, and an intrahepatic bile duct.
>> The intrahepatic ducts converge to form interlobular ducts. These form the right and left hepatic ducts, which then merge to form the common hepatic duct.
> The gallbladder:
>> Bile is stored and concentrated in the gallbladder.
>> The gallbladder consists of a rounded distal portion called the fundus, the body, and the neck, which empties into the cystic duct. The cystic duct merges with the common hepatic duct to form the common bile duct (CBD).
>> The gallbladder is supplied by the cystic artery, usually a branch of the right hepatic artery.
> The biliary tree:
>> The CBD merges with the pancreatic duct to form the ampulla of Vater, which at the major duodenal papilla empties into the duodenum through the sphincter of Oddi.
>> The head of the pancreas and its uncinate process are in close proximity to the CBD; a malignant lesion here can cause obstruction of the CBD.

INTERVENTIONAL RADIOLOGY

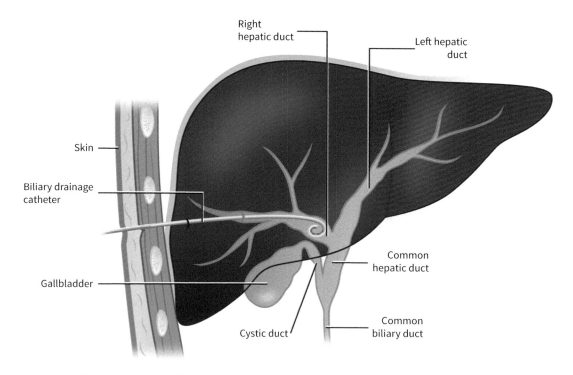

Figure 14.11 Percutaneous insertion of a drain into the biliary tree

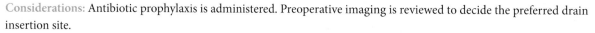

STEP-BY-STEP OPERATION

Anaesthesia: general or IV sedation with local.

Position: supine.

Considerations: Antibiotic prophylaxis is administered. Preoperative imaging is reviewed to decide the preferred drain insertion site.

1 The procedural site is infiltrated with local anaesthetic.
2 Ultrasound guidance is used to guide the puncture needle into the biliary tree.
3 Contrast and fluoroscopy are used to confirm the needle position within the biliary tree.
4 A guide wire is inserted through the needle to secure access.
5 An introducer sheath is inserted over a wire into the bile duct.

6 A wire and catheter are advanced through the sheath more centrally towards the liver hilum and, if possible, into the duodenum.
7 A drainage catheter is then fed over the guide wire to allow drainage of bile.
8 The guide wire is then removed, and the drainage catheter is connected to a drainage bag.
9 The drain is secured with dressings and sometimes a suture.

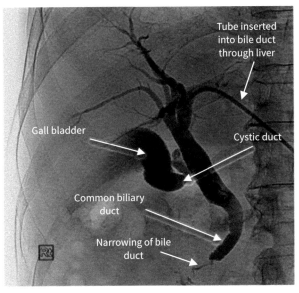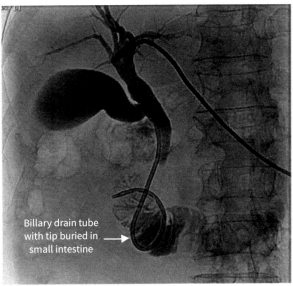

Figure 14.12 Intra-procedural imaging of the insertion of the percutaneous drain into the biliary tree, relieving obstruction

COMPLICATIONS

Early

> Failure to access a bile duct.
> Bleeding.
> Intraperitoneal bile leak.
> Puncture of pleura causing a pneumothorax or pleural bile leak.

Intermediate and late

> Sepsis (typically cholangitis) is a major complication (2.5%).
> Failure to relieve blockage.
> Obstruction/displacement of drain.

POSTOPERATIVE CARE

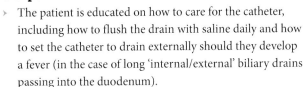

Inpatient

> Biliary output through the drain should be monitored to confirm relief of the obstruction.
> If the drain output is not adequate, a diagnostic cholangiogram can be performed to check drain position and patency.

Outpatient

> The patient is educated on how to care for the catheter, including how to flush the drain with saline daily and how to set the catheter to drain externally should they develop a fever (in the case of long 'internal/external' biliary drains passing into the duodenum).
> The catheter should be replaced every few months (in cases of long-term drainage).

SURGEON'S FAVOURITE QUESTION

What are the most common complications of gallstone disease?

In the gallbladder:
> Biliary colic.
> Acute cholecystitis.
> Mucocele.
> Empyema.
> Perforation of gallbladder.
> Gallbladder carcinoma.
> Pericholecystic abscess.
> Mirizzi syndrome.

In the CBD:
> Obstructive jaundice.
> Pancreatitis.
> Cholangitis.

In the gut:
> Gallstone ileus.

PERCUTANEOUS NEPHROSTOMY

Brendan S Kelly

DEFINITION

Insertion of a drain into the renal collecting system using the Seldinger technique with the aid of ultrasound and fluoroscopic guidance.

✓ INDICATIONS

- Complicated urinary tract obstruction (e.g., stone, tumour, trauma, retroperitoneal fibrosis where stenting is not possible).
- Urinary diversion—ureteric injury and urinary leak.
- Access for percutaneous procedures—stone treatment or ureteric stenting.
- Diagnostic testing—antegrade pyelography (rare).

✗ CONTRAINDICATIONS

Relative

- Uncorrected bleeding disorder or anticoagulation/antiplatelet therapy.
- Ureteral stenting may be preferred in simple obstruction.

ANATOMY

Gross anatomy

- The kidneys lie on either side of the vertebral column in the retroperitoneum.
- The renal pelvis is formed from the merger of the major calices of the kidney.
- The renal pelvis progressively narrows as it travels inferiorly and out of the hilum of the kidney.
- At the ureteropelvic junction (the narrowest point), the renal pelvis transitions to become the ureter, which descends into the pelvis to drain into the bladder.

Neurovasculature

- The right and left renal arteries arise as branches of the abdominal aorta just inferior to the origin of the superior mesenteric artery. The left renal artery commonly arises superior to the right renal artery. The right renal artery is longer and passes posterior to the inferior vena cava.
- As the renal artery courses towards the hilum of the kidneys, it gives off two branches: the ureteric branch of the renal artery and the inferior suprarenal artery. Within the hilum, these then divide into four branches: superior, anterior, posterior, and inferior segmental branches.
- The posterior portion of the kidney is the least vascular, the 'avascular plane of Brodel', and therefore is the safest point for access.
- Within the renal pelvis, interlobar/interlobular veins converge to form the renal vein, which runs anterior to the renal artery.
- The left renal vein crosses the midline anterior to the abdominal aorta. Both renal veins drain into the inferior vena cava.

Figure 14.13 Percutaneous nephrostomy

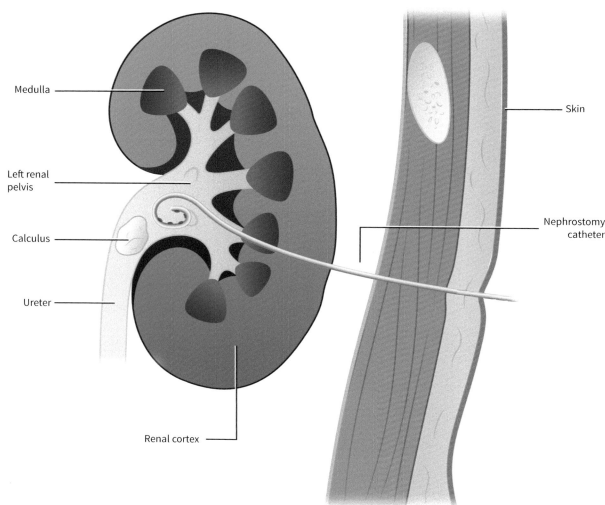

Medulla

Left renal pelvis

Calculus

Ureter

Renal cortex

Skin

Nephrostomy catheter

STEP-BY-STEP OPERATION

Anaesthesia: local with IV sedation.

Position: prone, lateral decubitus, or supine.

1 Using ultrasound guidance, the plane of Brodel is located.

2 Using an 18-gauge needle, a posterior minor calix in the plane of Brodel is punctured and a small amount of urine aspirated (this may be sent for analysis). The process of puncturing the calix is easier when the renal collecting system is dilated.

3 To confirm the position of the needle, a small volume of contrast is injected into the collecting system, and fluoroscopy is performed.

4 A guidewire is then passed through the needle and into the renal collecting system to secure access.

5 A series of dilators of increasing diameter are then passed over the wire to progressively widen the tract into the collecting system.

6 Once a tract is wide enough, an 8.5F or 10F pigtail catheter (depending on operator preference) is passed over the wire.

7 The pigtail catheter is then locked into position.

8 The pigtail catheter is connected to the draining catheter bag.

9 The insertion site is dressed.

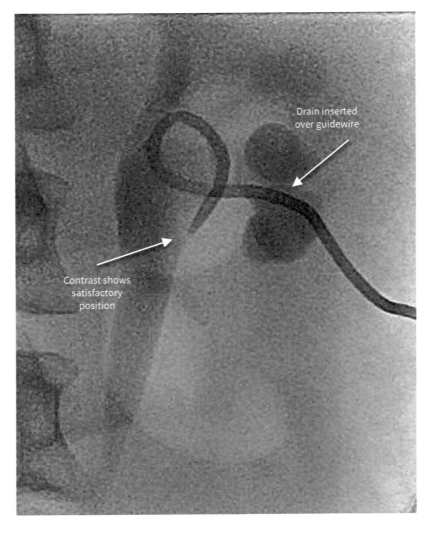

Figure 14.14 Radiographic imaging of a percutaneous nephrostomy

COMPLICATIONS

Early
- Haemorrhage—severe cases may require renal artery embolisation.
- Bowel injury and peritonitis.
- Urine leak.

Intermediate and late
- Infection—can progress to septic shock.
- Uncontrollable hypertension.
- Catheter displacement (~20%).

POSTOPERATIVE CARE

Inpatient
- A day-case procedure if a well patient with no complications

Outpatient
- The nephrostomy tube should be changed every 3 months.
- Removal of the nephrostomy tube depends upon the indication and reversibility of obstruction.

INTERVENTIONAL RADIOLOGY

 SURGEON'S FAVOURITE QUESTION

Explain the mechanism by which a parenchymal bleed can cause hypertension

Bleeding into the renal parenchyma increases the intracapsular pressure. This can cause constriction of the renal vasculature, resulting in reduced perfusion of the renal parenchyma. Reduced perfusion activates the renin-angiotensin-aldosterone system, resulting in constriction of the renal artery and increasing blood pressure. Increased blood pressure then leads to further bleeding, beginning a vicious cycle into uncontrollable hypertension.

RADIOLOGICALLY INSERTED GASTROSTOMY (RIG) OR GASTROJEJUNOSTOMY (RIGJ)

Brendan S Kelly

DEFINITION

The insertion of an enteral feeding tube into the stomach percutaneously using ultrasound and fluoroscopic guidance.

✓ INDICATIONS

> Enteral access is usually considered when it is anticipated that a patient will not be able to meet their nutritional needs by mouth for more than seven days.

✗ CONTRAINDICATIONS

> Uncorrected bleeding disorder or anticoagulation/ antiplatelet therapy.
> Abdominal wall abnormalities (e.g., anterior abdominal varices).
> Organomegaly obstructing access to the stomach/ jejunum.
> Large volume ascites.

ANATOMY

Gross anatomy

> The stomach has two curvatures (lesser and greater) and five parts (cardia, fundus, body, antrum, and pylorus).
> The acute angle between the cardia and the oesophagus is known as the cardiac notch or angle of His. It is formed by the fibres of the collar sling and the circular muscles surrounding the gastro-oesophageal junction. It forms a sphincter that prevents reflux.
> The stomach is attached to other structures by a series of ligaments:
>> Gastrocolic ligament—part of the greater omentum, connects the greater curvature of the stomach and the transverse colon.
>> Gastrosplenic ligament—connects the greater curvature of the stomach and the hilum of the spleen.
>> Gastrophrenic ligament—connects the fundus of the stomach to the diaphragm.
>> Hepatogastric ligament—connects the liver to the lesser curve of the stomach, forms part of the lesser omentum.

Histology

> The gastric mucosa contains:
>> Numerous gastric glands.
>> A two- or three-layer muscularis mucosae (aids in emptying the glands).
>> An intervening lamina propria.
> The smooth muscle of the muscularis externa is arranged in three layers:
>> Outer longitudinal.
>> Middle circular.
>> Inner oblique.
> When the stomach is empty and contracted, the mucosa and underlying submucosa are thrown into irregular, temporary folds called rugae. These rugae flatten when the stomach is full.

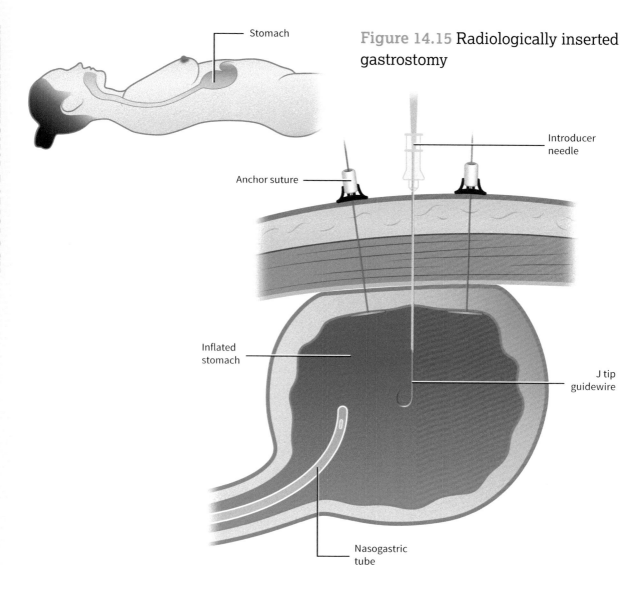

Figure 14.15 Radiologically inserted gastrostomy

STEP-BY-STEP OPERATION

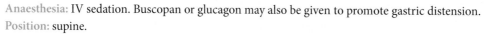

Anaesthesia: IV sedation. Buscopan or glucagon may also be given to promote gastric distension.

Position: supine.

Considerations: Oral barium may be administered the night before to visualise the colon. Here we describe the retrograde non-barium approach to a gastrostomy tube insertion.

1 Using a pre-inserted nasogastric tube, the stomach is inflated with air.
2 Lateral fluoroscopy can be used to identify a safe puncture site with no intervening transverse colon.
3 Using a needle through the anterior abdominal wall, the inflated stomach is punctured.
4 The position of the needle in the stomach is then confirmed by injecting contrast.
5 A gastropexy suture is inserted through the needle. This is repeated for a total of two to four sutures to ensure that the stomach is flush and fixed against the abdominal wall.
6 Another needle is inserted into the inflated stomach at the gastropexy site. The gastrostomy tube is then inserted into the stomach and a balloon inflated to keep it in position.
7 In the case of gastrojejunostomy tube insertion, a wire is passed through the gastrostomy site and is advanced into the jejunum. A long gastrojejunostomy tube can then be inserted over the wire.
8 The site of insertion is then cleaned and dressed.

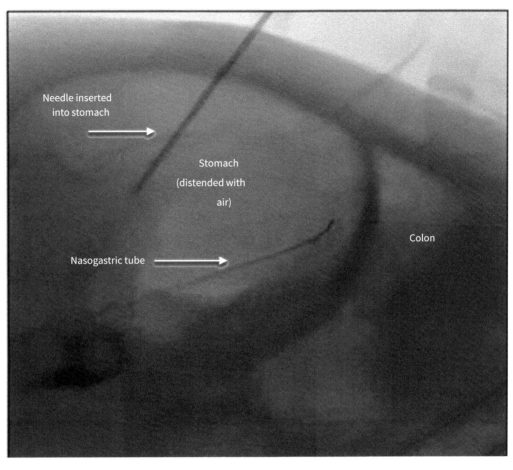

Figure 14.16 Intra-operative imaging to confirm the position of the needle in the stomach during a RIG

COMPLICATIONS

Early

- Gastric haemorrhage.
- Peritoneal leak around gastrostomy.
- Misplacement of tube outside stomach.
- Injury to liver, small or large intestine.

Intermediate and late

- Tube extrusion or accidental removal.
- Aspiration pneumonia after feeding gastrostomy.
- Gastro-cutaneous fistula.

POSTOPERATIVE CARE

Inpatient

- Patients must be monitored for signs of peritonitis (fever, severe abdominal pain, rigidity). This can occur if administered feeds or medications leak into the peritoneum.
- Feeding through the tube is normally initiated slowly, often beginning after 24 hours and increasing feeds by 50 ml hourly.

- Tube sites need to be checked daily for infection and patency.

Outpatient

- Routine tube changes every 3–6 months.
- Patient/family education on tube inspection and monitoring.

INTERVENTIONAL RADIOLOGY

 SURGEON'S FAVOURITE QUESTION

What is the immediate management if a long-term gastrostomy falls out?

For long-term gastrostomies, there will be an established tract. If the tube falls out, insertion of a Foley catheter (without inflation of the balloon) will maintain the tract until a formal gastrostomy catheter can be re-inserted.

OPHTHALMOLOGY

FARIHAH TARIQ

PHACOEMULSIFICATION (CATARACT SURGERY)

Tyson Chan and Farihah Tariq

DEFINITION

Removal of an opacified crystalline lens by emulsification (using ultrasound to break up the lens into smaller pieces) and subsequent implantation of an artificial intraocular lens.

✓ INDICATIONS

- No minimum level of vision is required to have a cataract operation. However, surgery is indicated when:
  - Symptoms of cataracts such as reduced vision, glare, and monocular diplopia interfere with the patient's activities of daily living.
  - Cataract hinders monitoring and treatment of a coexistent posterior segment pathology such as diabetic retinopathy.
  - Lens-induced disease such as a large cataract pushing forward the iris thereby causing secondary acute angle-closure glaucoma (phacomorphic glaucoma) or if there is leakage of lens material from a hypermature cataract which obstructs the trabecular meshwork causing secondary open angle glaucoma (phacolytic glaucoma). In some cases, there can be an inflammatory response to the lens proteins causing phacoanaphylactic uveitis.
  - Second eye surgery to balance the refractive power of both eyes (reduce anisometropia) and improve stereopsis.

✗ CONTRAINDICATIONS

Relative

- Active inflammatory conditions.
- Infections (e.g. untreated blepharitis).
- Unstable diabetic retinopathy.
- Recent contralateral phacoemulsification—second eye surgery should be delayed by at least 1 month to ensure healing and no complications.

Absolute

- Nil

ANATOMY

Gross anatomy

- The lens and cornea function to focus light onto the retina.
- The lens accounts for 30% of the eye's refractive power (15 dioptres), whilst the cornea is responsible for the remainder (43 dioptres).
- The lens is a transparent, ellipsoid biconvex-shaped structure that sits posterior to the iris and anterior to the vitreous body in a depression called the hyloid fossa.
- The lens is suspended via the zonular fibres, which connects to the ciliary body.
- Contraction of the ciliary muscles allow the lens to adapt its shape, enabling the eye to change focus from distance to near. This is known as accommodation.

- The lens consists of lens fibres that form the inner nucleus and outer cortex enveloped in an elastic capsule. Different types of cataracts form in each of the three layers.

Neurovasculature

- The lens is an epithelial structure with no direct innervation by nerves or blood vessels. It obtains its nutrients from the aqueous humour by passive diffusion.

Figure 15.1 Gross anatomy of the eye

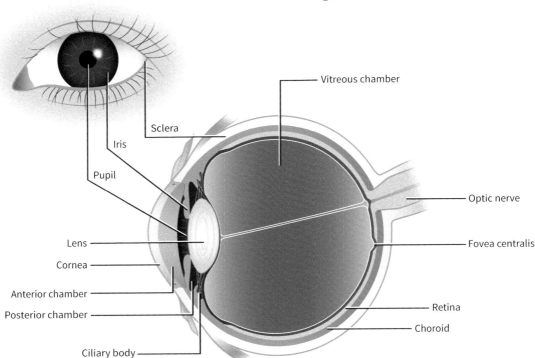

- Vitreous chamber
- Sclera
- Iris
- Pupil
- Optic nerve
- Lens
- Cornea
- Fovea centralis
- Anterior chamber
- Posterior chamber
- Retina
- Choroid
- Ciliary body

STEP-BY-STEP OPERATION

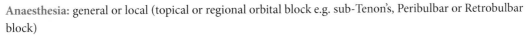

Anaesthesia: general or local (topical or regional orbital block e.g. sub-Tenon's, Peribulbar or Retrobulbar block)

Position: supine.

Considerations: The eye and surrounding structures are washed with 5% povidone-iodine, dried, and draped ensuring no lashes are in the surgical field. A speculum is inserted to keep the eye open.

1 The primary phaco incision is made using a keratome at the corneal margin, placed either temporally (laterally) or superiorly, approximately 3 mm in width whilst stabilising the globe with a micro-grooved forceps.

2 Viscoelastic, a viscous gel is inserted into the anterior chamber. This stabilises the anterior chamber during the next step, and protects the corneal endothelium from intraoperative trauma.

3 A smaller secondary incision known as paracentesis is made to accommodate additional instruments.

4 Next 'capsulorhexis' is performed, where a circular opening in the anterior capsule is made using a cystotome or rehixis forceps.

5 Balanced salt solution is injected between the lens and capsule edge separating the nucleus from the cortex known as hydrodissection.

6 Using a phaco probe and chopper instrument, the cataract is broken into smaller pieces using ultrasound energy (Phacoemulsification). These fragments and other remaining soft lens matter adherent to the capsule are aspirated and removed.

7 Viscoelastic is inserted into the capsular bag to open up the bag, creating space for the artificial lens. The lens is then inserted.

8 The viscoelastic gel is removed, and the anterior chamber is refilled with balanced salt solution.

9 Antibiotics (Cefuroxime) are given intracamerally (into the anterior chamber of the eye). Sutures are typically not required as the wounds are self-healing.

10 A clear shield is placed over the orbit to protect the eye.

OPHTHALMOLOGY

Figure 15.2
Phacoemulsification
and artificial lens
implantation

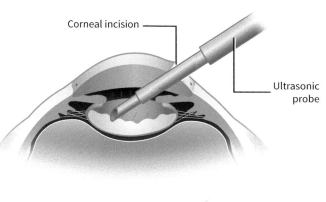

Corneal incision

Ultrasonic
probe

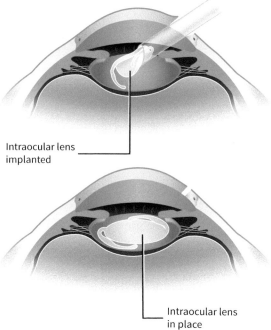

Intraocular lens
implanted

Intraocular lens
in place

COMPLICATIONS

Intraoperatively

> Rupture of posterior lens capsule with or without vitreous loss.
> Damage to the anterior capsule.
> Zonular dehiscence causing the capsule to become unstable.
> Loss of nuclear (lens) fragments into the vitreous chamber.
> Suprachoroidal haemorrhage—accumulation of blood between the choroid and the sclera.

Early

> Corneal oedema—swelling of cornea.
> Uveitis—inflammation of the uveal tract usually anterior.
> Increased intraocular pressure.
> Wound leak due to poorly constructed wounds.
> Iris prolapse.
> Endophthalmitis—inflammation of the intraocular cavity which may cause visual loss.

Intermediate and late

> Cystoid macular oedema—fluid accumulation in the retina at the macula.
> Rhegmatogenous retinal detachment—break or tear in the retina causing fluid accumulation between the neurosensory retina and the underlying retinal pigment epithelium.
> Corneal decompensation.
> Endophthalmitis.
> Lens-related problems e.g. decentred, subluxed or unstable.
> Posterior capsular opacification, where there is thickening of the residual posterior lens capsule, which may occur months to years following surgery. This is easily treated with Nd:YAG laser posterior capsulotomy.
> Visual loss.

POSTOPERATIVE CARE

Inpatient

> This procedure is typically performed as a day-case procedure.

> Eye shield on the post-operative eye should be worn at night for 5 nights to protect the eye from injury.

Outpatient

> Activities of daily living (excluding strenuous activity e.g. sports, heavy gardening, lifting for 2 weeks to decrease risk of complications associated with raised intraocular pressure and swimming for 2 weeks to decrease risk of infections) can be resumed in the evening following surgery.

> First post-operative day, reviews are only required if there are complications during surgery, or if there is concurrent pathology. Otherwise, patients are reviewed in clinic at four weeks or seen by their local optometrist. Practice varies between hospital and surgeons.

> Course of topical steroids e.g. dexamethasone 0.1% (1 drop four times a day for four weeks).

> Course of topical antibiotic drops e.g. chloramphenicol 0.5% (1 drop four times daily for two-four weeks).

> Patients should visit the optometrist 6 to 8 weeks post-operatively for refraction—new prescription for glasses.

🗨️ SURGEON'S FAVOURITE QUESTION

How do we select the correct intraocular lens for each patient?

Calculating the power of the new intraocular lens implant is known as biometry. This involves measuring the curvature of the cornea (keratometry) and using ultrasound to measure the length of the eye preoperatively. The values are put into a formula which computes the power of the lens.

VITRECTOMY

Huzaifa Malick

DEFINITION

Removal of the vitreous gel from the posterior segment and replacement with sterile saline or a tamponade such as gas or silicone oil.

✓ INDICATIONS

- Vitrectomy (pars plana vitrectomy) is performed when access to the posterior segment of the eye is necessary in the following circumstances:
  - › Rhegmatogenous or tractional retinal detachment
  - › Proliferative diabetic retinopathy
  - › Non-clearing vitreous haemorrhage
  - › Peeling of macular internal limiting membrane or epiretinal membrane
  - › Vitreomacular traction
  - › Endophthalmitis (inflammation of the intraocular cavity usually secondary to infection).
  - › Removal of retained lens fragments or a displaced intraocular lens following cataract surgery
  - › Intraocular foreign bodies from trauma
  - › Severe inflammatory changes within the vitreous
  - › Tumour biopsy

✗ CONTRAINDICATIONS

- Established non-reversible severe visual impairment or blindness.
- Retinoblastoma or choroidal melanoma (to avoid seeding).

ANATOMY

Gross anatomy

- The vitreous is a transparent gel-like structure occupying two-thirds of the globe.
- The outer zone is a denser collagenous layer and forms the anterior and posterior hyaloid face.
- The central zone constitutes the vitreous humour.
- The vitreous is strongly adherent to the retina at the margins of the vitreous base, the optic disc, the retinal vessels and the posterior lens capsule.
- The pars plana is part of the ciliary body and is found posterior to where the iris and sclera meet. This is a relatively avascular structure, thus making it a good point of entry for instruments during vitrectomy surgery.

Neurovasculature

- The choroid is the vascular layer of the posterior segment and provides nutrients to the retina.

Histology

- The retina is a complex 10 layered photosensory structure. The photoreceptors (rods and cones) convert light signal into electrical signal.
- Ganglion cells from the retina give rise to the optic nerve which deliver the signals ultimately to the occipital cortex.

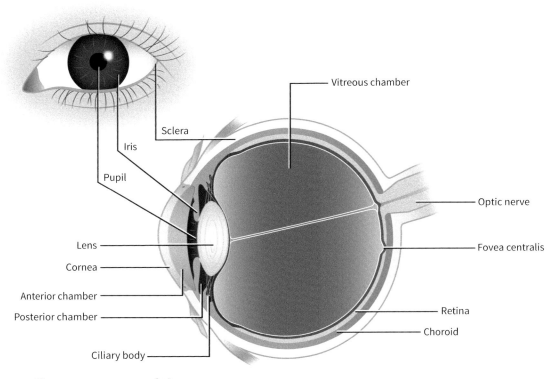

Figure 15.3 Gross anatomy of the eye

STEP-BY-STEP OPERATION

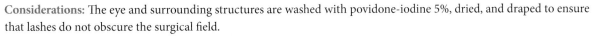

Anaesthesia: local.

Position: supine.

Considerations: The eye and surrounding structures are washed with povidone-iodine 5%, dried, and draped to ensure that lashes do not obscure the surgical field.

1 Access to the posterior segment is achieved using a trochar to pierce the sclera and choroid (sclerotomy). The sclerotomies are placed at three port sites via the pars plana (to minimise disruption to the eye):

  a For the infusion cannula.

  b For the light source.

  c For the vitrector.

2 The infusion cannula is used to achieve adequate intraocular pressure.

3 The vitrector and light source are then introduced. The infusion cannula maintains positive pressure of the globe by infusing fluid into the posterior chamber whilst the surgeon uses one hand to hold the light source and the other to hold the vitrector.

4 The vitrector is aimed towards the centre of the vitreous to achieve a core vitrectomy.

5 The vitrector is then placed lower into the posterior vitreous cavity to achieve a posterior vitrectomy. The light source is manoeuvred carefully with the other hand to ensure a good view at all times (infusion pressure must be monitored carefully, as vitrector use without adequate infusion will cause the eye to collapse).

6 Once the posterior vitreous is removed, the vitreous base is shaved (as its adherence to the retina prevents total removal)—this step is key in vitrectomy for a retinal detachment. Dye is utilised to help visualise any remaining vitreous.

7 Sterile saline (balanced salt solution—BSS), a tamponade (usually gas—octafluoropropane), or silicone oil is introduced.

8 The instruments are then removed.

9 Most 23-gauge and 25-gauge sclerotomies are self-sealing but require careful inspection to ensure no fluid leaks.

10 Subconjunctival antibiotics are injected, and the eye is shielded.

OPHTHALMOLOGY

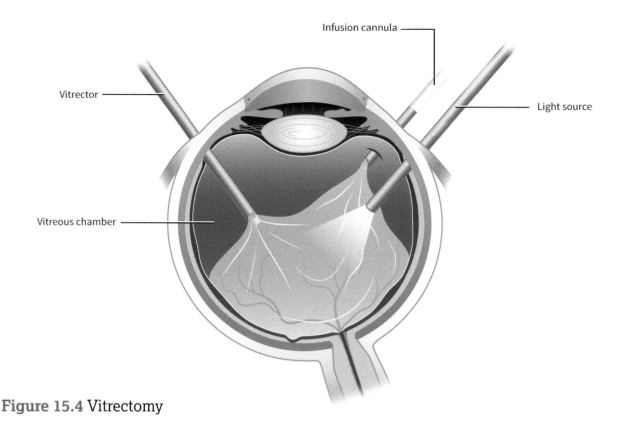

Figure 15.4 Vitrectomy

COMPLICATIONS

Early

> Iatrogenic retinal breaks or detachment.
> Choroidal haemorrhage.
> Endophthalmitis.

Intermediate and late

> Cataract.
> Glaucoma.

> Tamponade-associated problems—increased intraocular pressure, central retinal artery occlusion, and inverse hypopyon.
> Sympathetic ophthalmia—a bilateral, granulomatous uveitis that occurs after trauma to the eye.

POSTOPERATIVE CARE

Inpatient

> This procedure is typically performed as a day-case procedure.

Outpatient

> Patients who have had air or gas inserted will need to maintain a head-down posture for as long as possible over the following 7 days.

> Patients are reviewed in clinic on day 1 postoperatively and as needed thereafter.
> Corticosteroid, antibiotic, and mydriatic eye drops are prescribed for 3–4 weeks.

SURGEON'S FAVOURITE QUESTION

Why does the patient need to maintain a head-down posture postoperatively when a gas or air bubble is introduced?

Holding a head-down position will allow the air or gas bubble to rise and settle adjacent to the retina. This will help to hold the retina flat, (drain/prevent the reaccumulation of sub-retinal fluid before the retinopexy seals the break) and promote optimal healing.

TRABECULECTOMY

Farihah Tariq

DEFINITION
Creation of a fistula between the anterior chamber and the subconjunctival space to facilitate aqueous outflow from the eye to lower intraocular pressure.

✔ INDICATIONS

Trabeculectomy, also known as filtration surgery, is performed for chronic glaucoma in the following circumstances:

- If intraocular pressure is not controlled with maximal medical therapy or failed laser therapy.
- In patients where laser therapy is contraindicated.
- Patients who are non-compliant with medications.
- Patients with progressive glaucomatous optic nerve damage and/or loss of visual field.
- Ocular surface disease e.g. side effect of eye drops.

✗ CONTRAINDICATIONS

- Severe scarring on conjunctiva.
- Active neovascular glaucoma.
- Uveitic glaucoma.
- Active intraocular inflammation.
- Severe visual impairment.

ANATOMY

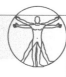

Gross anatomy

- The conjunctiva, a thin transparent mucous membrane, lines the sclera (bulbar conjunctiva) and the inside of the eyelid (palpebral conjunctiva). The junction between the bulbar and palpebral conjunctiva forms a fold known as the conjunctival fornix.
- The sclera is the white outer fibrous coat of the globe. As it continues anteriorly, it becomes transparent, which is called the cornea. The junction between the two is known as the limbus.
- The iridocorneal angle lies between the iris and the cornea. This drainage angle is where aqueous humour flows from the eye and into the trabecular meshwork.
- The trabecular meshwork is an array of collagenous tunnels overlying Schlemm's canal and involved in the drainage of the aqueous humour.
- Schlemm's canal are collecting ducts which channel the aqueous humour from the anterior chamber into the venous system via the episcleral vessels.
- Ciliary body is composed of the ciliary muscles and epithelium. This is the site of aqueous humour production. Contraction of the ciliary muscle facilitates outflow via the trabecular meshwork.

Neurovasculature

- The short ciliary nerve, a branch of the ciliary ganglion, contains parasympathetic fibres that innervate the sphincter pupillae and ciliary muscle, and sympathetic fibres that innervate the dilator pupillae muscle.
- The long ciliary nerve, a branch of the nasociliary nerve (a branch of the ophthalmic division of the trigeminal nerve), provides sensory innervation to the eyeball and cornea. It accompanies the short ciliary nerve from the ciliary ganglion.
- The eye is supplied by the central retinal artery, the anterior ciliary arteries, and the short and long posterior ciliary arteries. All are branches of the ophthalmic artery, a branch of the internal carotid artery.
- The cornea has no blood vessels and receives nutrients from passive diffusion from tear fluid and the aqueous humour.
- The venous drainage is primarily via the vortex and central retinal veins, which merge with the inferior and superior ophthalmic veins that drain posteriorly into the cavernous sinus.

Figure 15.5 Layers of the sclera and cornea and gross anatomy of the eye

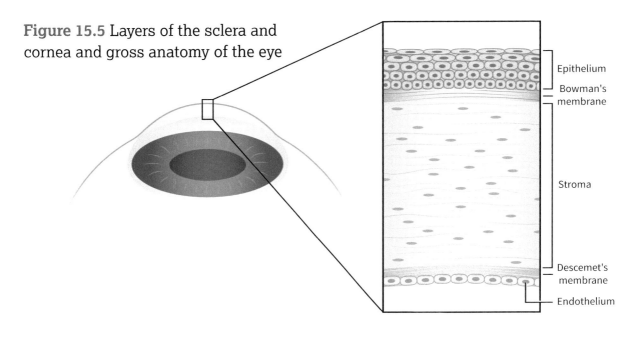

Epithelium
Bowman's membrane
Stroma
Descemet's membrane
Endothelium

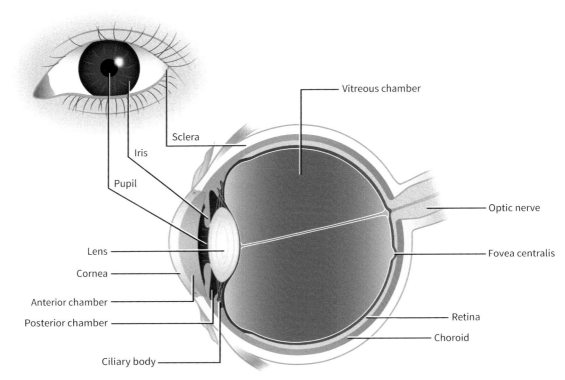

Vitreous chamber
Sclera
Iris
Pupil
Optic nerve
Lens
Cornea
Fovea centralis
Anterior chamber
Posterior chamber
Retina
Choroid
Ciliary body

STEP-BY STEP OPERATION

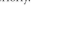

Anaesthesia: local or general.

Position: supine.

Considerations: The eye and surrounding structures are washed with 5% povidone-iodine, dried, and draped ensuring no lashes are in the surgical field. A speculum is inserted to keep the eye open.

1 A traction suture is placed in either the cornea or the superior rectus muscle to act as a hook and gain exposure of the surgical site at the superior globe.

2 The conjunctiva is incised and reflected backwards to expose the sclera below. This conjunctival flap formed can either be created at the fornix or superiorly.

3 Anti-scarring agent such as Mitomycin-C is used to prevent scarring and failure of the operation.

4 A partial thickness scleral flap is formed by incising two-thirds deep into the sclera.

5 A superotemporal opening called a paracentesis is then made in the cornea. This is required in subsequent steps when assessing the filter.

6 A section of sclerolimbal tissue is removed (a sclerostomy) thereby creating a fistula between the anterior chamber and subconjunctival space.

7 A peripheral iridectomy is performed, where a small piece of the iris is removed to prevent the iris moving forward and blocking the sclerostomy opening.

8 The partial thickness scleral flap is fixed back in place using either adjustable, releasable, or fixed sutures. The different types of sutures allow manipulation postoperatively to adjust drainage.

9 The flap is then assessed by injecting balanced salt solution via the paracentesis.

10 The conjunctiva is tightly sutured close to prevent retraction and leakage. Finally, subconjunctival steroid and antibiotic injections are administered.

Figure 15.6 Trabeculectomy

NORMAL

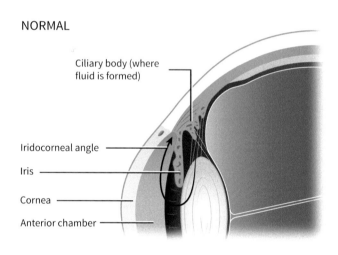

Ciliary body (where fluid is formed)

Iridocorneal angle

Iris

Cornea

Anterior chamber

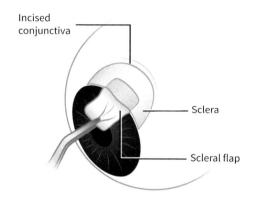

Incised conjunctiva

Sclera

Scleral flap

TRABECULECTOMY

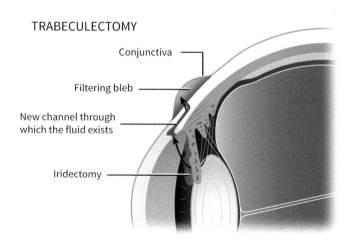

Conjunctiva

Filtering bleb

New channel through which the fluid exists

Iridectomy

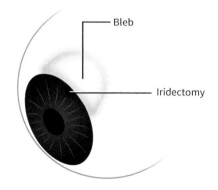

Bleb

Iridectomy

COMPLICATIONS

Early

- Infection—endophthalmitis or blebitis.
- Failure to control intra-ocular pressure (too high or too low).
- Bleeding—conjunctival, scleral, iris, or suprachoroidal haemorrhage.
- Shallow anterior chamber.
- Wound leak.
- Visual loss causing a "wipe out" in advanced glaucoma particularly if the intra-ocular pressure is too high or too low.

Late

- Shallow anterior chamber.
- Cataract.
- Ptosis.
- Filtration failure due to subconjunctival scarring forming a ring of steel.
- Bleb related complications—leakage, failure, cyst formation and blebitis.
- Infection.

POSTOPERATIVE CARE

Inpatient

- This procedure is typically performed as a day-case.

Outpatient

- Topical corticosteroids e.g. prednisolone acetate 1% or dexamethasone 0.1%—2 hourly for 2–4 weeks, then 4 tapering off over 2–3 months.

- Topical antibiotics e.g. chloramphenicol 0.5%—4 times a day for 1 month.
- Follow up in clinic on day 1 following surgery then at 1 week, then at regular intervals depending on results of the surgery.

💬 SURGEON'S FAVOURITE QUESTION

What is the purpose of using antimetabolite drugs in this type of surgery?

The body's natural response to damage is fibrosis and scarring. In trabeculectomy, the scarring can reduce the effectiveness of the newly formed channel; therefore antimetabolites such as mitomycin c and 5-fluorouracil can be used. These can be administered either intraoperatively or postoperatively, depending on the patient and their risk of scarring.

DACRYOCYSTORHINOSTOMY (DCR)

Huzaifa Malick

DEFINITION

Creation of a channel between the lacrimal sac and the nasal cavity by removing the intervening bony ostium to facilitate tear drainage.

✓ INDICATIONS

> Congenital lacrimal duct obstruction.
> Acquired lacrimal duct obstruction—secondary to ageing, chronic sinus, or nasal inflammation, dacryoliths (stones), and trauma.
> Functional obstruction secondary to facial nerve palsy or lacrimal pump failure.
> Chronic dacryocystitis.

✗ CONTRAINDICATIONS

> Atrophic rhinitis.
> Malignancy.
> Acute infection.

ANATOMY

> The nasolacrimal drainage system comprises:
> › Puncta.
> › Canaliculi.
> › Lacrimal sac.
> › Nasolacrimal duct.
> Tears drain into both the upper and lower puncta on the medial aspect of the upper and lower lids and then pass into the upper and lower canaliculi and into the common canaliculus.
> The canaliculi have an initial vertical segment that measures approximately 2 mm, followed by a horizontal segment that measures approximately 8 mm. The horizontal upper and lower canaliculi then converge to form the common canaliculus. The common canaliculus passes through the lacrimal fascia before entering the lacrimal sac.
> The lacrimal sac lies within the lacrimal fossa (a smooth concave depression in the lacrimal and maxillary bone that forms the medial wall of the orbit).

> The lacrimal bone is much thinner than the adjacent maxillary bone and is thus the chosen site of incision for DCR.
> The lacrimal sac is lined by a double-layered epithelium and has a fundus and a body. The fundus is the top half of the sac and extends approximately 4 mm above the medial canthal tendon. The body extends 10 mm below the fundus to the opening of the nasolacrimal canal.
> The nasolacrimal duct is approximately 18 mm long, with a 12 mm superior section inside the nasolacrimal canal (within the maxillary bone) and a 6 mm inferior membranous part that runs within the nasal mucosa and opens into the inferior nasal meatus.
> The nasolacrimal duct has several valves, the most important clinically being the valve of Hasner, at the opening of the nasolacrimal duct into the nasal cavity.

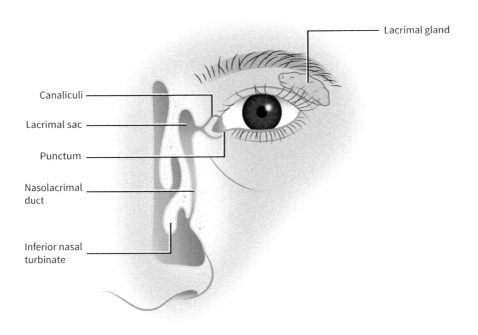

Figure 15.7 The nasolacrimal drainage system

STEP-BY-STEP OPERATION

Anaesthesia: general or local.

Position: supine.

Considerations: this surgery is a dual surgical specialty operation, with ENT surgeons using endoscopic assistance for the intranasal part of the surgery and Opthalmic surgeons working on the adnexal tissue around the eye.

1   The nose is packed with ribbon gauze soaked in adrenalised lignocaine (this serves to reduce nasal bleeding and keeps the nasal mucosa taut).

2   A J-shaped incision is made at the medial canthus to reveal fibres of orbicularis oculi (beneath the orbicularis oris, the medial palpebral ligament (MPL) is found).

3   The MPL is cut at its insertion point on the lacrimal crest (a bony projection on the frontal process of the maxilla).

4   The cut insertion site of the MPL ligament exposes a periosteal opening.

5   The periosteum is separated off the bone (with the aim of decreasing pain when it comes to cutting the bone).

6   The lacrimal sac is reflected laterally.

7   A rhinostomy is created by puncturing the floor of the lacrimal bone to access the nasal cavity with a sharp dissector. The bone fragments are removed with forceps.

8   The lacrimal sac is divided and flaps are fashioned on the lacrimal and nasal mucosa, which are then sutured together.

9   A silicone stent is passed through the lacrimal canaliculi into the lacrimal sac and past the anastomotic site.

10 The MPL is sutured back to its insertion point on the lacrimal crest. The orbicularis oculus muscle opening is sutured, and the skin is closed with non-absorbable fine sutures.

OPHTHALMOLOGY

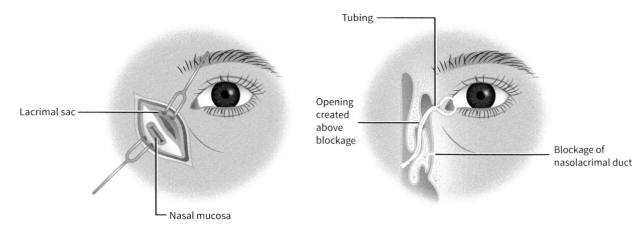

Figure 15.8 Exposure and cannulation of the nasolacrimal sac

COMPLICATIONS

Early

> Haemorrhage (epistaxis).

Intermediate and late

> Infection +/- wound breakdown.
> Silicone tube displacement.
> Granulomas at rhinostomy site.

> Rhinostomy fibrosis.
> Medial canthal asymmetry.
> Failed DCR due to closure of the ostium opening.

POSTOPERATIVE CARE

Inpatient

> DCR is typically performed as a day-case procedure.

Outpatient

> Ice packs to reduce swelling for approximately 24 hours.
> Patients are advised not to blow their nose.
> Prophylactic antibiotics for 10 days.

> Corticosteroid nasal spray and nasal decongestants for 10 days.
> Skin sutures are removed at 1 week.
> The silicone tube(s) is removed between 3 and 6 months postoperatively.

SURGEON'S FAVOURITE QUESTION

Why is a silicone stent left in situ postoperatively?

A silicone stent maintains the newly fashioned patent mucosal passageway into the nose by preventing premature closure of the anastomosis from scar tissue and fibrosis. It is usually left in situ for up to 6 months postoperatively.

HORIZONTAL STRABISMUS SURGERY

Conor Ramsden

DEFINITION

Adjustment of the horizontal recti muscles to realign the eyes by weakening (recession) or strengthening (resection) the muscles.

✓ INDICATIONS

Squint surgery is performed for functional or cosmetic reasons. Prior to surgery, correcting refractive error with nonoperative measures such as glasses, prisms and occlusion therapy should be explored. Alignment may be performed:

› To restore binocular single vision.
› To eliminate diplopia.

✗ CONTRAINDICATIONS

› Adults may not tolerate realignment, as they may be unable to process and combine the images after many years of misalignment. To predict this, orthoptists use a variety of tests. It can be useful to simulate the postoperative result preoperatively by using botulinum toxin to temporarily paralyse overacting muscles.

ANATOMY

Gross anatomy

› Six extraocular muscles (EOM) control eye movement, which include the four rectus and two oblique muscles.
› The oblique muscles originate from the bony wall of the orbit, whilst the recti muscles originate at the annulus of Zinn, a ring of fibrous tissue surrounding the optic nerve. The muscles travel anteriorly and insert into the sclera.
› The distance of insertion of the muscles in relation to the corneal limbus follows a rule called the spiral of Tillaux:
  › Medial rectus—5.5 mm.
  › Inferior rectus—6.6 mm.
  › Lateral rectus—6.9 mm.
  › Superior rectus—7.7 mm.

Neurovascular

› The superior oblique is supplied by the fourth cranial nerve (trochlear), the lateral rectus is supplied by the sixth cranial nerve (abducens), and all remaining EOM are supplied by the third cranial nerve (oculomotor).
› The ophthalmic artery supplies blood to all EOM. The rectus muscles carry the anterior ciliary arteries, which in turn supply blood to the anterior segment of the eye.

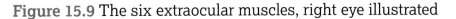

Figure 15.9 The six extraocular muscles, right eye illustrated

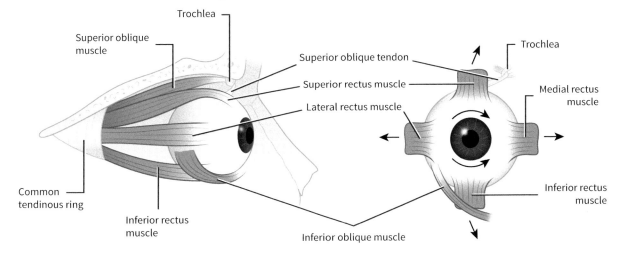

479

OPHTHALMOLOGY

STEP-BY-STEP OPERATION

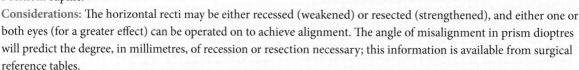

Anaesthesia: general.

Position: supine.

Considerations: The horizontal recti may be either recessed (weakened) or resected (strengthened), and either one or both eyes (for a greater effect) can be operated on to achieve alignment. The angle of misalignment in prism dioptres will predict the degree, in millimetres, of recession or resection necessary; this information is available from surgical reference tables.

1 Insert a traction suture into half depth of the sclera at the limbus; gentle traction on this will keep the globe stable whilst operating.

2 Perform a peritomy by opening the conjunctiva and Tenon's. With a spring scissors, cut along the border of the limbus for about 5mm, over the muscle to be operated on.

3 Insert a muscle hook under the muscle to isolate it.

The next steps depend on whether recession or resection is being performed:

4a Recession

  i The muscle is secured near its insertion with a suture.

  ii The muscle is then cut to disinsert it from the globe anterior to the sutures, and haemostasis is achieved.

  iii Measuring from the muscle stump, calipers set to the desired amount of recession are used to mark where the muscle is to be reinserted.

  iv Using the free ends of the suture, the muscle is reinserted into the marked point of the sclera at partial depth, taking extra care not to perforate the globe.

  v The conjunctiva is closed with absorbable sutures.

4b Resection

  i A second muscle hook is inserted posterior to the first hook, and the muscle is exposed by gentle traction along its length.

  ii The calipers are used to mark the desired amount of resection in millimetres. Posterior to this mark, the muscle is secured as described above in the recession procedure.

  iii A straight clamp is used to clamp the muscle anterior to the suture for a few moments.

  iv The muscle is cut anterior to the sutures, and haemostasis is achieved. The muscle stump attached to the globe is excised.

  v The cut muscle is reinserted at the original insertion using the long ends of the suture at partial thickness into the sclera and tied.

  vi The conjunctiva is closed with absorbable sutures.

5 Adjustable sutures are sometimes used for resections and recessions if the change in squint angle is not predictable. When the patient is awake, ocular alignment can be adjusted and the suture tied when the desired ocular alignment is achieved.

Recession

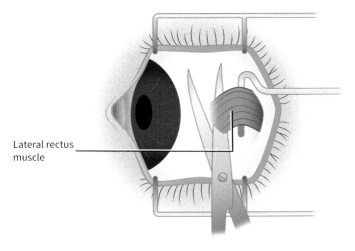

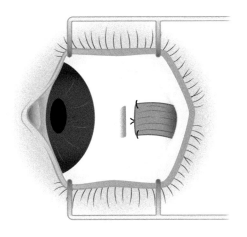

Lateral rectus
muscle

Resection

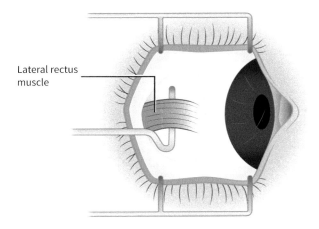

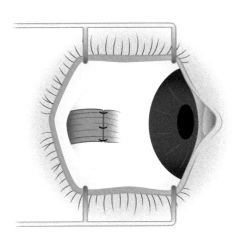

Lateral rectus
muscle

Figure 15.10 Resection and recession in horizontal strabismus surgery

COMPLICATIONS

Early

▸ Scleral perforation.
▸ Under- or overcorrection of strabismus.
▸ Postoperative diplopia.

Intermediate and late

▸ Slipped muscle.
▸ Anterior segment ischaemia (especially in three-muscle surgery).
▸ Infection.
▸ Scleritis.
▸ Discomfort due to exposed sutures (suture granuloma).

POSTOPERATIVE CARE

Inpatient

> Following surgery, the patient is reviewed the same day. If adjustable sutures have been used, ocular alignment is achieved by tightening or loosening the knots.

Outpatient

> Topical antibiotic and corticosteroid drops are prescribed 4 times a day for 1 month.
> Warn the patient that there may be some discomfort in the immediate post-op period.
> Patient is seen in clinic at 2 weeks to check the wound for any evidence of scleritis and then again at 2 months for postoperative results.

SURGEON'S FAVOURITE QUESTION

Why is it important to let the anaesthetist know when putting traction on the extraocular muscles?

It may stimulate a bradycardia or even asystole. This is known as the oculocardiac reflex.

Index

Page numbers followed by *f* indicate figures